CLINICAL HANDBOOK OF
NEPHROLOGY

CLINICAL HANDBOOK OF
NEPHROLOGY

ROBERT STEPHEN BROWN, MD

Associate Chief for Academic Affairs, Nephrology Division
Department of Medicine
Beth Israel Deaconess Medical Center;
Associate Professor of Medicine
Department of Medicine
Harvard Medical School
Boston, Massachusetts
United States

ELSEVIER

Elsevier
1600 John F. Kennedy Blvd.
Ste 1800
Philadelphia, PA 19103-2899

Notice

Executive Content Strategist: Nancy Anastasi Duffy
Senior Content Development Specialist: Priyadarshini Pandey
Publishing Services Manager: Shereen Jameel
Project Manager: Gayathri S
Design Direction: Amy L. Buxton

Printed in India

Last digit is the print number: 9   8   7   6   5   4   3   2   1

Working together
to grow libraries in
developing countries

www.elsevier.com • www.bookaid.org

Amtul Aala, MD
Instructor in Medicine
Harvard Medical School;
Transplant Nephrologist
Department of Medicine
Beth Israel Deaconess Medical Center
Boston, Massachusetts
United States

Robert Stephen Brown, MD
Associate Chief for Academic Affairs,
    Nephrology Division
Senior Physician
Department of Medicine
Beth Israel Deaconess Medical Center;

Associate Professor of Medicine
Harvard Medical School
Boston, Massachusetts
United States

Parvathy Geetha, MD
Nephrologist
Iowa Kidney Physicians
Des Moines, IA
United States

Alexander Goldfarb-Rumyantzev[†], MD, PhD, PhD
Lecturer, Harvard Medical School;
Department of Medicine, Division of
    Nephrology
Beth Israel Deaconess Medical Center
Boston, Massachusetts;

Medical Director
Clinical Development
Akebia Therapeutics, Inc
Cambridge, Massachusetts
United States

Periklis Kyriazis, MD
Assistant Professor of Medicine
Albert Einstein College of Medicine;
Transplant Nephrologist
Department of Medicine
Division of Nephrology
Montefiore Medical Center
Bronx, New York
United States

Stewart H. Lecker, MD, PhD
Assistant Professor of Medicine
Harvard Medical School;

Program Director, Nephrology Fellowship
Department of Medicine
Beth Israel Deaconess Medical Center
Boston, Massachusetts
United States

Alexander Morales, MD
Instructor in Medicine
Harvard Medical School;
Department of Medicine
Nephrology Division
Beth Israel Deaconess Medical Center
Boston, Massachusetts
United States

Subhash Paudel, MD
Nephrologist
Reliant Medical Group
Worcester, Massachusetts
United States

Nathan H. Raines, MD, MPH
Instructor in Medicine, Harvard Medical
    School;
Division of Nephrology
Department of Medicine
Beth Israel Deaconess Medical Center
Boston, Massachusetts
United States

[†]Deceased

Ruth Schulman, MD
Assistant Professor of Medicine
Boston University Chobanian & Avedisian
    School of Medicine;
Nephrology Division
Saint Elizabeth's Medical Center
Boston, Massachusetts
United States

Jeffrey H. William, MD
Assistant Professor of Medicine
Harvard Medical School;
Associate Program Director, Nephrology
    Fellowship
Department of Medicine
Division of Nephrology
Beth Israel Deaconess Medical Center
Boston, Massachusetts
United States

Mark E. Williams, MD
Director of Dialysis
Nephrology Division
Beth Israel Deaconess Medical Center;

Associate Professor of Medicine
Harvard Medical School;

Senior Staff Physician
Renal Division
Joslin Diabetes Center
Boston, Massachusetts
United States

Min Zhuo, MD, MPH
Associate Physician
Division of Renal Medicine
Brigham and Women's Hospital
Boston, Massachusetts
Associate Medical Director
Clinical Development
Visterra, Inc
Waltham, Massachusetts
United States

Nephrology, the subspecialty of internal medicine which covers the diagnosis and treatment of kidney diseases, hypertension, electrolyte and acid-base disorders, dialysis, and kidney transplantation, is often viewed as very difficult to master. Moreover, many major nephrology textbooks offer more information than students, residents, fellows, internists, family physicians, physician assistants, and nurse practitioners usually require. *Clinical Handbook of Nephrology* is an updated edition of *Nephrology Pocket*, a textbook published in 2014 by Börm Bruckmeier, which was used worldwide to provide clinicians with essential information regarding the diagnosis and treatment of renal disorders.

Clinical Handbook of Nephrology is structured to provide the data used to evaluate, understand, and manage most of the disorders commonly seen in the clinical practice of nephrology and which should be known to general medical caregivers. The book is in a format that can be easily used on hospital rounds and in office clinical care. The content of each of the 16 chapters is divided into subtopics that guide the reader directly to charts and algorithms to provide pertinent information quickly.

We feel sure you will find this to be a helpful reference that you will want to keep with you in your daily practice. We welcome your comments and suggestions as well.

Robert S. Brown, MD
Editor and Coauthor

ACKNOWLEDGMENTS

The editor and authors wish to acknowledge Börm Bruckmeier for providing *Nephrology Pocket*, the original textbook upon which this *Handbook* is based, and the editorial help of Nancy Duffy and Priyadarshini Pandey of Elsevier. Most of all, we are indebted to Alexander Goldfarb-Rumyantzev, MD, PhD, who provided the initial incentive to publish this *Handbook* but whose untimely accidental death on January 18, 2021, kept him from seeing its completion. In addition, we recognize that our roles as teachers of clinical medicine and nephrology to students, trainees, nurses, and young physicians at Harvard Medical School and the Beth Israel Deaconess Medical Center provided the inspiration for this book to augment their learning of renal and electrolyte disorders.

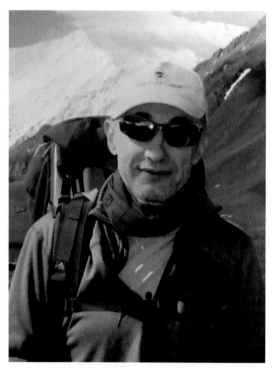

Alexander Goldfarb-Rumyantzev

Dedication

To my wife, Judy Brown, who puts up with my work after all these years; to the late Alex Goldfarb, my thoughtful and humorous coauthor and colleague; and to the late Frank Epstein, my mentor, colleague, and friend for 40 years who taught me to love nephrology.

Robert S. Brown, MD

CONTENTS

1   Introduction to Nephrology   1
Robert Stephen Brown

2   Symptoms, Signs, and Differential Diagnosis   5
Robert Stephen Brown ▪ Alexander Goldfarb-Rumyantzev

3   Renal Physiology   14
Robert Stephen Brown ▪ Alexander Morales ▪ Alexander Goldfarb-Rumyantzev

4   Water and Electrolyte Disorders   26
Robert Stephen Brown ▪ Alexander Goldfarb-Rumyantzev ▪ Alexander Morales

5   Acid-Base Disorders   49
Alexander Morales ▪ Alexander Goldfarb-Rumyantzev ▪ Robert Stephen Brown

6   Urinalysis and Diagnostic Tests   60
Robert Stephen Brown ▪ Alexander Goldfarb-Rumyantzev ▪ Ruth Schulman

7   Acute Kidney Injury   73
Robert Stephen Brown ▪ Alexander Goldfarb-Rumyantzev ▪ Nathan H. Raines

8   Glomerular Diseases   92
Robert Stephen Brown ▪ Alexander Goldfarb-Rumyantzev ▪ Subhash Paudel ▪
Stewart H. Lecker

9   Various Kidney Diseases: Interstitial, Cystic, Obstructive,
and Infectious Diseases   106
Robert Stephen Brown ▪ Alexander Goldfarb-Rumyantzev ▪ Parvathy Geetha ▪
Stewart H. Lecker

10   Kidney Disorders in Other Diseases   116
Robert Stephen Brown ▪ Alexander Goldfarb-Rumyantzev ▪ Periklis Kyriazis ▪
Stewart H. Lecker

11   Chronic Kidney Disease   132
Robert Stephen Brown ▪ Alexander Goldfarb-Rumyantzev ▪ Jeffrey H. William

12   Kidney Replacement Therapy: Dialysis   152
Mark E. Williams ▪ Alexander Goldfarb-Rumyantzev ▪ Robert Stephen Brown

13   Kidney Transplantation   230
Robert Stephen Brown ▪ Alexander Goldfarb-Rumyantzev ▪ Amtul Aala

14   Hypertension   260
Robert Stephen Brown ▪ Alexander Goldfarb-Rumyantzev ▪ Min Zhuo

15   Nephrolithiasis and Nephrocalcinosis   271
Robert Stephen Brown ▪ Alexander Goldfarb-Rumyantzev

16   Laboratory Values for Nephrology   283
Robert Stephen Brown ▪ Alexander Goldfarb-Rumyantzev

Index   299

CHAPTER 1

Introduction to Nephrology

Robert Stephen Brown

Nephrology, the subspecialty of internal medicine that covers the diagnosis and treatment of kidney diseases, hypertension, and electrolyte disorders, is often viewed as very difficult to master.

In *Clinical Handbook of Nephrology*, we break down the field of renal and electrolyte disorders into concise text, tables and algorithms that provide the reader with a simplified yet comprehensive approach to nephrology. While one cannot become a nephrologist in a month, this handbook has been designed to enable the reader to master the major areas of the specialty to a surprising degree of sophistication in the course of a 4-week period. Note that the reader should already have a basic knowledge of renal pathophysiology and function, body fluids, and metabolic disorders. However, a review of Chapter 3 will serve as a helpful memory refresher.

We suggest starting with a brief review of the first four chapters.

Week 1:   Chapter 1, Introduction to Nephrology
           Chapter 2, Symptoms, Signs, and Differential Diagnosis
           Chapter 3, Renal Physiology
           Chapter 4, Water and Electrolyte Disorders

Readers should then review the data in the remaining chapters specified for each week as follows:

Week 2:   Chapter 5, Acid-Base Disorders
           Chapter 6, Urinalysis and Diagnostic Tests
           Chapter 7, Acute Kidney Injury
           Chapter 8, Glomerular Diseases

Week 3:   Chapter 9, Various Kidney Diseases: Interstitial, Cystic, Obstructive, and Infectious
               Diseases
           Chapter 10, Kidney Disorders in Other Diseases
           Chapter 11, Chronic Kidney Diseases
           Chapter 12, Kidney Replacement Therapy: Dialysis

Week 4:   Chapter 13, Kidney Transplantation
           Chapter 14, Hypertension
           Chapter 15, Nephrolithiasis and Nephrocalcinosis
           Chapter 16, Lab Values for Nephrology

Before we get started, let's review the patient issues that will be the subject of most nephrology referrals or consultations.

1.1 Common Nephrology Consultations

Condition	Look For...	
• AKI or ARF • Etiology: prerenal, postrenal, intrinsic renal disease	• Cr increase with daily trend • Hx & Px for edema/volume depletion	• UA • Serum electrolytes, calcium phosphate • Urine chemistries (Cr, Na$^+$ for fractional excretion, Osm) • Renal US • UO
• CKD or chronic renal failure • Etiology of nephrotic syndrome, nephritis, or systemic diseases involving the kidneys	• Cr increase with weekly or monthly trend • Hx & Px for edema/volume depletion • UA • UO • Renal US	• Anemia • Cholesterol • Albumin • Ca^{++}/phos/bone disorders • Acidosis • PTH
• Evaluation of electrolyte disorders and volume status • Hypo/hypernatremia, hypo/hyperkalemia	• Hx & Px for edema/volume depletion • Cr • UO	• Urine "electrolytes" (U_{Na+}, U_{K+}, U_{Cl-}) • U_{Cr}, U_{Osm}
• Calcium, phosphate, and/or magnesium disorders	• Hyper/hypocalcemia • Hyper/hypophosphatemia • Hyper/hypoparathyroidism	• Vitamin D levels • Bone pathology • Dietary intake
• Nephrolithiasis, management and prevention	• Need for urological intervention • Stone composition • Crystalluria	• Blood tests (e.g., Cr, calcium, phosphate, uric acid, HCO_3) • 24-hour urine chemistries for supersaturation • Urine pH
• Need for HD, PD, CRRT, vascular access, or options counseling in ESKD or ARF patients	• Uremic symptoms • Volume overload/CHF • Uncontrollable hyperkalemia or acidosis • Low Cr clearance • Pericarditis	• Encephalopathy • Uremic coagulopathy
• Hypertension: controlled, uncontrolled, accelerated, or malignant	• Evaluate for secondary causes vs. "essential" causes and for end organ damage	• Management with specific drug indications
• Acid-base disorders	• Arterial or venous pH • Blood HCO_3 • $_pCO_2$	• Anion gap • Serum electrolytes
• Adjustment of medications in renal disease or kidney transplant patients	• Renal vs. hepatic excretion • Cr clearance or eGFR	• Knowledge of immunosuppressive drugs

AKI, Acute kidney injury; *ARF*, acute renal failure; *CHF*, congestive heart failure; *CKD*, chronic kidney disease; *Cr*, creatinine; *CRRT*, continuous renal replacement therapy; *ESKD*, end-stage kidney disease; *eGFR*, estimated glomerular filtration rate; *HD*, hemodialysis; *Hx & Px*, history and physical examination; *Osm*, osmolality; *PD*, peritoneal dialysis; *PTH*, parathyroid hormone; *UA*, urinalysis; *UO*, urine output; *US*, ultrasound.

1.2 Follow-Up Assessments of Nephrology Patients

- Etiology of renal disease based on test results
- Kidney function and trend
- Volume status, input and output (I&O)
- Electrolytes and acid-base status
- Hypertension (HTN)
- Anemia
- Calcium balance, hyperphosphatemia, hyperparathyroidism, bone disorders
- Appropriate doses of medications with renal excretion
- Systemic disease status, if present
- Need for dialysis, vascular access, and dialysis adequacy or kidney transplantation
- Nutritional status and hypoalbuminemia
- Concomitant conditions: cardiac, respiratory, infectious, gastrointestinal (GI), neurological diseases

1.3 General Overview of Renal Diseases

1.3.1 GLOMERULAR

1.3.1.1 Nephritic Syndromes

- Acute postinfectious glomerulonephritis (GN; immune complex deposition)
- Rapidly progressive glomerulonephritis (RPGN), crescentic GN
  - Immune complex deposition (e.g., bacterial endocarditis)
  - Antibody deposition (e.g., Goodpasture's syndrome)
  - Pauci-immune (e.g., Anti-neutrophil cytoplasmic autoantibody (ANCA)-positive associated vasculitis such as granulomatosis with polyangiitis [formerly Wegener's granulomatosis])
- Membranoproliferative glomerulonephritis (MPGN; immune complex deposition such as hepatitis C, systemic lupus erythematosus [SLE])
- Mesangial proliferative GN (immune complex deposition such as IgA nephropathy, SLE)

1.3.1.2 Nephrotic Syndromes

- Minimal-change disease (lipoid nephrosis or nil disease)
- Membranous nephropathy (immune complex deposition)
- Focal segmental glomerular sclerosis
- Collapsing glomerulopathy
- Secondary nephrotic syndrome (diabetes, tumors, HIV, amyloidosis, malaria, syphilis, drugs)

1.3.1.3 Vascular Syndromes

- Benign/malignant hypertensive nephrosclerosis
- Renal artery stenosis (arteriosclerosis, fibromuscular dysplasia)
- Renal artery occlusion (thrombosis, emboli)
- Renal arteriolar disease (Hemolytic uremic syndrome [HUS] and thrombotic thrombocytopenic purpura [TTP], thrombotic microangiopathy, preeclampsia, atherosclerosis)
- Vasculitis (polyarteritis nodosa, cryoglobulinemia, scleroderma)
- Bilateral renal vein thrombosis

1.3.1.4 Interstitial Syndromes

- Chronic pyelonephritis and other kidney infections (e.g., tuberculosis)
- Acute interstitial nephritis (e.g., allergic drug-induced)
- Chronic interstitial nephritis (e.g., analgesic nephropathy)

- Papillary necrosis
- Sarcoid nephritis, Sjögren's syndrome, interstitial nephritis
- Tubulointerstitial nephritis with uveitis (TINU) syndrome

1.3.1.5 Tubular Syndromes

- Ischemic or nephrotoxic AKI (e.g., acute tubular necrosis [ATN])
- Myoglobinuria, hemoglobinuria
- Hypercalcemic nephropathy, milk-alkali syndrome
- Crystal deposition: urate nephropathy, oxalosis, phosphate nephropathy
- Toxic nephropathies (lithium, heavy metals, "herbal" aristolochic acid nephropathy)

1.3.1.6 Other Syndromes

- Cystic kidney diseases (e.g., polycystic kidney disease)
- Diabetic nephropathy
- Obstructive nephropathy
- Renal-cell carcinoma, other infiltrative diseases
- Renal stones
- Multiple myeloma (light chain or cast nephropathy, amyloidosis)
- Tuberous sclerosis, hereditary kidney diseases

For additional data, see specific chapter headings in the table of contents.

CHAPTER 2

Symptoms, Signs, and Differential Diagnosis

Robert Stephen Brown ■ Alexander Goldfarb-Rumyantzev

2.1 Edema

2.1.1 RENAL

Probable Diagnosis	Symptoms/Signs	Diagnostic Procedures
Nephrotic syndrome	• Facial swelling • Swelling of the arms and legs, especially the ankles and feet • Pleural effusions • Foamy urination • Weight gain (water retention)	• Urine protein/Cr ratio or 24-hour urine protein • BUN • Serum Cr • Serum albumin • CrCl or eGFR • UA with sediment microscopy • Serum and urine protein electrophoresis • HIV, anti-PLA2R (for membranous nephropathy) and hepatitis antibodies • Renal biopsy
Nephritic syndrome (e.g., acute glomerulonephritis)	• Peripheral or periorbital edema • Hematuria • Oliguria • Headache, secondary to hypertension • Shortness of breath or dyspnea on exertion, secondary to heart failure • Possible flank pain, secondary to stretching of the renal capsule	• UA and urinary sediment for protein, RBCs, acanthocytes, WBCs, casts (e.g., RBC casts) • Serum electrolytes, BUN, Cr • Serological tests for C3, C4, ASLO, ANCA, anti-GBM, and hepatitis antibodies • Serum and urine protein electrophoresis • Renal US and renal biopsy
CKD	• Swelling: generalized (fluid retention), ankle, foot, and leg • High blood pressure • Nausea or vomiting • Loss of appetite • Metallic taste in mouth • Flank pain • Hyperkalemia, metabolic acidosis • Urination changes: oliguria, anuria, nocturia (excessive urination at night) • Fatigue	• Blood tests: Cr, BUN, electrolytes, CBC, calcium, phosphate, albumin • CrCl or eGFR • Urine tests: 24-hour urinary protein or urine protein to Cr ratio • Serum and urine protein electrophoresis • Arterial or venous blood gas, if serum bicarbonate is low • Renal US • Renal biopsy if indicated and kidneys are not contracted and small • Abdominal CT scan or MRI when indicated by US findings

ASLO, antistreptolysin O; *ANCA*, anti-neutrophil cytoplasmic autoantibody; *BUN*, blood urea nitrogen; *C3*, C3 complement; *C4*, C4 complement; *CBC*, complete blood count; *CKD*, chronic kidney disease; *Cr*, creatinine; *CrCl*, creatinine clearance; *eGFR*, estimated glomerular filtration rate; *GBM*, glomerular basement membrane; *PLA2R*, phospholipase-A2 receptor; *RBCs*, red blood cells; *UA*, urinalysis; *US*, ultrasound; *WBCs*, white blood cells.

2.1.2 CARDIOVASCULAR

Probable Diagnosis	Symptoms/Signs	Diagnostic Procedures
Congestive heart failure (CHF)	• Swelling (edema) of the ankles and legs or abdomen • Basilar lung crackles • S3 gallop • Dyspnea (shortness of breath) • Cough • Fatigue, weakness, faintness • Loss of appetite • Palpitations • Swollen (enlarged) liver or abdomen • Neck veins distended • Nocturia (increased urination at night) • Weight gain	• ECG • Echocardiogram (echo) • Chest X-ray • Cardiac catheterization and angiography, if indicated • Blood test: BNP level
Cardiomyopathy (largely similar to CHF)	• Shortness of breath or dyspnea with physical exertion • Chest pain • Fatigue (tiredness) • Swelling in the ankles, feet, legs, abdomen, and veins in the neck • Dizziness, fainting • Lightheadedness • Arrhythmias (irregular heartbeats) • Heart murmurs	• Physical examination (tachypnea, tachycardia, hypertension or hypotension, hypoxia, JVD, pulmonary edema (lung crackles and/or wheezes), S3 gallop • BNP • Chest X-ray, MRI • Cardiac catheterization

BNP, Brain natriuretic peptide; CHF, congestive heart failure; ECG, electrocardiogram; JVD, jugular venous distension.

2.1.3 ENDOCRINE

Probable Diagnosis	Symptoms/Signs	Diagnostic Procedures
Cushing syndrome	• Round, red, full face (moon face) • Cervical fat pads • Comedones (acne) • Purplish pink stretch marks (abdominal striae) • Fatigue, headache, weak muscles • High blood pressure, high blood sugars, hypokalemia • Polydipsia and polyuria • Loss of libido, depression	• Clinical evaluation • Serum and salivary cortisol level, ACTH levels • Dexamethasone suppression test • 24-hour urinary measurement for cortisol • Abdominal CT or MRI scan of adrenal glands and MRI of pituitary gland • Bone density test
Hypothyroidism	• Puffy face and hands, and swelling of the legs • Increased sensitivity to cold • Fatigue or feeling slowed down • Joint or muscle pain • Coarse hair or brittle fingernails • Dry skin • Muscle cramps	• Clinical evaluation • TFTs • TRH test • MRI of the brain
Hyperthyroidism	(see 2.2 Hypertension)	

ACTH, Adrenocorticotropic hormone; TFTs, thyroid function tests; TRH, thyroid releasing hormone.

2.1.4 OTHERS

Probable Diagnosis	Symptoms/Signs	Diagnostic Procedures
Cirrhosis	• Swelling or fluid buildup of the legs (edema) and in the abdomen (ascites) • Confusion or problems thinking (hepatic encephalopathy) • Loss of appetite • Nausea and vomiting • Nosebleeds or bleeding gums • Pale or clay-colored stools • Small, red, spider-like blood vessels on the skin (spider angiomas) • Yellow color in the skin, mucus membranes, or eyes (jaundice) • Impotence, loss of libido	• Clinical history (alcoholism, obesity, hepatitis B or C, type 2 diabetes) • CBC, LFTs • Abdominal US • CT or MRI of the abdomen, hepatic fibrosis scan • Endoscopy to check abnormal variceal veins in the esophagus or stomach • Liver biopsy confirming cirrhosis/etiology • Levels of AFP • Wilson's disease, hemochromatosis studies, if indicated
Preeclampsia	• Swelling of face or legs • Severe headaches • Hypertension • Hyperreflexia • Blurry vision, flashing lights, or floaters • Vomiting, pain in the upper abdomen • Decrease in urine output	• CBC with differential and platelet count • Check for proteinuria • 24-hour urine collection for CrCl and total protein • Fetal US • sFLT-1 level or sFLT-1:PlGF ratio when diagnosis is unclear • LFTs (acute fatty liver of pregnancy)

AFP, Alpha-fetoprotein; *CBC*, complete blood count; *CrCl*, creatinine clearance; *LFTs*, liver function tests; *US*, ultrasound.

2.2 Hypertension

Probable Diagnosis	Symptoms/Signs	Diagnostic Procedures
CKD	(see 2.1.1 Renal)	
Hyperthyroidism	• High blood pressure • Difficulty concentrating • Fatigue • Frequent bowel movements • Goiter (visibly enlarged thyroid gland) or thyroid nodules • Heat intolerance • Increased appetite • Increased sweating • Itching (overall) • Lack of menstrual periods • Nausea and vomiting • Pounding, rapid, or irregular pulse • Protruding eyes (exophthalmos)	• Clinical evaluation • TFTs, thyroid scan • Radioactive iodine uptake • Blood glucose (hyperglycemia)

Continued on following page

Probable Diagnosis	Symptoms/Signs	Diagnostic Procedures
Cushing syndrome	(see 2.1.3 Endocrine)	
Primary hyperaldosteronism (Conn's syndrome)	• Hypertension • Muscle weakness • Polydipsia • Polyuria • Hypokalemia	• Blood test: plasma aldosterone/renin ratio • 24-hour urinary excretion of aldosterone test • Serum electrolytes for hypokalemia, metabolic alkalosis • Saline suppression test of aldosterone • MRI of adrenal glands • Adrenal vein sampling (to distinguish adenoma from bilateral hyperplasia) • Spironolactone therapeutic trial

CKD, Chronic kidney disease; *TFTs*, thyroid function tests.

2.3 Polyuria (UO >3000 mL/24 hr)

Probable Diagnosis	Symptoms/Signs	Diagnostic Procedures
CKD	(see 2.1.1 Renal)	
DI (central DI, nephrogenic DI)	• Polyuria, polydipsia • Unexplained weakness • Lethargy • Muscle pains • Irritability	• Urinalysis with specific gravity, osmolality • Serum sodium, urine sodium • Fluid deprivation test if not already hypernatremic • Desmopressin urine concentration test
Primary hyperaldosteronism	(see 2.2 Hypertension)	
Psychogenic or primary polydipsia	• Excessive water-drinking in the absence of a physiological stimulus to drink • Polyuria • Anxiety • History of psychiatric illnesses	• Fluid deprivation test • Serum sodium and osmolality • Urinary osmolality and sodium
Diabetes mellitus, hyperglycemia	• Frequent urination • Increased thirst • Headaches • Fatigue (weak, tired feeling) • Obesity or weight loss	• Blood sugar levels, HbA1c • Urine for glucose, ketones • Glucose tolerance test
Diuretics	• Recent initiation of diuretic for volume overload (e.g., due to heart failure or peripheral edema) • Patients who are likely to surreptitiously use diuretics for weight loss (e.g., those with eating disorders or concerns about weight, athletes, adolescents)	• Clinical evaluation of volume status • Serum electrolytes and osmolality • Urine osmolality, sodium, potassium and chloride • Urine diuretic screen, if indicated

CKD, Chronic kidney disease; *DI*, diabetes insipidus.

2.4 Hematuria

Probable Diagnosis	Symptoms/Signs	Diagnostic Procedures
Glomerulonephritis	(see 2.1.1 Renal)	
UTI	• Pain or burning upon urination • Cloudy or foul-smelling urine • A strong, persistent urge to urinate • Passing frequent, small amounts of urine • Urine that appears red, bright pink, or cola-colored (a sign of blood in the urine) • Pelvic pain in women	• UA, CBC • Urine and blood cultures • Pelvic exam in women • Vaginal discharge tested for STD organisms (e.g., *Neisseria* and *Chlamydia*) • Special culture media • Urinary tract radiology when indicated
Kidney stone	• Flank pain that is severe and colicky in nature • Pain often accompanied by restlessness, nausea, and vomiting • Hematuria, gross or microscopic • Stone passage: may be felt, but best to strain urine to catch stone	• Serum electrolytes, calcium, phosphate, Cr • UA to look for hematuria, infection, crystals • Stone analysis • Noncontrast CT is preferable imaging • Abdominal X-ray (KUB), IVP, or US can be helpful if CT unavailable
Bladder cancer	• Abdominal pain • Hematuria • Painful urination • Urinary frequency • Urinary urgency • Urine leakage (incontinence) • Weight loss • Fatigue	• Abdominal and pelvic CT scan, MRI scan • Cystoscopy • Bladder biopsy • UA, urine cytology
Drug side effects or overdose: aspirin, warfarin, or antiplatelet agents (e.g., clopidogrel)	• Abdominal pain with cramping • Hematuria • Unusual bleeding (nose, mouth, vagina, or rectum) • Burning, itching, numbness, prickling, "pins and needles," or tingling feelings • Difficulty breathing or swallowing • Dizziness, faintness, headache • Increased menstrual flow or vaginal bleeding	• History: warfarin overdose more common than other anticoagulant drug causes • Coagulation tests • Anatomical studies for causes indicated even with anticoagulation-associated hematuria • Clinical evaluation

CBC, Complete blood count; *Cr*, creatinine; *IVP*, intravenous pyelogram; *KUB*, kidney, ureter, and bladder x-ray; *STD*, sexually transmitted disease; *UA*, urinalysis; *US*, ultrasound; *UTI*, urinary tract infection.

2.5 Metallic Taste

Probable Diagnosis	Symptoms/Signs	Diagnostic Procedures
CKD	(see 2.1.1 Renal)	
Vitamin B12 deficiency	• Tingling, numbness in fingers and toes • Weakness, tiredness, or light-headedness • Memory loss, disorientation, depression • Loss of appetite • Palpitations and breathing • Sore tongue	• Clinical evaluation • CBC with differential and RBC MCV • Serum vitamin B12 level
Pregnancy	• Fatigue/tiredness • Nausea/morning sickness • Backaches • Headache • Frequent urination • Itchy skin during pregnancy, especially on the abdomen, thighs, breasts, and arms	• Blood test: PAPP-A screening, hCG • AFP screening • US (abdomen and pelvis)
Oral health and sinus problems (plaque, gingivitis, periodontitis, tooth decay and abscesses)	• Bleeding gums • Gums that are tender when touched, but otherwise painless • Mouth sores • Swollen gums	• Clinical evaluation • Dental X-rays
Drug side effects or overdose (clarithromycin, metronidazole, cisplatin, carboplatin, metformin, paxlovid (nirmatrelvir/ritonavir))	• Nausea • Headaches • Loss of appetite • Rash	• Medical history • Blood testing as indicated

AFP, Alpha-fetoprotein; *CBC,* complete blood count; *CKD,* chronic kidney disease; *hCG,* human chorionic gonadotropin; *MCV,* mean corpuscular volume; *PAPP-A,* pregnancy-associated plasma protein; *RBC,* red blood cell; *US,* ultrasound.

2.6 Weakness, Fatigue, and Lethargy

Probable Diagnosis	Symptoms/Signs	Diagnostic Procedures
CKD	(see 2.1.1 Renal)	
Hypothyroidism	(see 2.1.3 Endocrine)	
Anemia	• Fatigue, lethargy, weakness • Dyspnea on exertion, progressing to dyspnea at rest • Lightheadedness • Dizziness • Fainting • Chest pain, angina • Palpitations	• Lab tests: CBC, iron level, transferrin level, ferritin, vitamin B12, LFTs, folate, BUN, Cr • Bone marrow biopsy • Lung examination • Systolic heart murmur may be present

Probable Diagnosis	Symptoms/Signs	Diagnostic Procedures
Autoimmune disease	• Fatigue, lethargy, weakness • Fever • Malaise • Skin or joint findings	• CBC, CRP, ESR • Antinuclear antibody tests • Autoantibody tests
Depression	• Fatigue, lethargy, weakness • Feels helpless, hopeless • Loss of appetite • Anger • Irritability • Loathing of life	• Lab tests to rule out other medical conditions causing depression: TFTs, calcium, serum electrolytes, LFTs, BUN, Cr • CT scan or MRI of the brain • EEG, ECG
Adrenal insufficiency (Addison's disease)	(see 2.9 Hyperkalemia)	

BUN, blood urea nitrogen; *CBC*, complete blood count; *CKD*, chronic kidney disease; *Cr*, creatinine; *CRP*, C-reactive protein; *ECG*, electrocardiogram; *EEG*, electroencephalogram; *ESR*, erythrocyte sedimentation rate; *LFTs*, liver function tests; *TFTs*, thyroid function tests.

2.7 Shortness of Breath

Probable Diagnosis	Symptoms/Signs	Diagnostic Procedures
Pleural effusion	• Pleuritic chest pain • Lung field that is dull to percussion • Diminished breath sounds	• Chest X-ray, chest CT • Thoracentesis
CHF	(see 2.1.2 Cardiovascular)	
Anemia	(see 2.6 Weakness, Fatigue, and Lethargy)	
CKD	(see 2.1.1 Renal)	
Pneumonia	• Fever, chills, cough, purulent sputum • Dyspnea, tachycardia	• Chest X-ray
Pneumothorax	• Unilateral diminished breath sounds • Dyspnea • Subcutaneous emphysema (air under the skin) may be present • May follow injury or occur spontaneously (especially in tall, thin patients or patients with COPD)	• Chest X-ray
Pulmonary embolism	• Pleuritic pain • Dyspnea • Palpitations, tachycardia • Cough, sweating • Hemoptysis • Hypotension (shock)	• CT angiography • V/Q scan • Doppler or duplex study of extremities for deep vein thrombosis • ABG for hypoxemia • D dimor level
COPD exacerbation	• Cough • Dyspnea • Poor air movement • Pursed-lip breathing • Accessory muscle use for breathing	• Clinical evaluation • Chest X-ray • ABG for hypoxemia, hypercarbia • Pulmonary function testing

Continued on following page

Probable Diagnosis	Symptoms/Signs	Diagnostic Procedures
Asthma, broncho-spasm, reactive airway disease	• Wheezing, poor air exchange • Arising spontaneously or after stimulus (e.g., cold, exercise, allergen) • Sometimes pulsus paradoxus	• Clinical evaluation • Sometimes pulmonary function testing or bedside peak flow measurement
Foreign body inhalation	• Sudden cough or stridor	• Chest X-ray (inspiratory and expiratory) • Sometimes bronchoscopy
Restrictive lung disease	• Progressive dyspnea	• Chest X-ray • Pulmonary function testing
Interstitial lung disease	• Fine crackles on auscultation • Progressive dyspnea	• High-resolution chest CT

ABG, arterial blood gas; *CHF*, Congestive heart failure; *COPD*, chronic obstructive pulmonary disease; *D-dimer*, protein fragment from blood clot degradation; *V/Q scan*, pulmonary ventilation and perfusion scan.

2.8 Changes in Urination

2.8.1 BURNING ON URINATION, URGENCY, AND FREQUENCY

Probable Diagnosis	Symptoms/Signs	Diagnostic Procedures
UTI	(see 2.4 Hematuria)	
Bladder cancer	(see 2.4 Hematuria)	
Interstitial cystitis	• Urgency • Frequency • Suprapubic pain • Dyspareunia	• UA • Cystoscopy • Biopsy of the bladder

UA, urinalysis; *UIT*, urinary tract infection.

2.9 Hyperkalemia

Probable Diagnosis	Symptoms/Signs	Diagnostic Procedures
CKD	(see 2.1.1 Renal)	
Acidosis	• Rapid breathing • Confusion • Lethargy • Shortness of breath	• ABG or VBG • Serum electrolytes • Urine pH • Pulmonary function testing • Chest X-ray
Glomerulonephritis	(see 2.4 Hematuria)	
Adrenal insufficiency (Addison's disease)	• Fatigue, weakness • Weight loss • GI symptoms • Hypotension • Hyperpigmentation • Hyponatremia • Hyperkalemia • Hypoglycemia	• Serum cortisol (morning or stressed) • Plasma ACTH (morning level) • Cosyntropin stimulation test

Probable Diagnosis	Symptoms/Signs	Diagnostic Procedures
Hypoaldosteronism	• Metabolic acidosis, nonanion gap, with hyperkalemia	• Blood and Urine electrolytes and Osm for transtubular K^+ gradient (TTKG) and anion gap • Plasma renin, aldosterone and cortisol levels

ABG, Arterial blood gas; *CKD*, chronic kidney disease; *GI*, gastrointestinal; *Osm*, osmolarity; *TTKG*, transtubular potassium gradient; *VBG*, venous blood gas.

2.10 Rash or Itchy, Dry Skin

Probable Diagnosis	Symptoms/Signs	Diagnostic Procedures
CKD	(see 2.1.1 Renal)	
Liver disease	• Nausea • Vomiting • Abdominal pain • Jaundice • Fatigue, weakness, and weight loss • Itching due to deposits of bile salts	• LFTs, CBC, serum electrolytes, INR • Hepatitis viral serological testing • Radiology: CT scan, US, or MRI, hepatic fibrosis scan • Liver biopsy
Psoriasis	• Irritated, red, scaling patches or plaques of skin (dry and covered with silver, flaky scales) • Red patches may appear anywhere on the body, including the scalp • Pitting of fingernails • Joint pain	• Physical examination • Medical and family history • Skin biopsy • X-rays (if joint pains)
Eczema	• Blisters with oozing and crusting • Itchy and dry skin	• Medical and family history • Skin biopsy • Allergy skin testing
Pregnancy	(see 2.5 Metallic Taste)	
Drug allergy (antibiotics, antifungal and many others)	• Red, itchy, and raised swellings on the skin (e.g., hives or palpable purpura) • Fever • Muscle and joint aches	• Medical history • CBC (e.g., eosinophil count for eosinophilia) • Skin biopsy

CBC, Complete blood count; *CKD*, chronic kidney disease; *INR*, international normalized ratio; *LFTs*, liver function tests; *US*, ultrasound.

CHAPTER 3

Renal Physiology

Robert Stephen Brown ■ Alexander Morales ■ Alexander Goldfarb-Rumyantzev

3 Renal Physiology[1,2]

The kidney has multiple functions, including the following:
- Excretory function—elimination of small molecular "wastes" from the body
- Maintaining electrolyte balance
- Maintaining acid-base balance
- Maintaining appropriate body volumes and tonicity (osmolarity)
- Endocrine function—production of erythropoietin, renin, 1,25-dihydroxyvitamin D (calcitriol), and prostaglandins (not discussed here)
- Gluconeogenesis (not discussed here)

3.1 ANATOMY OF THE KIDNEY

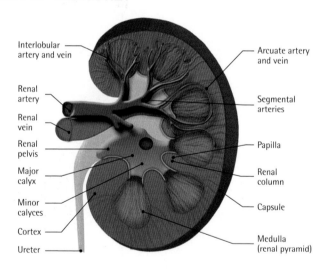

Interlobular artery and vein

Renal artery

Renal vein

Renal pelvis

Major calyx

Minor calyces

Cortex

Ureter

Arcuate artery and vein

Segmental arteries

Papilla

Renal column

Capsule

Medulla (renal pyramid)

3.2 ANATOMY OF A NEPHRON

Each kidney has about one million nephrons with a structure depicted in simplified fashion below. The nephrons are in close contact with the renal vasculature as the efferent arteriolar outflow of blood from the glomeruli perfuses the tubules in the kidney cortex. These arterioles form the vasa recta, capillary loops which extend into the renal medulla adjacent to the Loop of Henle and are important to maintain sodium reabsorption in the thick ascending limb necessary to both dilute the urine and maintain osmotic concentrations in the renal papillae needed to concentrate the urine.[1,2]

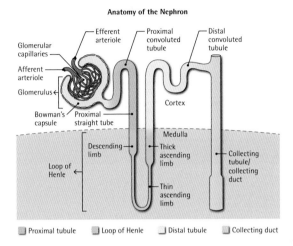

Anatomy of the Nephron

3.3 PHYSIOLOGY OF GLOMERULAR FILTRATION

- The renal blood flow is approximately 20% of the cardiac output at rest (1–1.2 L/min).
- The glomerular filtration rate (GFR) normally is approximately 120 mL/min or about 170–180 L/day.
- The filtration fraction, GFR/RPF (renal plasma flow), is approximately 20%, or about 10% of renal blood flow is filtered.
- GFR is determined by the pressure gradient across the glomerular capillary wall and glomerular basement membrane (GBM), the permeability of the GBM (filtration coefficient), and the filtration area.[3,4]
- The pressure gradient driving glomerular filtration is the sum of the net hydraulic pressure (glomerular capillary hydrostatic pressure of ~55–60 mmHg less capsular hydrostatic pressure of ~15 mmHg or a net of ~40–45 mmHg) favoring filtration counteracted by the blood colloid osmotic pressure (~30 mmHg). As blood traverses the glomerular capillaries, filtration pressure equilibrium is reached as the fluid loss from the capillary lowers the hydraulic pressure and increases the colloid osmotic pressure, as shown below.[1,2]

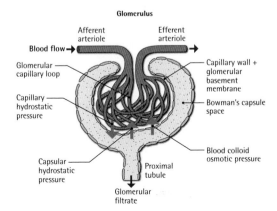

Glomerulus

The rate of glomerular filtration can be regulated by changing intraglomerular pressure, which is primarily regulated by changing the tonus of the afferent and efferent arterioles (i.e., in the afferent arteriole, constriction reduces the flow and intraglomerular pressure, and dilation increases the flow and intraglomerular pressure, whereas constriction of the efferent arteriole will increase intraglomerular pressure to maintain GFR even when blood flow is reduced).[1]

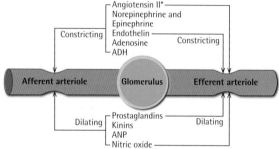

Regulation of Glomerular Filtration Rate

*Angiotensin II has a greater effect on the efferent arteriole than on the afferent arteriole, so it will initially serve to maintain GFR at low BP.
ADH, antidiuretic hormone; *ANP*, atrial natriuretic peptide.

3.4 AUTOREGULATION OF GFR

Autoregulation of GFR is a mechanism that maintains relatively constant renal blood flow and GFR despite changes in systemic arterial pressure. This mechanism fails at very low (MAP <50 mmHg) and very high (MAP >150 mmHg) arterial pressures, in which case renal blood flow, and to a lesser extent, GFR, decreases or increases, respectively. These autoregulatory factors, some of which are noted above, tend to maintain GFR at normal or near normal levels over a wide range of arterial blood pressures.[1,4,5]

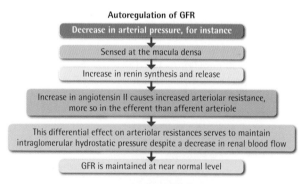

Autoregulation of GFR

Decrease in arterial pressure, for instance

Sensed at the macula densa

Increase in renin synthesis and release

Increase in angiotensin II causes increased arteriolar resistance, more so in the efferent than afferent arteriole

This differential effect on arteriolar resistances serves to maintain intraglomerular hydrostatic pressure despite a decrease in renal blood flow

GFR is maintained at near normal level

3.5 TUBULAR FUNCTION OF THE NEPHRON, AT A GLANCE

The glomerular filtrate of approximately 170 to 180 L/day allows the excretion of large quantities of small molecular waste products that are freely filtered and not reabsorbed by the tubules. The glomerular filtrate enters the renal tubules, and since the final urinary volume is about 1 to 1.5 L/day, about 99% of the fluid volume and the requisite amounts of electrolytes, glucose, amino acids, and proteins must be reabsorbed by the tubules to maintain body balance.[1,4] This process depends upon the active renal tubular cell transport of sodium, an energy-requiring process that creates the osmotic and electrostatic forces which drive the reabsorptive transport of electrolytes and water and the secretion of other molecules, such as hydrogen ions, potassium, and uric acid.[1] A general depiction of this function is shown below.

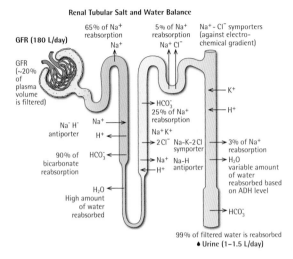

Renal Tubular Salt and Water Balance

3.6 RENAL HANDLING OF SODIUM

Under common conditions, over 99% of the filtered sodium is reabsorbed overall, 65% in the proximal tubule with bicarbonate and chloride as "accompanying" anions, and to a much lesser degree, sodium is co-transported with glucose, phosphate, and amino acids.[1,2,6,7] In the collecting ducts, sodium reabsorption is accomplished by exchange for secretion of hydrogen and potassium cations.[1,4,8,9] The reabsorption of sodium and water to maintain homeostasis of body volumes is dependent upon the GFR, as well as glomerulotubular balance to increase or decrease sodium reabsorption in parallel with the GFR. A number of regulatory hormones impart changes in the GFR and glomerulotubular balance to effect sodium and water handling, thereby maintaining volume and osmotic balance.

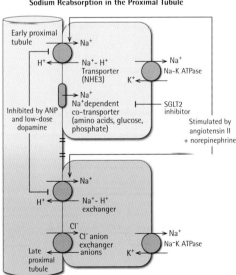

Sodium Reabsorption in the Proximal Tubule

Sodium Reabsorption in the Loop of Henle

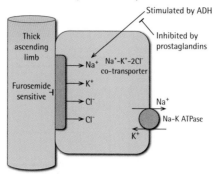

Sodium Reabsorption in the Distal Tubule

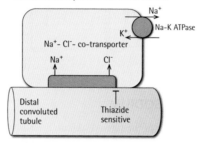

Sodium Reabsorption in the Collecting Duct

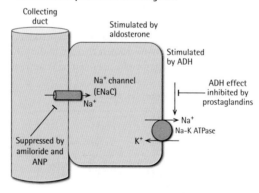

Kidney Regulation of Sodium Balance
Mechanism of increased sodium reabsorption

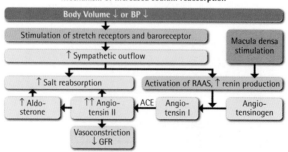

Mechanism of decreased sodium reabsorption

↑BP, ↑atrial distention

↑ GFR, ↑ ANP production, ↓ aldosterone

↓ Na⁺ reabsorption in proximal tubule + collecting duct

3.7 ACID-BASE REGULATION

To maintain normal blood pH, the kidney must first reabsorb the filtered bicarbonate. This takes place mainly in the proximal tubule in a process largely coupled to sodium reabsorption and hydrogen ion (H+) secretion which is dependent upon carbonic anhydrase by the mechanisms shown below.[1,10] Since most human diets produce metabolic acids to excrete, after reabsorption of bicarbonate takes place, additional hydrogen ions are secreted into the urine to be excreted as "titratable" acid (mainly as phosphates and sulfates at urine pH levels that can be reduced below 5), and by ammonium ions.[1,4,10] Alkalinization of the urine by bicarbonate secretion, though also shown below, can take place but is usually unnecessary.

Bicarbonate Reabsorption

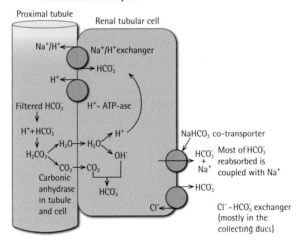

Bicarbonate Secretion

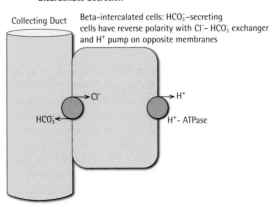

3.8 RENAL ACID EXCRETION[1,10,11]

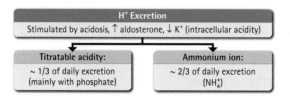

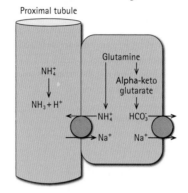

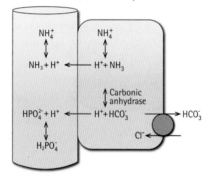

3.9 POTASSIUM HOMEOSTASIS[1,12]

Total body stores of potassium amount to about 3000 mEq, most of which is intracellular, as in muscle cells and in bone, while only about 60 mEq or 2% of potassium is in the extracellular fluid.[1] Since maintenance of the potassium electrical gradient across heart muscle cell membranes is so important, precise regulation of potassium distribution between the intracellular and extracellular fluid compartments is essential. The major factors increasing cellular uptake of potassium are insulin and beta-sympathetic catecholamines (epinephrine), which stimulate the Na-K ATPase transporter, and alkalosis with low intracellular $H+$ ion that will lower serum K^+. Conversely, low-insulin, alpha-sympathetic catecholamines, or acidosis, will raise serum K^+, as shown below. In addition, the ultimate regulation of total body potassium depends upon renal excretion of the approximately 100 mEq/day of dietary potassium required to maintain proper potassium balance. About 90% of the roughly 700 mEq/day of potassium filtered by the glomeruli is reabsorbed in the proximal tubule. Typically, there is an excess of potassium from dietary sources which can subsequently be excreted in the distal nephron. However, in states of low potassium balance (such as those that can be seen in gastrointestinal losses), distal K conservation can occur.[1,4] The major factors affecting potassium excretion are aldosterone, distal tubular Na+ delivery, urine flow rate, and acid-base status, as shown below. In addition, potassium adaptation stimulated by increased K+ in the diet or high serum K+ causes both increased intracellular uptake of K+ by muscle cells and increased renal K+ excretion to protect against worsening hyperkalemia (with the opposite occurring in cases of a low K+ diet and low serum K+ levels to protect against hypokalemia).

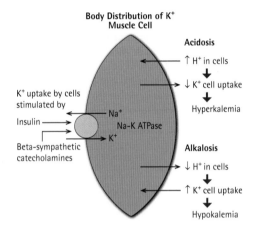

Body Distribution of K+
Muscle Cell

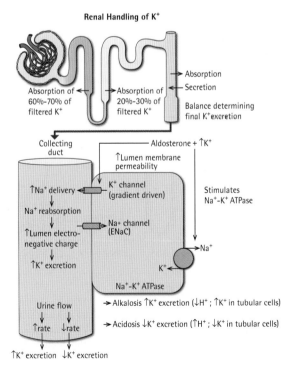

Renal Handling of K+

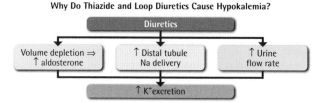

Why Do Thiazide and Loop Diuretics Cause Hypokalemia?

3.10 DIURETIC SITES OF ACTION IN THE NEPHRON[13]

The three major classes of diuretics used for enhancing sodium excretion are thiazide diuretics, loop diuretics, and potassium-sparing diuretics (either aldosterone antagonists or epithelial sodium channel blockers). Other drugs have diuretic action, but are used for more specific purposes, such as carbonic anhydrase inhibitors (to cause bicarbonaturia or alkalinize the urine), osmotic diuretics (to enhance urinary excretion of poisons or for central nervous system edema), low-dose dopamine (for congestive heart failure and acute kidney injury (AKI), but probably no longer indicated for AKI treatment), and ADH antagonists (to induce a water diuresis to correct hyponatremia). Their sites of action in the renal tubule are shown in the diagram below.

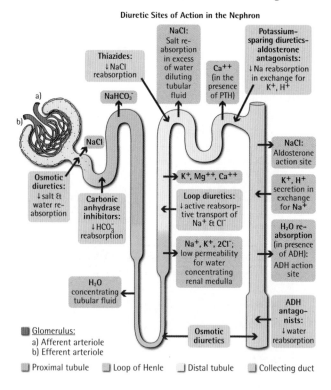

Diuretic Sites of Action in the Nephron

3.11 RENAL HANDLING OF CALCIUM

Since calcium is partially bound to albumin, about 6 mg/dL of calcium is filtered, amounting to about 10,800 mg/day in the 180 L/day of glomerular filtrate. With intestinal absorption, and therefore, renal excretion amounting to about 200 mg/day, 98% of the filtered calcium is reabsorbed by the tubules. In the proximal tubule and the Loop of Henle, about 80% of the calcium is reabsorbed, largely paralleling sodium reabsorption.[1,14,15] In the distal tubule where about 15% of the calcium is reabsorbed, hormonal regulation controls calcium reabsorption to achieve body balance by the mechanisms shown below.

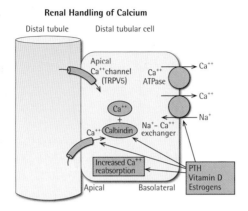

Renal Handling of Calcium

3.12 RENAL HANDLING OF PHOSPHATE

Phosphate is filtered at the glomerulus and reabsorbed mainly in the proximal tubule along with sodium, and has a fractional excretion of about 15% to 20%. Excretion can vary depending upon dietary phosphate intake.[1,15] Phosphate excretion is under the regulation of the hormones PTH (parathyroid hormone) and FGF23 (fibroblast growth factor 23)-Klotho complex, which exert a phosphaturic action by blocking renal tubular phosphate reabsorption, as shown below.

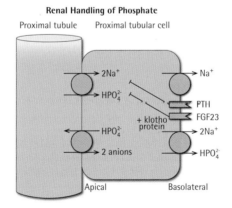

Renal Handling of Phosphate

3.13 RENAL HANDLING OF WATER

A simplified schema of the tubular water reabsorption mechanisms to reduce the urine volume to approximately 1% of the filtered fluid volume is depicted here. The first mechanism is the passive water reabsorption in the proximal tubule, Loop of Henle, and distal tubule based on the isoomolar, cortical, and hyperosmolar medullary environments. The second mechanism is the ADH-dependent water reabsorption occurring mainly in the collecting duct, which determines the final urine concentration.[1,16,17]

Passive Water Reabsorption

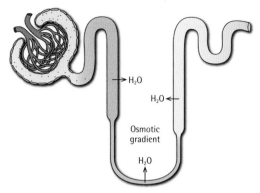

ADH-Mediated Water Reabsorption

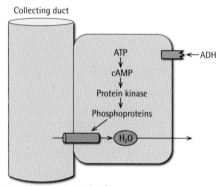

Urine osmolarity 50–1200 mOsm/L
ADH↓⟹↑urine volume with decreased osmolarity
ADH↑ increases water reabsorption and urine osmolarity with decreased urine volume

References

1. Rose B, Post T. *Clinical Physiology of Acid-Base and Electrolyte Disorders*. 5th ed. McGraw-Hill; 2001: 35-49, 72-102, 147, 148-153, 287-296.
2. Eaton D, Pooler J. Chapter 1 Renal Functions Basic Processes, and Anatomy; Chapter 2 Renal Blood Flow and Glomerular Filtration; Chapter 6 Basic Renal Processes for Sodium, Chloride, and Water. *Vander's Renal Physiology*. 8th ed. McGraw-Hill; 2013:1-15; 1-13; 1-20.
3. Deen WM, Bridges CR, Brenner BM, Myers BD. Heteroporous model of glomerular size selectivity: application to normal and nephrotic humans. *Am J Physiol*. 1985;249(3 Pt 2):F374–F389. doi:10.1152/ajprenal.1985.249.3.F374.
4. Rennke HG, Denker BM. *Renal Pathophysiology: The Essentials*. 5th ed. Wolters Kluwer; 2020:vi, 1-67, 154-173.
5. Cupples WA, Braam B. Assessment of renal autoregulation. *Am J Physiol Renal Physiol*. 2007; 292(4):F1105–F1123. doi:10.1152/ajprenal.00194.2006.
6. Brown E, Heerspink HJL, Cuthbertson DJ, Wilding JPH. SGLT2 inhibitors and GLP-1 receptor agonists: established and emerging indications. *Lancet*. 2021;398(10296):262–276. doi:10.1016/S0140-6736(21)00536-5.
7. Wright EM. SGLT2 inhibitors: physiology and pharmacology. *Kidney360*. 2021;2(12):2027–2037. doi:10.34067/KID.0002772021.

8. Frömter E, Rumrich G, Ullrich KJ. Phenomenologic description of Na1, Cl2 and HCO-3 absorption from proximal tubules of the rat kidney. *Pflugers Arch.* 1973;343(3):189–220. doi:10.1007/BF00586045.

9. Eladari D, Chambrey R, Peti-Peterdi J. A new look at electrolyte transport in the distal tubule. *Annu Rev Physiol.* 2012;74:325–349. doi:10.1146/annurev-physiol-020911-153225.

10. Danziger J, Zeidel M, Parker M. *Renal Physiology: A Clinical Approach.* Lippincott Williams & Wilkins; 2012:155-178.

11. Wagner CA, Imenez Silva PH, Bourgeois S. Molecular pathophysiology of acid-base disorders. *Semin Nephrol.* 2019;39(4):340–352. doi:10.1016/j.semnephrol.2019.04.004.

12. Clase CM, Carrero JJ, Ellison DH, et al. Potassium homeostasis and management of dyskalemia in kidney diseases: conclusions from Kidney Disease: Improving Global Outcomes (KDIGO) Controversies Conference. *Kidney Int.* 2020;97(1):42–61. doi:10.1016/j.kint.2019.09.018.

13. Ellison DH. Clinical pharmacology in diuretic use [published correction appears in *Clin J Am Soc Nephrol.* 2019;14(11):1653–1654]. *Clin J Am Soc Nephrol.* 2019;14(8):1248–1257. doi:10.2215/CJN.09630818.

14. Lambers TT, Bindels RJM, Hoenderop, JGJ. Coordinated control of renal Ca^{2+} handling. *Kidney Int.* 2006;69(4):650–654. doi:10.1038/sj.ki.5000169.

15. Blaine J, Chonchol M, Levi M. Renal control of calcium, phosphate, and magnesium homeostasis. *Clin J Am Soc Nephrol.* 2015;10(7):1257–1272. doi:10.2215/CJN.09750913.

16. Schrier RW. *Renal and Electrolyte Disorders.* 8th ed. Lippincott Williams & Wilkins; 2017:viii, pp1-96.

17. Schrier RW. Body water homeostasis: clinical disorders of urinary dilution and concentration. *J Am Soc Nephrol.* 2006;17(7):1820–1832. doi:10.1681/ASN.2006030240.

CHAPTER 4

Water and Electrolyte Disorders

Robert Stephen Brown ▧ Alexander Goldfarb-Rumyantzev ▧
Alexander Morales

4.1 Water Distribution Between Body Compartments[1-6]

The diagram below illustrates water distribution between intracellular and extracellular body compartments, the latter including interstitial and intravascular spaces.

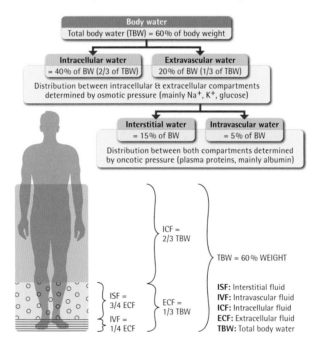

4.2 Sites of Electrolyte Reabsorption

The simplified diagram below illustrates important sites of electrolyte reabsorption in the nephron and where Na^+ reabsorption can be inhibited by diuretics.[1-7]

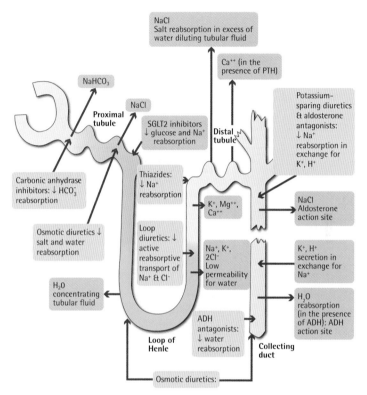

ADH, Antidiuretic hormone; SGLT2, sodium-glucose co-transporter 2.

4.3 Hypernatremia[8,9]

Causes of hypernatremia are divided into three categories based on the patient's volume status, as shown in the diagram below. Hypernatremia occurs in only 0.1% to 0.2% of hospitalized patients. It is always associated with hypertonicity (hyperosmolality).

4.3.1 HYPERNATREMIA: CAUSES

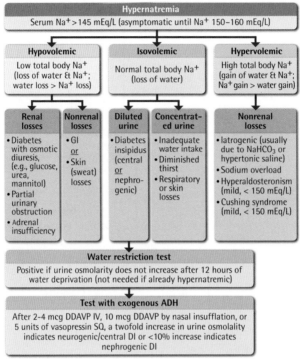

ADH, Antidiuretic hormone; GI, gastrointestinal; DDAVP, 1-deamino-8-D-arginine vasopressin or desmopressin; DI, diabetes insipidus; SQ, subcutaneous.

4.3.2 HYPERNATREMIA CLINICAL MANIFESTATIONS

The clinical manifestations of hypernatremia depend upon rapidity of onset, duration, and magnitude of hypernatremia.

Alteration of brain water content with brain volume loss:

- In severe cases (generally with serum Na^+ >160 mmol/L): substantial brain shrinkage, traction of the venous sinuses and intracerebral veins leading to rupture and hemorrhage
- In less severe cases: nonspecific symptoms (nausea, muscle weakness, fasciculations, decreased mental status)

Complications of aggressive treatment:

- Adaptation to hypernatremia results in the uptake of idiogenic osmoles by brain cells, resulting in brain edema when overly rapid rehydration takes place (causing seizures, decreased mental status).
- However, the complications as a result of overly rapid correction of chronic hypernatremia (in <48 hr) are described predominantly in pediatric patients.[10,11]

4.3.3 TREATMENT OF HYPERNATREMIA

For practical purposes one can imagine that the body maintains the homeostasis of the basic components in the following order of priority:

1. Circulatory volume
2. Osmotic equilibrium
3. Electrolyte concentration

Similarly, in the treatment of electrolyte disorders, therapeutic measures should be directed at the same aspects in the same order (e.g., attempts to correct the circulatory volume should take priority and precede correction of sodium concentration and osmolality).

Helpful points in treating hypernatremia:

- In patients with hypovolemia, start with volume expansion with normal (isotonic) saline or lactated Ringers solution, then correct water deficit either with oral water replacement or with intravenous (IV) half-normal saline or dextrose 5% in water.
- In patients with hypervolemia, treat with water + loop diuretic to avoid pulmonary or cerebral edema. Recall that only about 10% of "free" water, typically provided with 5% dextrose intravenously, is maintained intravascularly, and thus contribution to additional volume overload is modest.
- Replace calculated water deficit (see formula below) plus ongoing losses (urinary, gastrointestinal [GI]) plus insensible losses (no more than half of the calculated water deficit in the first 24 hr to prevent cerebral edema).
- Reduce Na^+ concentration by ≤ 1 mmol/L/hr (≤ 1 mEq/L/hr) if symptomatic initially, but do not reduce Na^+ by more than 12 mmol/L/day.
- When symptoms are resolved, replace the remaining water deficit within 24 to 48 hours.
- In acute hypernatremia (<48 hr duration), the water deficit should be corrected rapidly to prevent cerebral hemorrhage or acute osmotic demyelination.
- Worsening neurological status after initial improvement suggests brain edema. Discontinue water replacement.
- Central diabetes insipidus (CDI)—treat with desmopressin (DDAVP)
- Nephrogenic diabetes insipidus (NDI): Thiazides inhibit urinary diluting capacity and cause mild intravascular volume depletion, which decreases water delivery to the collecting duct, which in turn decreases polyuria for symptomatic benefit.
- Amiloride for lithium-induced NDI: Like thiazides, amiloride decreases polyuria, but spares excessive K^+ wasting and may diminish lithium toxicity (by blocking lithium entry into collecting duct cells in exchange for Na^+).

Water deficit to correct in hypernatremia:

Water deficit to correct in hypernatremia (assuming distribution volume of Na^+ to be 0.6 of the body mass):

$$\text{Water deficit} \left(L\right) = \frac{\text{Serum } Na^+ \left(\text{mmol}/L\right) - 140}{140} \times 0.6 \times \text{Body mass}\left(kg\right)$$

4.4 Hyponatremia[8,9]

Hyponatremia is relatively common, occurring in 1% to 2% of hospitalized patients. Unlike hypernatremia (which is always associated with hypertonicity), hyponatremia can be associated with hypotonicity, isotonicity, or hypertonicity. To identify the cause of hyponatremia one has to collect the following information: plasma osmolality, patient volume status, urine sodium concentration, and urine osmolality (Uosm), the latter which reflects antidiuretic hormone (ADH) secretion.[8,9,12–16]

Plasma Osmolality

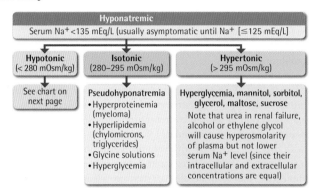

Volume Status and Urine Na⁺

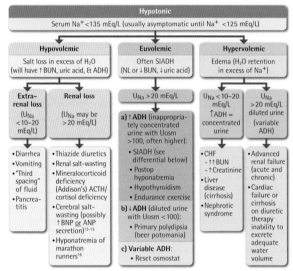

ACTH, Adrenocorticotropic hormone; *ADH*, antidiuretic hormone; *ANP*, atrial natriuretic peptide; *BNP*, brain natriuretic peptide; *BUN*, blood urea nitrogen; *CHF*, congestive heart failure; *NL*, normal; *SIADH*, syndrome of inappropriate antidiuretic hormone secretion.

Helpful points for syndrome of inappropriate antidiuretic hormone secretion (SIADH):

- A low ADH level results in diluted urine, so Uosm <100 mOsm/Kg (e.g., in primary polydipsia/"beer potomania").
- SIADH is the most common cause of euvolemic hyponatremia. SIADH is hard to distinguish from cerebral salt wasting as volume status might be difficult to estimate, but cerebral salt wasting is usually due to intracranial hemorrhage and much less common. It does not have strict diagnostic criteria or lab tests associated with it, though management is often similar to SIADH. Both can be treated with 3% (hypertonic) saline, making differentiation in an urgent clinical scenario of little importance.[13,17]
- Diagnostic criteria for SIADH: hypoosmolarity (serum osmolarity <280 mOsm/kg); hyponatremia (Na⁺ ≤134 mEq/L) with clinical euvolemia; urinary Na⁺ >40 mEq/L; inappropriately concentrated urine (Uosm >100 mOsm/kg); and normal adrenal, thyroid, cardiac, renal, and hepatic function, frequently with hypouricemia.[9,12]

Differential Diagnosis of SIADH

SIADH is the most frequent cause of hyponatremia in a hospitalized patient. It is important to identify the underlying cause of SIADH, as it may be due to serious or even urgent medical conditions, or may recur.

Malignant neoplasia:
- Carcinoma (bronchogenic, duodenal, pancreatic, ureteral, prostatic, bladder)
- Lymphoma and leukemia
- Thymoma, mesothelioma, and Ewing's sarcoma

Central nervous system (CNS) disorders:
- Trauma, subarachnoid hemorrhage, and subdural hematoma
- Infection (encephalitis, meningitis, brain abscess)
- Tumors
- Porphyria
- Stroke
- Vasculitis

Pulmonary disorders:
- Tuberculosis
- Pneumonia
- Vasculitis
- Mechanical ventilators with positive pressure
- Lung abscess

Drugs:
- Desmopressin
- Vasopressin
- Chlorpropamide
- Thiazide diuretics
- Oxytocin
- Haloperidol
- Phenothiazines
- Tricyclic antidepressants
- High-dose cyclophosphamide
- Selective serotonin reuptake inhibitors (SSRIs) and serotonin and norepinephrine reuptake inhibitors (SNRIs)
- Vinblastine/vincristine
- Nicotine

Other:
- "Idiopathic" SIADH
- Hypothyroidism
- HIV infection
- Guillain-Barre syndrome
- Multiple sclerosis
- Nephrogenic SIADH[18] (hereditary V2 receptor mutation[19])

4.4.1 CLINICAL MANIFESTATIONS OF HYPONATREMIA

Symptoms of hyponatremia depend on:
- the degree and rapidity of onset,
- underlying CNS status, and
- other metabolic factors such as:
  - hypoxia,

- acidosis,
- hypercalcemia, and
- hypercapnia.

The underlying mechanism of symptoms is hypoosmolar encephalopathy (brain edema from water shift):

- Mild symptoms: headache, nausea
- More severe symptoms (usually with Na^+ <125 mmol/L): confusion, obtundation, focal neurological deficits, seizures

4.4.2 TREATMENT OF HYPONATREMIA

As in the case of hypernatremia, the therapeutic measures aimed to correct hyponatremia should be directed at correcting the circulatory volume first and then at correcting the sodium concentration. If the hyponatremia developed rapidly (<24 hr), it should be corrected rapidly; if it developed slowly, it should be corrected slowly to decrease the risk of a CNS demyelinating syndrome.

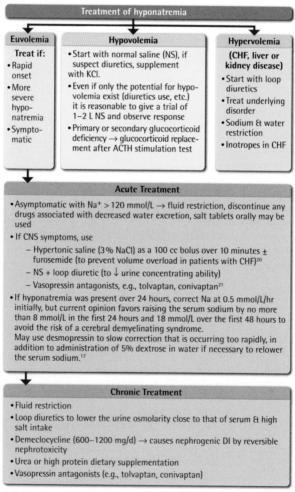

Treatment of hyponatremia

Euvolemia	Hypovolemia	Hypervolemia
Treat if: • Rapid onset • More severe hypo-natremia • Sympto-matic	• Start with normal saline (NS), if suspect diuretics, supplement with KCl. • Even if only the potential for hypo-volemia exist (diuretics use, etc.) it is reasonable to give a trial of 1–2 L NS and observe response • Primary or secondary glucocorticoid deficiency → glucocorticoid replace-ment after ACTH stimulation test	**(CHF, liver or kidney disease)** • Start with loop diuretics • Treat underlying disorder • Sodium & water restriction • Inotropes in CHF

Acute Treatment

- Asymptomatic with Na^+ > 120 mmol/L → fluid restriction, discontinue any drugs associated with decreased water excretion, salt tablets orally may be used
- If CNS symptoms, use
  - Hypertonic saline (3% NaCl) as a 100 cc bolus over 10 minutes ± furosemide (to prevent volume overload in patients with CHF)[20]
  - NS + loop diuretic (to ↓ urine concentrating ability)
  - Vasopressin antagonists, e.g., tolvaptan, conivaptan[21]
- If hyponatremia was present over 24 hours, correct Na at 0.5 mmol/L/hr initially, but current opinion favors raising the serum sodium by no more than 8 mmol/L in the first 24 hours and 18 mmol/L over the first 48 hours to avoid the risk of a cerebral demyelinating syndrome. May use desmopressin to slow correction that is occurring too rapidly, in addition to administration of 5% dextrose in water if necessary to relower the serum sodium.[17]

Chronic Treatment

- Fluid restriction
- Loop diuretics to lower the urine osmolarity close to that of serum & high salt intake
- Demeclocycline (600–1200 mg/d) → causes nephrogenic DI by reversible nephrotoxicity
- Urea or high protein dietary supplementation
- Vasopressin antagonists (e.g., tolvaptan, conivaptan)

ACTH, Adrenocorticotropic hormone; *ADH*, antidiuretic hormone; *CHF*, congestive heart failure; *CNS*, central nervous system; *DI*, diabetes insipidus.

Additional considerations for using 3% NaCl:

- Stop infusion if symptoms are abolished, or if serum Na^+ has risen to ≥ 125 mEq/L.
- Correct serum Na^+ at 0.5 mEq/L/hr (max 1 mOsm/kg/hr), initially raising Na^+ not more than 8 mEq/L over the first 24 hours and 18 mEq/L over the first 48 hours.
- Rapid osmolality correction can cause demyelination syndrome, as well as pontine and extrapontine myelinolysis, with substantial neurological morbidity and mortality.
- Overly rapid correction or overcorrection can occur with vasopressin antagonists as well.[22,23]

Calculations to establish the rate of 3% NaCl infusion

Calculations are based on the following assumptions: although NaCl is distributed mainly in the extracellular space, the distribution volume of NaCl is total body water, or therefore, roughly $0.6 \times$ body mass in kg. The calculations below are crude approximations since they do not account for the rate of Na^+ and water excretion or potassium losses.

As 1 liter of 3% NaCl has 512 mmol of Na^+ (0.512 mmol/mL), if the rate of correction of serum Na+ is to be 0.5 mmol/L/hr, the rate of infusion of 3% NaCl infusion in mL/hr will be $= 0.5/0.512 \times 0.6$ body mass (in kg).

Calculation of total Na deficit to correct hyponatremia

$$\text{Calculated } Na^+ \text{ Deficit (mmol)} = 0.6\big(\text{Body mass}[\text{kg}]\big) \times \big(140 - \text{Serum } Na^+ [\text{mmol/L}]\big)$$

If volume depletion is present, replace estimated volume deficit in liters with normal saline in addition.

Relative risk versus benefit in treatment of hyponatremia:

	Risk of Uncorrected Hyponatremia	Risk of Demyelination
Rapid onset, symptoms	Higher	Lower
Slow onset, asymptomatic	Lower	Higher

4.5 Hypokalemia[24]

Similar to other electrolytes, hypokalemia can be explained by either lower intake, higher excretion, or intracellular redistribution of potassium. To identify the cause of hypokalemia, the following tests are very helpful: urine potassium, and for concentrated urines (Uosm >300 mOsm/kg), the transtubular potassium gradient (TTKG; described below), urine chloride, and plasma bicarbonate.

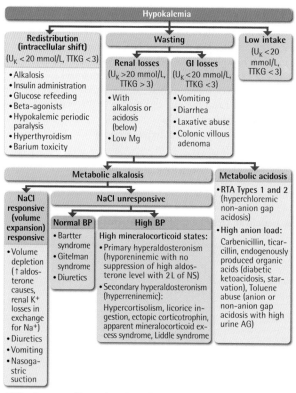

BP, Blood pressure; GI, gastrointestinal; NS, normal saline, RTA, renal tubular acidosis; TTKG, transtubular potassium gradient.

Transtubular Potassium Gradient (TTKG)[25–27]

The concept of TTKG helps to identify renal wasting of potassium (high TTKG), as opposed to GI losses or intracellular shift (low TTKG). TTKG compensates for a high urinary concentration, above 300 mOsm/kg, which raises the U_K concentration by removing tubular fluid from the final urine, but without excreting more potassium.

Note that this formula is valid only when Uosm >300 mOsm/kg and U_{Na}^+ >25 mEq/L, and should not be used to "correct" for dilute urines.

$$\text{TTKG} = \frac{\text{Urine}_K}{\text{Plasma}_K} \div \frac{\text{Urine}_{Osm}}{\text{Plasma}_{Osm}} = \frac{U_K}{P_K} \times \frac{P_{Osm}}{U_{Osm}}$$

TTKG < 3: GI loss, intercellular redistribution with renal K conservation

TTKG < 8: Inadequate renal K excretion when hyperkalemic

TTKG > 5: Renal K wasting when hypokalemic

TTKG > 8: Denotes appropriate renal and aldosterone effect when hyperkalemic

An alternative is to use the urine potassium-to-urine creatinine ratio[28]:

- $U_K/U_{creatinine}$ <2.5 mEq/mmol—GI loss, intracellular redistribution with renal K conservation when hypokalemic
- $U_K/U_{creatinine}$ >4 mEq/mmol—renal K wasting when hypokalemic
- $U_K/U_{creatinine}$ >15 to 20 mEq/mmol—denotes appropriate renal and aldosterone effect when hyperkalemic
- $U_K/U_{creatinine}$ <15 mEq/mmol—denotes inadequate renal tubular K excretion when hyperkalemic

4.5.1 CLINICAL MANIFESTATIONS OF HYPOKALEMIA

- ECG changes (prominent U-wave, T-wave flattening, ST depression)
- Skeletal muscle weakness to the point of paralysis[25]
- Respiratory arrest, which may occur with severe hypokalemia
- Decreased motility of the smooth muscle (ileus), urinary retention
- Rhabdomyolysis, which may occur with severe hypokalemia[29]
- Nephrogenic DI (hypokalemia interfering with concentrating mechanism in the distal nephron)

4.5.2 TREATMENT OF HYPOKALEMIA

- Oral or IV K^+ (oral is safer)
- IV (for K^+ <3.0 mmol/L) not more than 10 mmol/hr; recheck K^+ every 2 to 3 hours
- Magnitude of K^+ replacement cannot be calculated from serum K^+ but is often >200 mmol when serum K^+ <3.0 mEq/L

4.6 Hyperkalemia

4.6.1 CAUSES OF HYPERKALEMIA

Increased intake:
- Use of salt substitutes or K^+ supplements (usually in the setting of CKD)

Redistribution from cells:
- Shift of K^+ out of cells due to acidosis, depolarizing paralytic agents (e.g., succinylcholine), or decreased functioning of Na-K-ATPase related to hypoxia, insulin deficiency, beta blockade, or severe digitalis toxicity
- Cell destruction due to crush injuries, rhabdomyolysis, burns, and hemolysis
- Receipt of old or improperly administered blood or massive blood transfusion[30]

Inadequate excretion:
- Renal failure
- Hypoaldosteronism or adrenal insufficiency
- Renal tubular defects: Type 4 renal tubular acidosis (RTA), interstitial renal diseases
- Medications: aliskiren, angiotensin converting enzyme inhibitor (ACEI), angiotensin receptor blocker (ARB) aldosterone receptor antagonists, amiloride, trimethoprim, calcineurin inhibitors[31-33]
- Pseudohypoaldosteronism (PHA)

4.6.2 CLINICAL MANIFESTATIONS OF HYPERKALEMIA

- Skeletal muscle weakness to the point of paralysis and respiratory failure
- ECG changes[34]:
  - Peaking of T-wave
  - First-degree atrioventricular (AV) block

- Widening of QRS
- ST depression
- Shallow P-waves → atrial standstill
- Biphasic waves → ventricular standstill

4.6.3 ACUTE TREATMENT OF HYPERKALEMIA

- Stabilize the myocardium with intravenous (IV) calcium gluconate 2 to 3 g over 2 to 3 minutes or calcium chloride 1 g over 1 minute (be sure that calcium chloride does not infiltrate, as it may cause tissue necrosis). Repeat once in 5 minutes if no ECG improvement of severe changes (e.g., widened QRS, atrial or ventricular standstill).
- Shift K^+ to the intracellular space[35]:
  - Insulin at doses of 10 units IV (K^+ decreases in 15–30 min) with dextrose (to avoid hypoglycemia)
  - Beta-agonists such as inhaled albuterol (K^+ decreases in 30 min): are as effective as insulin for lowering serum potassium and have a longer duration of action, but may promote arrhythmia[35]
  - Sodium bicarbonate 50 to 150 mEq IV (K^+ decreases in 1–4 hr): supported only by studies with weak and equivocal results, but useful when acidotic[35,36]
- Remove potassium from the body:
  - Diuresis, ideally coupled with saline administration if no volume overload
  - Gastrointestinal (GI) K-binding resins for acute management: sodium zirconium cyclosilicate 10 g suspension orally or sodium polystyrene sulfonate 15 g orally (preferably without sorbitol to protect against GI toxicity with possible GI perforation) and repeat in 1 to 2 hours; or 30 to 50 g rectally and repeat in 6 hours[37,38,38A]
  - Patiromer[39,38A] with a delayed onset of action: not commonly used for acute hyperkalemia management, but, like sodium zirconium cyclosilicate, can be used for chronic K^+ removal (8.4 g/day initially up to 25.2 g/day) and performs better than sodium polystyrene sulfonate
  - Dialysis in refractory or severe hyperkalemia with cardiac arrythmia

Regulation of Calcium and Phosphate Balance[40–43]

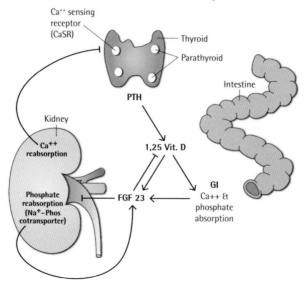

Role of Parathyroid Hormone (PTH), Vitamin D and Fibroblast Growth Factor 23 (FGF 23) on Calcium and Phosphate Balance

4.7 Hypercalcemia[44–47]

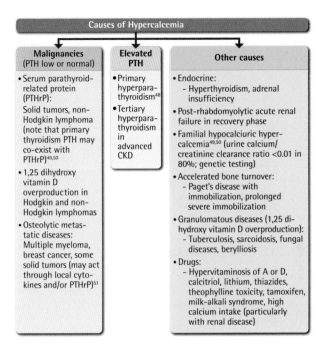

Calcium, phosphate, and PTH in hyperparathyroidism, malignancy, and vitamin D excess syndromes:

	Ca^{++}	Phosphate	PTH
Primary hyperparathyroidism: adenoma (85%), hyperplasia (15%), or carcinoma (<1%) of the parathyroid glands	↑	↓	↑
Malignancy (PTH-rP or osteolysis)	↑	↓	↓
1,25 dihydroxy vitamin D overproduction (e.g., sarcoidosis)	↑	↑	↓

4.7.1 CLINICAL MANIFESTATIONS OF HYPERCALCEMIA

Cardiovascular:
- Dysrhythmia
- ECG changes (short corrected QT interval, broad T-waves, first-degree atrioventricular (AV) block)
- Digoxin sensitivity
- Hypertension

Gastrointestinal:
- Anorexia
- Nausea/vomiting
- Constipation
- Abdominal pain
- Pancreatitis

Genitourinary:
- Polyuria
- Polydipsia
- Nephrolithiasis

Musculoskeletal:
- Muscle weakness
- Hyporeflexia
- Bone pain
- Fractures

Neurological:
- Insomnia
- Delirium
- Dementia
- Psychosis
- Lethargy
- Somnolence
- Coma

4.7.2 TREATMENT OF HYPERCALCEMIA

- Acute treatment if total calcium >14 or altered mental status/ECG changes[52,53]
- Normal saline 2.5–4 L/day[54] + furosemide 10 to 40 mg IV every 6 hours (only if developing evidence of volume overload, such as increasing edema or respiratory distress)
- Calcitonin (Miacalcin)[55]
- Bisphosphonates (pamidronate, zoledronic acid)
- Denosumab (useful when renal function precludes use of a bisphosphonate)[56]
- Calcimimetics in those with high PTH (e.g., cinacalcet)[52]
- Glucocorticoids (especially in hematological malignancies and sarcoidosis)[57]
- Estrogens, raloxifene
- Dialysis can be considered in a last-resort scenario with low- or no-calcium dialysate if severe, as in hypercalcemia of malignancy

4.7.3 INDICATIONS FOR PARATHYROIDECTOMY

Criteria for Parathyroidectomy in Patients With Hyperparathyroidism

In patients with asymptomatic primary hyperparathyroidism[58]:
- Serum calcium >1 mg/dL (0.25 mmol/L) above the upper limit of normal
- Creatinine clearance <60 mL/min; attributed to calcemic nephropathy
- Development of kidney stone clinically or by imaging
- Bone mineral density (BMD) T-score <−2.5 determined by dual-energy X-ray absorptiometry (DEXA) scan at lumbar spine, hip, femoral neck
- Vertebral fracture

In secondary/tertiary hyperparathyroidism in end-stage kidney disease (ESKD)[59,60]:
- Severe hypercalcemia resistant to medical or dialysis treatment
- High total alkaline phosphatase accompanied by specific radiological and/or histomorphological changes of renal osteopathy
- Hyperphosphatemia resistant to treatment with extraskeletal soft-tissue calcifications
- Calciphylaxis
- Symptomatic disease: pruritus, myopathy osteitis
- Marked hyperparathyroidism (PTH level >10 times upper normal limit) resistant to calcimimetic treatment

4.8 Hypocalcemia[61,62]

4.8.1 CLINICAL MANIFESTATIONS OF HYPOCALCEMIA

- Muscle spasms, cramps, and tremors
- Hyperactive reflexes
- Diarrhea
- Tingling of the fingers, toes, lips, and face
- Tetany
- Positive Trousseau's sign: carpopedal spasm (hand spasm when B/P cuff inflated above arterial pressure for 3–4 min).
- Positive Chvostek's sign (twitching of the circumoral muscles with tapping lightly over the facial nerve)
- Seizures
- ECG changes/arrhythmia

4.8.2 TREATMENT OF HYPOCALCEMIA[61,63]

- Monitor labs for other disturbances such as hypokalemia, hyperphosphatemia, hypomagnesemia, and alkalosis.
- Utilize a cardiac monitor.
- Follow seizure precautions and quiet room to decrease external stimuli with severe hypocalcemia or seizure presentation.
- Administer oral calcium supplements and/or vitamin D for mild to moderate hypocalcemia.
- Give oral calcium between meals to increase intestinal absorption.
- Give oral calcitriol in hypoparathyroidism (usually surgical after parathyroidectomy or total thyroidectomy) given rapid onset of action.
- Administer IV calcium for severe hypocalcemia via slow IV bolus followed by slow IV drip.
- Watch for infiltration, as calcium chloride can cause necrosis and tissue sloughing (calcium gluconate is safer to infuse). Never give calcium intramuscularly (IM) or subcutaneously (SC).
- Check Chvostek's sign every hour when giving IV calcium until resolution.
- Teach patient about foods and fluids high in calcium.

4.9 Hypophosphatemia

4.9.1 Causes of Hypophosphatemia

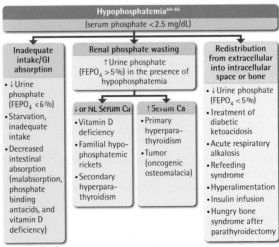

FEPO$_4$, Fractional excretion of phosphate; NL, normal.

Treatment of Hypophosphatemia

Oral phosphate supplementation is adequate for mild to moderate hypophosphatemia, but IV replacement with 20 to 30 mmol of potassium phosphate can be considered when there is cardiac or respiratory compromise, anemia, or phosphate levels <1.0 mg/dL (0.32 mmol/L).[67]

4.10 Hyperphosphatemia

4.10.1 CAUSES OF HYPERPHOSPHATEMIA[68,69]

Elevated Intake	Decreased Renal Excretion	Redistribution From Intracellular to Extracellular Space
• Phosphate containing laxatives or enemas (can cause severe acute kidney injury due to phosphate nephropathy)	• Renal failure (Stage >4) • Vitamin D toxicity • Bisphosphonates • Hypoparathyroidism • Acromegaly • Familial tumoral calcinosis	• Rhabdomyolysis • Tumor lysis syndrome • Diabetic ketoacidosis • Lactic acidosis • Severe hemolytic reaction

4.10.2 TREATMENT OF HYPERPHOSPHATEMIA

Treatment is usually undertaken for patients with renal failure to reduce serum phosphate to <5.5 mg/dL (1.8 mmol/L)[70–72]:

- Dietary phosphate restriction
- Oral phosphate binders to limit intestinal absorption:
  - Calcium carbonate or acetate, usually limited to ≤1.5 g/day of calcium
  - Sevelamer
  - Lanthanum carbonate
  - Ferric citrate
  - Sucroferric oxyhydroxide
  - Aluminum hydroxide; limit use to short-term acute kidney injury (AKI) of <1 month to avoid aluminum toxicity
- Drugs targeting intestinal phosphate transporters to decrease absorption (not commonly used):
  - Nicotinic acid and nicotinamide[73]
  - Tenapanor[72,74]
- Dialysis
- Correction of secondary hyperparathyroidism in ESKD

Fractional Excretion of Phosphate

Urine phosphate can be measured either in a 24-hour urine sample or as a fractional phosphate excretion in a random urine sample:

$$FE_{PO_4} = \frac{\left(\text{urine phosphate} \times \text{serum creatinine}\right)}{\left(\text{serum phosphate} \times \text{serum creatinine}\right)} \times 100\%$$

FE_{PO4} usually varies between 5% and 20%, but may increase to >80% with secondary hyperparathyroidism of renal failure.

4.11 Magnesium: Effects in the Body

Magnesium is the fourth most common cation in the body, and the second most common intracellular cation.[2,75-77] Magnesium (Mg) has the following important actions:

- Vasodilatation by direct action on blood vessels (Mg acts as a calcium antagonist) and antisympathetic activity
- Negative inotropic effect
- Bronchodilation
- Tocolytic effect
- Renal vasodilation and diuresis
- Cofactor for many intracellular enzymes
- Responsible for the maintenance of transmembrane gradients of sodium and potassium

Renal Handling of Magnesium[77,77A]

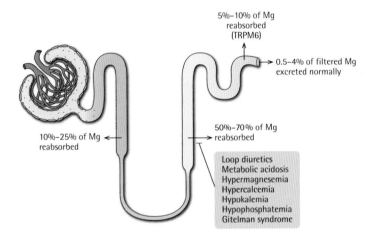

5%–10% of Mg reabsorbed (TRPM6)

0.5–4% of filtered Mg excreted normally

50%–70% of Mg reabsorbed

10%–25% of Mg reabsorbed

Loop diuretics
Metabolic acidosis
Hypermagnesemia
Hypercalcemia
Hypokalemia
Hypophosphatemia
Gitelman syndrome

4.12 Hypomagnesemia

4.12.1 CAUSES OF HYPOMAGNESEMIA[78,79]

- **Low intake or poor GI absorption:**
  - Celiac disease
  - Inflammatory bowel disease
  - Proton pump inhibitors[80] (especially in patients also taking diuretics)
- **Increased loss:**
  - GI loss: diarrhea, vomiting, laxative use
  - Renal loss: tubular defect (congenital or acquired), diabetes, alcohol, drugs affecting tubular absorption (diuretics, aminoglycosides, amphotericin, cisplatin, pentamidine, cyclosporine), hypercalcemia
  - Skin loss: excessive sweating
- **Higher requirements:**
  - Pregnancy[81]
  - Growth

4.12.2 CLINICAL MANIFESTATIONS OF HYPOMAGNESEMIA[76,78]

- Neurological: nystagmus, convulsions, numbness
- Fatigue
- Muscle spasms, cramps, or muscle weakness
- Cardiac arrhythmias
- Hypocalcemia, hypokalemia from renal wasting
- Cardiac or respiratory arrest, if severe

The diagnosis of GI versus renal losses of Mg in hypomagnesemic patients can be made by calculating the fractional excretion of magnesium (FEMg) as follows[82]:

$$FE_{Mg} = \frac{U_{Mg} \times P_{Cr}}{0.7^* \times P_{Mg} \times U_{Cr}} \times 100$$

*Factoring the plasma or serum Mg level by 0.7 is because of the protein-bound Mg of about 30% which is not filtered by the kidney. The FEMg in hypomagnesemic patients with extra renal Mg losses was found to be 0.5-2.7%, while in those with renal Mg wasting, the FEMg was 4-48%[82].

Treatment of Hypomagnesemia

For mild hypomagnesemia, oral Mg replacement is preferred, though some patients may experience diarrhea with magnesium salts. When serum magnesium concentration is below 1.0 mEq/L (0.5 mmol/L or 1.2 mg/dL) in ill patients, IV replacement of Mg to achieve a goal Mg of ≥2 mEq/L can be initiated using a "rule of thumb" estimation that 1 g of IV MgSO₄ should raise the serum Mg by ~0.15 mEq/L.[83]

4.13 Hypermagnesemia[78,84]

4.13.1 CAUSES OF HYPERMAGNESEMIA

- Iatrogenic causes (e.g., parenteral magnesium)
- Excessive use of magnesium-containing laxatives and antacids, often in the setting of acute or chronic kidney disease.

4.13.2 EFFECTS OF HYPERMAGNESEMIA

- Depressed CNS, muscle weakness, areflexia (usually with serum Mg >6 mg/dL or 2.5 mmol/L or 5.0 mEq/L)
- Depressed cardiac conduction, widened QRS complexes, prolonged P-R interval

4.13.3 TREATMENT OF HYPERMAGNESEMIA

- Forced diuresis
- Dialysis
- Intravenous calcium

4.14 Magnesium: Therapeutic Use

- Preeclampsia and eclampsia[75,85]
- Cardiac arrhythmias (torsades de pointes, digoxin toxicity, any serious ventricular or atrial arrhythmias especially accompanied by hypokalemia)[75,86,87]
- Asthma[88]
- Refractory hypokalemia in the context of hypomagnesemia
- Tocolytic agent to suppress premature labor [88A]

4.15 Polyuria (Urine Output >3000 mL/24 hr) Workup[89]

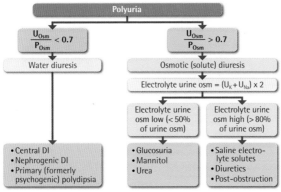

DI, Diabetes insipidus; *Osm*, osmolality.

4.16 Diuretic Therapy[90–95]

	Loop Diuretics	Thiazides	Amiloride/Triamterene
Mechanism	Block Na^+- K^+- $2Cl^-$ cotransporter	Block electroneutral Na^+ - Cl^- cotransporter	Block apical Na^+ channels
Water and Na^+	Impair urinary concentration ability: Water is excreted in excess of sodium	Impair the ability to dilute urine and excrete a water load while diuresing sodium	
Other electrolytes	Loss of K^+ and Mg^{++}, increased urinary Ca^{++} excretion	Loss of K^+ and Mg^{++}, urinary Ca^{++} retention	Impair the excretion of K^+ and H^+ in exchange for Na^+ absorption

Diuretic Sites of Action[96–98]

The three major classes of diuretics used for enhancing sodium excretion are:

- thiazide diuretics (e.g., hydrochlorothiazide),
- loop diuretics (e.g., furosemide), and
- potassium-sparing diuretics, either aldosterone antagonists (e.g., spironolactone) or sodium channel blockers (e.g., amiloride).

Other drugs have diuretic action, but are used for more specific purposes, such as:

- carbonic anhydrase inhibitors (e.g., acetazolamide, to cause bicarbonaturia or alkalinize the urine to correct metabolic alkalosis),
- osmotic diuretics (e.g., mannitol, mainly to enhance urinary excretion of poisons or for CNS edema),
- low-dose dopamine for congestive heart failure (CHF), and
- ADH antagonists (e.g., tolvaptan, to induce a water diuresis to correct hyponatremia).

Their sites of action in the renal tubule are described above and shown in the diagram of the nephron in Chapter 3.

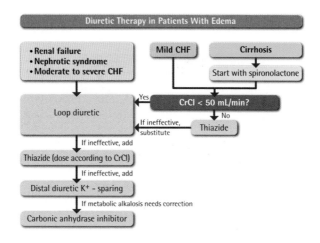

References

1. Danziger J, Zeidel M, Parker M. *Renal Physiology: A Clinical Approach*. Lippincott Williams & Wilkins; 2012.
2. Rose B, Post T. *Clinical Physiology of Acid-Base and Electrolyte Disorders*. 5th ed. McGraw-Hill; 2001.
3. Schrier RW. *Renal and Electrolyte Disorders*. 8th ed. Lippincott Williams & Wilkins; 2017:viii, pp1–96.
4. Rennke HG, Denker BM. *Renal Pathophysiology: The Essentials*. 5th ed. Wolters Kluwer; 2020.
5. Eaton DC, Pooler JP. *Vander's Renal Physiology*. 9th ed. LANGE Medical Books/McGraw Hill, Medical Pub. Division; 2018.
6. Jameson JL, Loscalzo J. *Harrison's Nephrology and Acid-Base Disorders*. 3rd ed. McGraw-Hill Education Medical; 2017.
7. Eladari D, Chambrey R, Peti-Peterdi J. A new look at electrolyte transport in the distal tubule. *Annu Rev. Physiol.* 2012;74:325–349. doi:10.1146/annurev-physiol-020911-153225.
8. Winn Seay N, Lehrich RW, Greenberg A. Diagnosis and management of disorders of body tonicity-hyponatremia and hypernatremia: core curriculum 2020. *Am J Kidney Dis.* 2020;75(2):272–286. doi:10.1053/j.ajkd.2019.07.014.
9. Offenstadt G, Das V. Hyponatremia, hypernatremia: a physiological approach. *Minerva Anestesiol.* 2006;72(6):353–356.
10. Lien YH, Shapiro JI, Chan L. Effects of hypernatremia on organic brain osmoles. *Journal Clin Invest.* 1990;85(5):1427–1435. doi:10.1172/JCI114587.
11. Sterns RH. Disorders of plasma sodium—causes, consequences, and correction. *N Engl J Med.* 2015 1;372(1):55–65. doi:10.1056/NEJMra1404489.
12. Hannon MJ, Thompson CJ. The syndrome of inappropriate antidiuretic hormone: prevalence, causes and consequences. *Eur J Endocrinol.* 2010;162 suppl 1:S5–S12. doi:10.1530/EJE-09-1063.
13. Sterns RH, Silver SM. Cerebral salt wasting versus SIADH: what difference? *J Am Soc Nephrol.* 2008; 19(2):194–196. doi:10.1681/ASN.2007101118.
14. Kalita J, Singh RK, Misra UK. Cerebral salt wasting is the most common cause of hyponatremia in stroke. *J Stroke Cerebrovasc Dis.* 2017;26(5):1026–1032. doi:10.1016/j.jstrokecerebrovasdis.2016.12.011
15. Cui H, He G, Yang S, et al. Inappropriate antidiuretic hormone secretion and cerebral salt-wasting syndromes in neurological patients. *Front Neurosci.* 2019;13:1170. doi:10.3389/fnins.2019.01170.
16. Noakes TD. Overconsumption of fluids by athletes. *BMJ.* 2003;327(7407):113–114. doi:10.1136/bmj.327.7407.113.
17. Sterns RH. Treatment of severe hyponatremia. *Clin J Am Soc Nephrol.* 2018;13(4):641–649. doi:10.2215/CJN.10440917.
18. Feldman BJ, Rosenthal SM, Vargas GA, et al. Nephrogenic syndrome of inappropriate antidiuresis. *N Engl J Med.* 2005;352(18):1884–1890. doi:10.1056/NEJMoa042743.

19. Valenti G, Tamma G. The vasopressin-aquaporin-2 pathway syndromes. *Handb Clin Neurol.* 2021; 181:249–259. doi:10.1016/B978-0-12-820683-6.00018-X.

20. Garrahy A, Dineen R, Hannon AM, et al. Continuous versus bolus infusion of hypertonic saline in the treatment of symptomatic hyponatremia caused by SIAD. *J Clin Endocrinol Metab.* 2019;104(9): 3595–3602. doi:10.1210/jc.2019-00044.

21. Schrier RW, Gross P, Gheorghiade M, et al. Tolvaptan, a selective oral vasopressin V2-receptor antagonist, for hyponatremia. *N Engl J Med.* 2006;355(20):2099–2112. doi:10.1056/NEJMoa065181.

22. Morris JH, Bohm NM, Nemecek BD, et al. Rapidity of correction of hyponatremia due to syndrome of inappropriate secretion of antidiuretic hormone following tolvaptan. *Am J Kidney Dis.* 2018; 71(6):772–782. doi:10.1053/j.ajkd.2017.12.002.

23. Kim Y, Lee N, Lee KE, Gwak HS. Risk factors for sodium overcorrection in non-hypovolemic hyponatremia patients treated with tolvaptan. *Eur J Clin Pharmacol.* 2020;76(5):723–729. doi:10.1007/s00228-020-02848-6.

24. Palmer BF, Clegg DJ. Physiology and pathophysiology of potassium homeostasis: core curriculum 2019. *Am J Kidney Dis.* 2019;74(5):682–695. doi:10.1053/j.ajkd.2019.03.427.

25. Lin S-H, Lin Y-F, Chen D-T, Chu P, Hsu C-W, Halperin ML. Laboratory tests to determine the cause of hypokalemia and paralysis. *Arch Intern Med.* 2004;164(14):1561–1566.doi:10.1001/archinte.164. 14.1561.

26. Choi MJ, Ziyadeh FN. The utility of the transtubular potassium gradient in the evaluation of hyperkalemia. *J Am Soc Nephrol.* 2008;19(3):424–426. doi:10.1681/ASN.2007091017.

27. Ethier JH, Kamel KS, Magner PO, Lemann J Jr, Halperin ML. The transtubular potassium concentration in patients with hypokalemia and hyperkalemia. *Am J Kidney Dis.* 1990;15(4):309–315. doi:10.1016/s0272-6386(12)80076-x.

28. Kamel KS, Halperin ML. Intrarenal urea recycling leads to a higher rate of renal excretion of potassium: an hypothesis with clinical implications. *Curr Opin Nephrol Hypertens.* 2011;20(5):547–554. doi:10.1097/MNH.0b013e328349b8f9.

29. Khan FY. Rhabdomyolysis: a review of the literature. *Neth J Med.* 2009;67(9):272–283.

30. Sihler KC, Napolitano LM. Complications of massive transfusion. *Chest.* 2010;137(1):209–220. doi:10.1378/chest.09-0252.

31. Harel Z, Gilbert C, Wald R, et al. The effect of combination treatment with aliskiren and blockers of the renin-angiotensin system on hyperkalaemia and acute kidney injury: systematic review and meta-analysis. *BMJ.* 2012;344:e42. doi:10.1136/bmj.e42.

32. Clase CM, Carrero J-J, Ellison DH, et al. Potassium homeostasis and management of dyskalemia in kidney diseases: conclusions from a Kidney Disease: Improving Global Outcomes (KDIGO) Controversies Conference. *Kidney Int.* 2020;97(1):42–61. doi:10.1016/j.kint.2019.09.018.

33. Nappi JM, Sieg A. Aldosterone and aldosterone receptor antagonists in patients with chronic heart failure. *Vasc Health Risk Manag.* 2011;7:353 363. doi:10.2147/VHRM.S13779

34. Littmann L, Gibbs MA. Electrocardiographic manifestations of severe hyperkalemia. *J Electrocardiol.* 2018;51(5):814–817. doi:10.1016/j.jelectrocard.2018.06.018.

35. Elliott MJ, Ronksley PE, Clase CM, Ahmed SB, Hemmelgarn BR. Management of patients with acute hyperkalemia. *CMAJ.* 2010;182(15):1631–1635. doi:10.1503/cmaj.100461.

36. Allon M, Shanklin N. Effect of bicarbonate administration on plasma potassium in dialysis patients: interactions with insulin and albuterol. *Am J Kidney Dis.*1996;28(4):508–514. doi:10.1016/s0272-6386 (96)90460-6.

37. Packham DK, Rasmussen HS, Lavin PT, et al. Sodium zirconium cyclosilicate in hyperkalemia. *N Engl J Med.* 2015;372(3):222–231. doi:10.1056/NEJMoa1411487.

38. Peacock WF, Rafique Z, Vishnevskiy K, et al. Emergency potassium normalization treatment including sodium zirconium cyclosilicate: a phase II, randomized, double-blind, placebo-controlled study (ENERGIZE). *Acad Emerg Med.* 2020;27(6):475–486. doi:10.1111/acem.13954.

38A. Meaney CJ, Beccari MV, Yang Y, Zhao J. Systematic review and meta-analysis of patiromer and sodium zirconium cyclosilicate: a new armamentarium for the treatment of hyperkalemia. *Pharmacotherapy.* 2017;37(4):401–411. doi: 10.1002/phar.1906.

39. Desai NR, Rowan CG, Alvarez PJ, Fogli J, Toto RD. Hyperkalemia treatment modalities: a descriptive observational study focused on medication and healthcare resource utilization. *PloS One.* 2020;15(1): e0226844. doi:10.1371/journal.pone.0226844.

40. Peacock M. Calcium metabolism in health and disease. *Clin J Am Soc Nephrol*. 2010;5 suppl 1:S23–S30. doi:10.2215/CJN.05910809.

41. Lambers TT, Bindels RJM, Hoenderop JGJ. Coordinated control of renal Ca2+ handling. *Kidney Int*. 2006;69(4):650–654. doi:10.1038/sj.ki.5000169.

42. Goltzman D, Mannstadt M, Marcocci C. Physiology of the calcium-parathyroid hormone-vitamin D axis. *Front Horm Res*. 2018;50:1–13. doi:10.1159/000486060.

43. Song L. Calcium and bone metabolism indices. *Adv Clin Chem*. 2017;82:1–46. doi:10.1016/bs.acc.2017.06.005.

44. Richter B, Faul C. FGF23 actions on target tissues—with and without klotho. *Front Endocrinol (Lausanne)*. 2018;9:189. doi:10.3389/fendo.2018.00189.

45. Carroll MF, Schade DS. A practical approach to hypercalcemia. *Am Fam Physician*. 2003;67(9): 1959–1966.

46. Goltzman D. Nonparathyroid hypercalcemia. *Front Horm Res*. 2019;51:77–90. doi:10.1159/000491040.

47. Barstow C, Braun M. Electrolytes: calcium disorders. *FP Essent*. 2017;459:29–34.

48. Masi L. Primary hyperparathyroidism. *Front Horm Research*. 2019;51:1–12. doi:10.1159/000491034.

49. Varghese J, Rich T, Jimenez C. Benign familial hypocalciuric hypercalcemia. *Endocr Pract*. 2011;17 suppl 1:13–17. doi:10.4158/EP10308.RA.

50. Lee JY, Shoback DM. Familial hypocalciuric hypercalcemia and related disorders. *Best Pract Res Clin Endocrinol Metab*. 2018;32(5):609–619. doi:10.1016/j.beem.2018.05.004.

51. Goldner W. Cancer-related hypercalcemia. *J Oncol Pract*. 2016;12(5):426–432. doi:10.1200/JOP.2016.011155.

52. Makras P, Papapoulos SE. Medical treatment of hypercalcaemia. *Hormones (Athens)*. 2009;8(2):83–95. doi:10.14310/horm.2002.1225.

53. Maier JD, Levine SN. Hypercalcemia in the intensive care unit: a review of pathophysiology, diagnosis, and modern therapy. *J Intensive Care Med*. 2015;30(5):235–252. doi:10.1177/0885066613507530.

54. Hosking DJ, Cowley A, Bucknall CA. Rehydration in the treatment of severe hypercalcaemia. *Q J Med*. 1981;50(200):473–481.

55. Khan A, Gurnani PK, Peksa GD, Whittier WL, DeMott JM. Bisphosphonate versus bisphosphonate and calcitonin for the treatment of moderate to severe hypercalcemia of malignancy. *Ann Pharmacother*. 2021;55(3):277–285. doi:10.1177/1060028020957048.

56. Cicci JD, Buie L, Bates J, van Deventer H. Denosumab for the management of hypercalcemia of malignancy in patients with multiple myeloma and renal dysfunction. *Clin Lymphoma Myeloma Leuk*. 2014;14(6)e207–e211. doi:10.1016/j.clml.2014.07.005

57. Khan A, Grey A, Shoback D. Medical management of asymptomatic primary hyperparathyroidism: proceedings of the third international workshop. *J Clin Endocrinol Metab*. 2009;94(2):373–381. doi:10.1210/jc.2008-1762.

58. Bilezikian JP, Brandi ML, Eastell R, et al. Guidelines for the management of asymptomatic primary hyperparathyroidism: summary statement from the Fourth International Workshop. *J Clin Endocrinol Metab*. 2014;99(10):3561–3569. doi:10.1210/jc.2014-1413.

59. Schlosser K, Zielke A, Rothmund M. Medical and surgical treatment for secondary and tertiary hyperparathyroidism. *Scand J Surg*. 2004;93(4):288–297. doi:10.1177/145749690409300407.

60. Tang JA, Friedman J, Hwang MS, Salapatas AM, Bonzelaar LB, Friedman M. Parathyroidectomy for tertiary hyperparathyroidism: a systematic review. *Am J Otolaryngol*. 2017;38(5):630–635. doi:10.1016/j.amjoto.2017.06.009.

61. Pepe J, Colangelo L, Biamonte F, et al. Diagnosis and management of hypocalcemia. *Endocrine*. 2020;69(3):485–495. doi:10.1007/s12020-020-02324-2.

62. Bilezikian JP, Brandi ML, Cusano NE, et al. Management of hypoparathyroidism: present and future. *J Clin Endocrinol Metab*. 2016;101(6):2313–2324. doi:10.1210/jc.2015-3910.

63. Cooper MS, Gittoes NJL. Diagnosis and management of hypocalcaemia. *BMJ*. 2008;336(7656): 1298–1302. doi:10.1136/bmj.39582.589433.BE.

64. Assadi F. Hypophosphatemia: an evidence-based problem-solving approach to clinical cases. *Iran J Kidney Dis*. 2010;4(3):195–201.

65. Gaasbeek A, Meinders AE. Hypophosphatemia: an update on its etiology and treatment. *Am J Med*. 2005;118(10):1094–1101. doi:10.1016/j.amjmed.2005.02.014.

66. Liamis G, Milionis HJ, Elisaf M. Medication-induced hypophosphatemia: a review. *QJM*. 2010; 103(7):449–459. doi:10.1093/qjmed/hcq039.
67. Felsenfeld AJ, Levine BS. Approach to treatment of hypophosphatemia. *Am J Kidney Dis*. 2012;60(4):655–661. doi:10.1053/j.ajkd.2012.03.024.
68. Lee R, Weber TJ. Disorders of phosphorus homeostasis. *Curr Opin Endocrinol Diabetes Obes*. 2010; 17(6):561–567. doi:10.1097/MED.0b013e32834041d4.
69. Goyal R, Jialal I. Hyperphosphatemia. In: *StatPearls [Internet]*. Treasure Island (FL): StatPearls Publishing; 2022.
70. Scialla JJ, Kendrick J, Uribarri J, et al. State-of-the-art management of hyperphosphatemia in patients with CKD: an NKF-KDOQI controversies perspective. *Am J Kidney Dis*. 2021;77(1):132–141. doi:10.1053/j.ajkd.2020.05.025.
71. Vervloet MG, van Ballegooijen AJ. Prevention and treatment of hyperphosphatemia in chronic kidney disease. *Kidney Int*. 2018;93(5):1060–1072. doi:10.1016/j.kint.2017.11.036.
72. Ketteler M, Block GA, Evenepoel P, et al. Executive summary of the 2017 KDIGO Chronic Kidney Disease-Mineral and Bone Disorder (CKD-MBD) Guideline Update: what's changed and why it matters. *Kidney Int*. 2017;92(1):26–36. doi:10.1016/j.kint.2017.04.006.
73. Müller D, Mehling H, Otto B, et al. Niacin lowers serum phosphate and increases HDL cholesterol in dialysis patients. *Clin J Am Soc Nephrol*. 2007;2(6):1249–1254. doi:10.2215/CJN.01470307.
74. Ketteler M, Liangos O, Biggar PH. Treating hyperphosphatemia—current and advancing drugs. *Expert Opin Pharmacother*. 2016;17(14):1873–1879. doi:10.1080/14656566.2016.1220538.
75. Fawcett WJ, Haxby EJ, Male DA. Magnesium: physiology and pharmacology. *Br J Anaesth*. 1999; 83(2):302–320. doi:10.1093/bja/83.2.302.
76. Saris NE, Mervaala E, Karppanen H, Khawaja JA, Lewenstam A. Magnesium. An update on physiological, clinical and analytical aspects. *Clin Chim Acta*. 2000;294(1–2):1–26. doi:10.1016/s0009-8981(99)00258-2.
77. Xi Q, Hoenderop JGJ, Bindels RJM. Regulation of magnesium reabsorption in DCT. *Pflugers Arch*. 2009 May;458(1):89–98. doi:10.1007/s00424-008-0601-7.
77A. Maeoka Y, McCormick JA. NaCl cotransporter activity and Mg2+ handling by the distal convoluted tubule. *Am J Physiol Renal Physiol*. 2020;319(6):F1043–F1053. doi: 10.1152/ajprenal.00463.2020.
78. Van Laecke S. Hypomagnesemia and hypermagnesemia. *Acta Clin Belg*. 2019;74(1):41–47. doi:10.1080/17843286.2018.1516173.
79. Ahmed F, Mohammed A. Magnesium: the forgotten electrolyte—a review on hypomagnesemia. *Med Sci (Basel)*. 2019;7(4):56. doi:10.3390/medsci7040056.
80. Srinutta T, Chewcharat A, Takkavatakarn K, et al. Proton pump inhibitors and hypomagnesemia: a meta-analysis of observational studies. *Medicine*. 2019;98(44):e17788. doi:10.1097/MD.0000000000017788.
81. Morton A. Hypomagnesaemia and pregnancy. *Obstet Med*. 2018;11(2):67–72. doi:10.1177/1753495X17711478.
82. Elisaf M, Panteli K, Theodorou J, Siamopoulos KC. Fractional excretion of magnesium in normal subjects and in patients with hypomagnesemia. *Magnes Res*. 1997;10(4):315–320.
83. Hammond DA, Stojakovic J, Kathe N, et al. Effectiveness and safety of magnesium replacement in critically ill patients admitted to the medical intensive care unit in an academic medical center: a retrospective, cohort study. *J Intensive Care Med*. 2019;34(11–12):967–972. doi:10.1177/0885066617720631.
84. Cascella M, Vaqar S. Hypermagnesemia. In: *StatPearls [Internet]*. Treasure Island (FL): StatPearls Publishing; 2022.
85. Vigil-De Gracia P, Ludmir J. The use of magnesium sulfate for women with severe preeclampsia or eclampsia diagnosed during the postpartum period. *J Matern Fetal Neonatal Med*. 2015;28(18): 2207–2209. doi:10.3109/14767058.2014.982529.
86. Fox C, Ramsoomair D, Carter C. Magnesium: its proven and potential clinical significance. *South Med J*. 2001;94(12):1195–1201.
87. Guerrera MP, Volpe SL, Mao JJ. Therapeutic uses of magnesium. *Am Fam Physician*. 2009;80(2):157–162.
88. Irazuzta JE, Chiriboga N. Magnesium sulfate infusion for acute asthma in the emergency department. *J Pediatr (Rio J)*. 2017;93 suppl 1:19–25. doi:10.1016/j.jped.2017.06.002.
88A. Haas DM, Caldwell DM, Kirkpatrick P, McIntosh JJ, Welton NJ. Tocolytic therapy for preterm delivery: systematic review and network meta-analysis. *BMJ*. 2012;345:e6226. doi: 10.1136/bmj.e6226.

89. Ranieri M, Di Mise A, Tamma G, Valenti G. Vasopressin-aquaporin-2 pathway: recent advances in understanding water balance disorders. *F1000Res.* 2019;8:F1000 Faculty Rev-149. doi:10.12688/f1000research.16654.1.

90. Wile D. Diuretics: a review. *Ann Clin Biochem.* 2012;49(Pt 5):419–431. doi:10.1258/acb.2011.011281.

91. Bernstein PL, Ellison DH. Diuretics and salt transport along the nephron. *Semin Nephrol.* 2011;31(6): 475–482. doi:10.1016/j.semnephrol.2011.09.002.

92. Brater DC. Update in diuretic therapy: clinical pharmacology. *Semin Nephrol.* 2011;31(6):483–494. doi:10.1016/j.semnephrol.2011.09.003.

93. Palmer BF. Metabolic complications associated with use of diuretics. *Semin Nephrol.* 2011;31(6): 542–552. doi:10.1016/j.semnephrol.2011.09.009.

94. Sarafidis PA, Georgianos PI, Lasaridis AN. Diuretics in clinical practice. Part I: mechanisms of action, pharmacological effects and clinical indications of diuretic compounds. *Expert Opin Drug Saf.* 2010;9(2):243–257. doi:10.1517/14740330903499240.

95. Sarafidis PA, Georgianos PI, Lasaridis AN. Diuretics in clinical practice. Part II: electrolyte and acid-base disorders complicating diuretic therapy. *Expert Opin Drug Saf.* 2010;9(2):259–273. doi:10.1517/14740330903499257.

96. Kassamali R, Sica DA. Acetazolamide: a forgotten diuretic agent. *Cardiol Rev.* 2011;19(6):276–278. doi:10.1097/CRD.0b013e31822b4939.

97. Sica DA, Carter B, Cushman W, Hamm L. Thiazide and loop diuretics. *J Clin Hypertens (Greenwich).* 2011;13(9):639–643. doi:10.1111/j.1751-7176.2011.00512.x.

98. Epstein M, Calhoun DA. Aldosterone blockers (mineralocorticoid receptor antagonism) and potassium-sparing diuretics. *J Clin Hypertens (Greenwich).* 2011;13(9):644–648. doi:10.1111/j.1751-7176.2011.00511.x.

99. Sica DA, Moser M. Diuretic therapy in cardiovascular disease. In: *Hypertension.* Elsevier; 2007:213–230.

CHAPTER 5

Acid-Base Disorders

Alexander Morales ■ Alexander Goldfarb-Rumyantzev ■
Robert Stephen Brown

5.1 Introduction

This chapter discusses how to use arterial or venous blood gas results and routine serum electrolytes to identify an acid-base disorder.[1,2]

5.1.1 Henderson-Hasselbalch Equation

Interpretations of blood gas findings start with the Henderson-Hasselbalch equation:

$$pH = pK_a + \log \frac{[Base]}{[Acid]} \text{ where } pK_a \text{ is the negative log of the acid dissociation constant}$$

The blood buffering system uses bicarbonate as the base and carbonic acid as the acid; therefore, this equation can be rewritten as follows:

$$pH = pK_a + \log \frac{[HCO_3^-]}{[H_2CO_3]}$$

Using a pK_a value of 6.1 for carbonic acid, and a conversion factor of 0.03 to express the acid concentration in terms of partial arterial pressure of CO_2 ($paCO_2$), which is measured in arterial blood gases (ABGs), this is finally rewritten as follows:

$$pH = 6.1 + \log \frac{[HCO_3^-]}{0.03 p_a CO_2}$$

Since this final expression includes a logarithm, which is difficult for quick bedside calculation, several simple approximations may be used, as discussed on the pages that follow.

Note that at a normal pH of 7.4, the concentration of the base $[HCO_3^-]$ of about 25 mEq/L is 20 times that of carbonic acid with a concentration of 1.2 mEq/L (or a pCO_2 of 40 mmHg).

5.2 ACID-BASE DISORDER DIAGNOSTIC ALGORITHM

This algorithm provides an interpretation of ABGs in conjunction with plasma chemistry.

To use this algorithm:

1. Examine the pH and identify acidemia or alkalemia.
2. Using the bicarbonate (HCO_3^-) concentration obtained from serum electrolytes and the pCO_2 from the ABG, identify whether the primary cause of the disorder is metabolic or respiratory (see ABG algorithm below).
3. Perform a calculation to examine whether a primary respiratory disorder has appropriate metabolic compensation, or whether a primary metabolic disorder has appropriate respiratory compensation (refer to the compensation table on the next page)[3-5]

If neither case is true, a second primary disorder—considered to be a "complex" (meaning more than just one) acid-base disorder rather than a "simple" (meaning a single) acid-base disorder—is underlying the observed changes.[6]

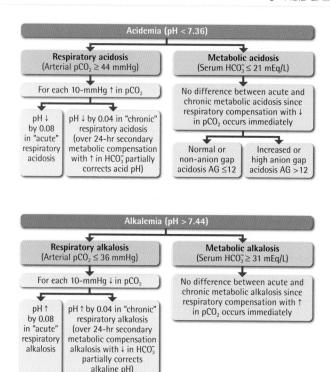

Compensation for Respiratory Alkalosis

Acute

When acute, expect serum HCO_3^- to fall about 2 mEq/L for each 10-mmHg decrease in pCO_2 for normal metabolic compensation.

Chronic

When over 24 hours, expect serum HCO_3^- to fall about 5 mEq/L for each 10-mmHg decrease in pCO_2 for normal metabolic compensation.

Compensation for Respiratory Acidosis

Acute

When acute, expect serum HCO_3^- to rise about 1 mEq/L for each 10-mmHg increase in pCO_2 for normal metabolic compensation.

Chronic

When over 24 hours, expect serum HCO_3^- to rise about 3.5 mEq/L for each 10-mmHg increase in pCO_2 for normal metabolic compensation.

Compensation for Metabolic Alkalosis

There are three common ways to evaluate for normal respiratory compensation response (±2 mmHg):

1. Expect pCO_2 to rise 0.7 mmHg for each 1 mEq/L rise in serum HCO_3^- for normal respiratory compensation.
2. pCO_2 should be equal to serum HCO_3^- + 15 mmHg up to a pCO_2 of about 60 when the pCO_2 rises no further.
3. The easy way: pCO_2 should be equal to the last 2 digits of the pH up to pH 7.60.

Compensation for Metabolic Acidosis

There are three common ways to evaluate for normal respiratory compensation response (±2 mmHg):

1. Expect pCO_2 to decrease 1.2 mmHg for each 1 mEq/L fall in HCO_3^-.
2. pCO_2 should be equal to 1.5 times (HCO_3^-) + 8.
3. The easy way: pCO_2 should be equal to the last 2 digits of the pH down to pH 7.10.

5.2.1 Useful Tips

- Acid-base disorders do not compensate completely, so if the pH is acidic, assume acidosis; if it is alkaline, assume alkalosis.
- In interpreting serum bicarbonate level:
  - If HCO_3^- is ↑, there is either a primary metabolic alkalosis or compensation for a respiratory acidosis.
  - If HCO_3^- is ↓, there is either a primary metabolic acidosis or compensation for a respiratory alkalosis.
  - If HCO_3^- is normal, either there is a normal acid-base state or a complex (double or triple) disorder may be present.
- An ↑ anion gap almost always indicates a metabolic acidosis.
- Serum K^+ concentration may be helpful. If K^+ is ↓, there is usually an alkalosis; if K^+ is ↑, there is usually an acidosis.
- When blood urea nitrogen (BUN) and creatinine levels are ↑, renal failure may be associated with a metabolic acidosis that often has a normal anion gap when mild, and an increased anion gap when renal failure is more severe.
- Liver failure is usually associated with metabolic acidosis.

5.3 Metabolic Acidosis

5.3.1 CAUSES OF METABOLIC ACIDOSIS

- Once the diagnosis of metabolic acidosis is established, the next step is to identify the cause.
- To identify the cause, assess whether the metabolic acidosis is associated with a normal anion gap (10 ± 2 mEq/L) or an abnormally high anion gap, as shown in the algorithm below.
- An increased anion gap indicates the presence of unmeasured acids which may be endogenous (e.g., lactic acid) or exogenous (e.g., oxalic acid from ethylene glycol poisoning).[7,8]
- Metabolic acidosis with a normal anion gap is caused by either loss of bicarbonate (from the gastrointestinal [GI] tract or in the urine) or failure to excrete acid [H^+] by the kidneys.

5.3.2 SERUM OSMOLAR GAP

Using the serum or plasma osmolar gap will help to differentiate between a nonosmolar gap (usually endogenous) and a high osmolar gap (exogenous toxin) acidosis.[9] The osmolar gap is determined by comparing the measured serum or plasma osmolality to the calculated serum osmolality.

Serum osmolality:

Calculated serum osmolality (Osm, to compare with measured S_{Osm} for assessment of an osmolar gap):

$$S_{Osm} = 2(Na^+) + \frac{Glucose\,(mg/dL)}{18} + \frac{BUN\,(mg/dL)}{2.8}$$

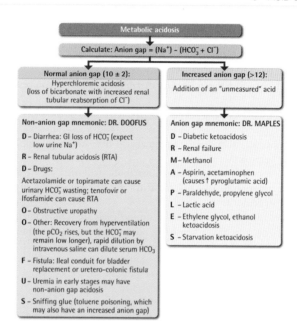

5.3.2.1 Non-Anion Gap Metabolic Acidosis

5.3.2.1.1 Renal Tubular Acidosis Versus GI Losses. In metabolic acidosis associated with a normal anion gap, the low serum bicarbonate is either due to loss of bicarbonate from the GI tract from diarrhea, or from failure of the kidneys to conserve bicarbonate or to regenerate bicarbonate by excreting acid.[8] The differential diagnosis between these two conditions is based on showing a normal renal response to acidemia in GI losses. First, the urine pH should be acidic. Second, the urine anion gap should be negative, indicating the presence of the unmeasured urinary cation, NH_4^+, which provides additional acid excretion.[6–8] If renal tubular NH_4^+ secretion is impaired, the urinary anion gap remains positive or around zero. Remember that calculating a urine anion gap has no role in an increased anion gap metabolic acidosis because there is an unmeasured anion in the urine that obscures the quantity of the unmeasured NH_4^+ cation.[10,11]

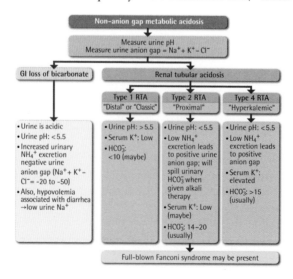

5.3.3 TYPES OF RENAL TUBULAR ACIDOSIS

The patterns of renal tubular acidosis (RTA) of Types 1, 2, and 4 are described in the charts above and below.[15,16] Type 3, RTA (a mixture of Types 1 and 2), was associated with renal insufficiency and is no longer recognized. Localization of the defect in the nephron is described on the table below.

Distal (Type 1)[12]	Proximal (Type 2)[13]	Hyperkalemic (Type 4)[14]
Features		
• Selective deficit of H^+ secretion in the distal nephron with increased K^+ secretion $\Rightarrow$ alkalotic urine with hyperchloremia and hypokalemia • May often be associated with secondary hypercalciuria, hypocitraturia, and nephrolithiasis	• Inability to reabsorb filtered HCO_3^- with bicarbonate wasting (e.g., carbonic anhydrase inhibitors) $\Rightarrow$ hyperchloremia, normal or low serum K^+, acidic urine: pH <5.5 once serum bicarbonate is low • Not associated with nephrolithiasis except after HCO_3^- replacement therapy or when carbonic anhydrase inhibitors cause proximal tubular HCO_3^- wasting	• Is often called hyporeninemic hypoaldosteronism (though often renin level is not low) • ↓Aldosterone $\Rightarrow$ impaired renal tubular Na^+ reabsorption leading to impaired K^+ and H^+ secretion with impaired ability to generate NH_4^+ $\Rightarrow$ ↓NH_4^+ excretion $\Rightarrow$ hyperchloremia, hyperkalemia, acidic urine • Can also be caused by tubulointerstitial renal diseases (e.g., lupus nephritis), causing unresponsiveness to aldosterone
Underlying causes		
• Familial • Toluene toxicity • Sjögren's syndrome • Rheumatoid arthritis • Active cirrhosis • Obstructive uropathy and SLE may cause Type 1 RTA with hyperkalemia	• Multiple myeloma with light chain nephropathy • Heavy metals • Tenofovir • Ifosfamide • Hereditary in children	• Diabetic or hypertensive nephropathy (usually with hypoaldosteronism) • Tubulointerstitial diseases • Potassium-sparing diuretics, ACE inhibitors, ARBs, and trimethoprim can cause drug-induced Type 4 RTA

ACE, Angiotensin-converting-enzyme; ARB, angiotensin receptor blocker; RTA, renal tubular acidosis; SLE, systemic lupus erythematosus.

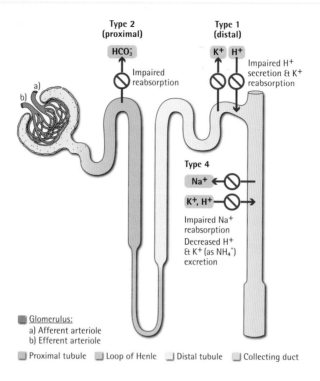

Glomerulus:
a) Afferent arteriole
b) Efferent arteriole

▨ Proximal tubule ▨ Loop of Henle ▨ Distal tubule ▨ Collecting duct

5.3.4 TYPES OF LACTIC ACIDOSIS

Lactic acidosis is one of the most common types of metabolic acidosis associated with an increased anion gap. The diagram below illustrates underlying causes of lactic acidosis of type A (caused by tissue hypoxia) and type B (associated with other causes of increased lactate generation or decreased excretion).[7,17–26]

Type A	Type B
Tissue hypoxia • Circulatory insufficiency (shock, heart failure) • Severe anemia • Cholera • Sepsis • Tumor lysis syndrome • Regional ischemia, burns	Lactate overproduction and/or decreased hepatic re-moval of lactate • Hypoglycemia (glycogen storage disease) • Seizures • Diabetes mellitus • Ethanol • Hepatic failure • Malignancy • Medications: carboplatin, antiretrovirals, salicylates, metformin • Mitochondrial enzyme defects and inhibitors (CO, cyanide) • Thiamine deficiency (cofactor in oxidative phos-phorylation) • D-lactic acidosis

Treatment of lactic acidosis:
- Treat underlying condition (e.g., restore tissue perfusion)
- Avoid vasoconstrictors, but need caution to avoid fluid overload from volume expansion
- Bicarbonate therapy for pH <7.1 (be aware that bicarbonate stimulates phosphofructokinase ⇒ leading to enhanced lactate production, can increase pCO_2, and cause overshoot alkalosis after lactate converts to bicarbonate)[27,28]

5.3.5 ALKALINIZING THERAPY

Alkalinizing therapy for severe acidemia, of which sodium bicarbonate is the most commonly used agent, should be considered in non-anion gap metabolic acidosis and when pH is <7.1.

Bicarbonate administration guidelines:
- Goal: return pH to ≥7.2 and serum bicarbonate to >8 to 10 (goal is pH 7.45–7.5 in case of salicylate poisoning to enhance excretion).[29]
- Calculate bicarbonate deficit initially using a distribution volume of bicarbonate of 0.5 × body weight in kg. This is an approximation due to the need to alkalinize both HCO_3^- and other buffers.
- Administer sodium bicarbonate as continuous infusion in severe acidemia.
- Check bicarbonate level after ≥30 minutes have elapsed since completion of the infusion.

Potential complications of bicarbonate therapy:
- Fluid overload
- Alkalemia occurring as postrecovery respiratory alkalosis or as "overshoot" metabolic alkalosis (in lactic acidosis, when lactate is converted to bicarbonate)
- Hypernatremia, hyperosmolality
- May promote precipitation of calcium phosphate and can induce or exacerbate hypocalcemia
- May increase pCO_2 with paradoxical worsening of intracellular acidosis[30]

Alternative alkalinizing agents to NaHCO$_3$:
Carbicarb[31]—Sodium bicarbonate + Sodium carbonate
- Limits generation of CO_2
- Minimal ↑ in pCO_2

THAM—0.3N tromethamine[31] buffers metabolic and respiratory acids (but rarely used):
Since THAM is a proton acceptor[32] (THAM + H^+ → THAM$^+$), carbonic acid is buffered as follows: THAM + H_2CO_3 → THAM$^+$ + HCO_3^-.
- Limits CO_2 generation
- Side effects: hyperkalemia, hypoglycemia, ventilatory depression, local injury in cases of extravasation, hepatic necrosis in neonates

5.4 Metabolic Alkalosis

5.4.1 CAUSES OF METABOLIC ALKALOSIS

Metabolic alkalosis is caused by H^+ and Cl^- loss, or bicarbonate accumulation.[33]

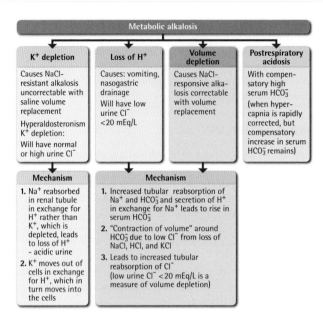

5.4.2 DIAGNOSTIC WORKUP

Diagnostic workup into causes of metabolic alkalosis is based on the following tests: urine chloride and potassium concentrations, and arterial blood pressure.[1,6,33]

The figure below shows an algorithm of the workup process:

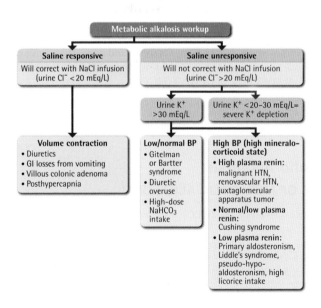

5.4.3 TREATMENT OF METABOLIC ALKALOSIS

- Saline for NaCl-responsive metabolic alkalosis due to volume depletion or GI losses
- Potassium chloride for K and Cl depletion in saline-resistant metabolic alkalosis (plus saline for diuretic overuse if volume contracted)
- Acetazolamide to lower high serum bicarbonate posthypercapnia or when hypervolemic
- HCl 0.3N rarely used (needs central intravenous catheter infusion)

5.5 Acid-Base Disorders

5.5.1 POTASSIUM AND ACID-BASE BALANCE INTERRELATION

The diagram below illustrates the association between alkalosis and hypokalemia and between acidosis and hyperkalemia.

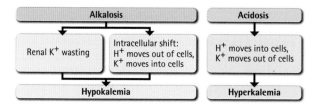

5.5.2 "COMPLEX" (DOUBLE OR TRIPLE) ACID-BASE DISORDERS

A single patient may have two or even three primary acid-base disorders. For example, a primary respiratory alkalosis from overbreathing and a concomitant anion gap metabolic acidosis may be seen with sepsis or salicylate toxicity.[34,35] It is also possible to have a primary metabolic acidosis (e.g., diabetic ketoacidosis) and a simultaneous primary metabolic alkalosis (e.g., vomiting with HCl loss). These two metabolic disturbances can be diagnosed using the anion gap. In an increased anion gap metabolic acidosis, a "hidden" metabolic alkalosis can be discovered with the "delta/delta" concept. It is based on the assumption that for a given increase in the anion gap (Δ AG), there is a concomitant decrease in bicarbonate concentration (Δ HCO_3) from the added unmeasured acid titrating away the bicarbonate.[7,8,36]

The Delta/Delta calculation:

$$\Delta\,AG = \text{Measured AG} - \text{Normal AG}\ (10-12\ \text{mEq/L}) = \text{Unmeasured anions}$$
$$\Delta\,HCO_3 = \text{Normal}\ HCO_3\ (24\ \text{mEq/L}) - \text{measured}\ HCO_3 = \text{Fall in}\ HCO_3$$

If $\Delta AG/\Delta HCO_3 > 2$, it suggests a concomitant metabolic alkalosis.

Looked at another way, if the unmeasured anions in the large anion gap metabolic acidosis were rapidly metabolized to HCO_3, the patient would have a high serum bicarbonate level and become alkalotic. This would indicate the concomitance of both a metabolic acidosis and alkalosis. Were such a patient to also overbreathe or underbreathe, the added primary respiratory disorder (respiratory alkalosis or acidosis) would give rise to a triple acid-base disturbance.

It is important to note that because there are other buffers besides serum bicarbonate, the AG often increases somewhat more than the serum bicarbonate falls, so the $\Delta AG/\Delta HCO_3$ is usually >1; therefore, between 1 and 2 is usual, in a simple increased anion gap metabolic acidosis.

However, if the AG is significantly less than the fall in serum bicarbonate, it suggests that there may be a concomitant primary non-anion gap metabolic acidosis from loss of HCO_3 (e.g., from diarrhea). This can be calculated as follows:

$\Delta AG/\Delta HCO_3$ <1 suggests a combined normal anion gap acidosis in addition to the high anion gap metabolic acidosis.[8,37]

References

1. Rose B, Post T. *Clinical Physiology of Acid-Base and Electrolyte Disorders.* 5th ed. McGraw-Hill; 2001:535–680.
2. Hamm LL, Nakhoul N, Hering-Smith KS. Acid-base homeostasis. *Clin J Am Soc Nephrol.* 2015;10(12):2232–2242. doi:10.2215/CJN.07400715.
3. Adrogué HJ, Madias NE. Secondary responses to altered acid-base status: the rules of engagement. *J Am Soc Nephrol.* 2010;21(6):920–923. doi:10.1681/ASN.2009121211.
4. Bushinsky DA, Coe FL, Katzenberg C. Arterial pCO$_2$ in chronic metabolic acidosis. *Kidney Int.* 1982;22(3):311–314. doi:10.1038/KI.1982.172.
5. Fulop M. A guide for predicting arterial CO$_2$ tension in metabolic acidosis. *Am J Nephrol.* 1997;17(5): 421–424. doi:10.1159/000169134.
6. Narins RG, Emmett M. Simple and mixed acid-base disorders: a practical approach. *Medicine (Baltimore).* 1980;59(3):161–187. doi:10.1097/00005792-198005000-00001.
7. Emmett M, Narins RG. Clinical use of the anion gap. *Medicine (Baltimore).* 1977;56(1):38–54. doi:10.1097/00005792-197756010-00002.
8. Reddy P, Mooradian AD. Clinical utility of anion gap in deciphering acid-base disorders. *Int J Clin Pract.* 2009;63(10):1516–1525. doi:10.1111/J.1742-1241.2009.02000.X.
9. Kraut JA, Xing SX. Approach to the evaluation of a patient with an increased serum osmolal gap and high-anion-gap metabolic acidosis. *Am J Kidney Dis.* 2011;58(3):480–484. doi:10.1053/j.ajkd.2011. 05.018.
10. Kamel KS, Halperin ML. Use of urine electrolytes and urine osmolality in the clinical diagnosis of fluid, electrolytes, and acid-base disorders. *Kidney Int Reports.* 2021;6(5):1211–1224. doi:10.1016/j.ekir.2021. 02.003.
11. Uribarri J, Oh MS. The urine anion gap: common misconceptions. *J Am Soc Nephrol.* 2021;32(5):1025–1028. doi:10.1681/ASN.2020101509.
12. Soares SBM, de Menezes Silva LAW, de Carvalho Mrad FC, Simões e Silva AC. Distal renal tubular acidosis: genetic causes and management. *World J Pediatr.* 2019;15(5):422–431. doi:10.1007/S12519-019-00260-4.
13. Kashoor I, Batlle D. Proximal renal tubular acidosis with and without Fanconi syndrome. *Kidney Res Clin Pract.* 2019;38(3):267–281. doi:10.23876/J.KRCP.19.056.
14. Batlle D, Arruda J. Hyperkalemic forms of renal tubular acidosis: clinical and pathophysiological aspects. *Adv Chronic Kidney Dis.* 2018;25(4):321–333. doi:10.1053/j.ackd.2018.05.004.
15. Soleimani M, Rastegar A. Pathophysiology of renal tubular acidosis: core curriculum 2016. *Am J Kidney Dis.* 2016;68(3):488–498. doi:10.1053/J.AJKD.2016.03.422.
16. Palmer BF, Kelepouris E, Clegg DJ. Renal tubular acidosis and management strategies: a narrative review. *Adv Ther.* 2021;38(2):949–968. doi:10.1007/S12325-020-01587-5.
17. Blohm E, Lai J, Neavyn M. Drug-induced hyperlactatemia. *Clin Toxicol (Phila).* 2017;55(8):869–878. doi:10.1080/15563650.2017.1317348.
18. Hashim H, Sahari NS, Sazlly Lim SM, Hoo FK. Fatal tenofovir-associated lactic acidosis: a case report. *Iran Red Crescent Med J.* 2015;17(10):e19546. doi:10.5812/IRCMJ.19546.
19. Pedrós C, Ávila M, Gómez-Lumbreras A, Manríquez M, Morros R. Lactic acidosis associated with metformin in patients with moderate to severe chronic kidney disease: study protocol for a multicenter population-based case-control study using health databases. *BMC Nephrol.* 2019;20(1):193. doi:10.1186/ S12882-019-1389-8.
20. Garcia-Alvarez M, Marik P, Bellomo R. Sepsis-associated hyperlactatemia. *Crit Care.* 2014;18(5):503. doi:10.1186/S13054-014-0503-3.
21. Reddy AJ, Lam SW, Bauer SR, Guzman JA. Lactic acidosis: clinical implications and management strategies. *Cleve Clin J Med.* 2015;82(9):615–624. doi:10.3949/CCJM.82A.14098.
22. Brivet FG, Slama A, Prat D, Jacobs FM. Carboplatin: a new cause of severe type B lactic acidosis secondary to mitochondrial DNA damage. *Am J Emerg Med.* 2011;29(7):842.e5–842.e7. doi:10.1016/J.AJEM. 2010.07.005.
23. Claessens YE, Chiche JD, Mira JP, Cariou A. Bench-to-bedside review: severe lactic acidosis in HIV patients treated with nucleoside analogue reverse transcriptase inhibitors. *Crit Care.* 2003;7(3):226–232. doi:10.1186/CC2162.

24. Lalau JD, Lacroix C, Compagnon P, et al. Role of metformin accumulation in metformin-associated lactic acidosis. *Diabetes Care*. 1995;18(6):779–784. doi:10.2337/DIACARE.18.6.779.

25. Ruiz JP, Singh AK, Hart P. Type B lactic acidosis secondary to malignancy: case report, review of published cases, insights into pathogenesis, and prospects for therapy. *ScientificWorldJournal*. 2011;11:1316–1324. doi:10.1100/TSW.2011.125.

26. Uppal N, Workeneh B, Rondon-Berrios H, Jhaveri K. Electrolyte and acid-base disorders associated with cancer immunotherapy. *Clin J Am Soc Nephrol*. 2022;17(6):922–933. doi:10.2215/CJN.14671121.

27. Jaber S, Paugam C, Futier E, et al. Sodium bicarbonate therapy for patients with severe metabolic acidaemia in the intensive care unit (BICAR-ICU): a multicentre, open-label, randomised controlled, phase 3 trial. *Lancet*. 2018;392(10141):31–40. doi:10.1016/S0140-6736(18)31080-8.

28. Kraut JA, Kurtz I. Use of base in the treatment of severe acidemic states. *Am J Kidney Dis*. 2001;38(4):703–727. doi:10.1053/AJKD.2001.27688.

29. Mirrakhimov AE, Ayach T, Barbaryan A, Talari G, Chadha R, Gray A. The role of sodium bicarbonate in the management of some toxic ingestions. *Int J Nephrol*. 2017;2017:7831358. doi:10.1155/2017/7831358.

30. Kraut JA, Madias NE. Treatment of acute metabolic acidosis: a pathophysiologic approach. *Nat Rev Nephrol*. 2012;8(10):589–601. doi:10.1038/NRNEPH.2012.186.

31. Kraut JA, Madias NE. Lactic acidosis: current treatments and future directions. *Am J Kidney Dis*. 2016;68(3):473–482. doi:10.1053/J.AJKD.2016.04.020.

32. Nahas GG, Sutin KM, Fermon C, et al. Guidelines for the treatment of acidaemia with THAM. *Drugs*. 1998;55(2):191–224. doi:10.2165/00003495-199855020-00003.

33. Emmett M. Metabolic alkalosis: a brief pathophysiologic review. *Clin J Am Soc Nephrol*. 2020;15(12):1848–1856. doi:10.2215/CJN.16041219.

34. Singh V, Khatana S, Gupta P. Blood gas analysis for bedside diagnosis. *Natl J Maxillofac Surg*. 2013;4(2):136. doi:10.4103/0975-5950.127641.

35. Palmer BF, Clegg DJ. Salicylate toxicity. *N Engl J Med*. 2020;382(26):2544–2555. doi:10.1056/NEJMRA2010852/SUPPL_FILE/NEJMRA2010852_DISCLOSURES.PDF.

36. Yan MT, Chau T, Cheng CJ, Lin SH. Hunting down a double gap metabolic acidosis. *Ann Clin Biochem*. 2010;47(Pt 3):267–270. doi:10.1258/ACB.2010.009213.

37. Rastegar A. Clinical utility of Stewart's method in diagnosis and management of acid-base disorders. *Clin J Am Soc Nephrol*. 2009;4(7):1267–1274. doi:10.2215/CJN.01820309.

CHAPTER 6

Urinalysis and Diagnostic Tests

Robert Stephen Brown ▪ Alexander Goldfarb-Rumyantzev ▪ Ruth Schulman

URINALYSIS

Urine examination is an invaluable tool in patient evaluation and diagnosis. Easy to obtain but often overlooked, the voided urine offers clues to the diagnosis of kidney conditions and helps with the prognosis in cardiovascular disease and diabetes.

A complete urinalysis consists of visual inspection for color and turbidity, a dipstick exam, and a microscopic exam of the centrifuged urinary sediment. While the dipstick is a "waived" test that can be done in any office, the microscopic exam requires Clinical Laboratory Improvement Amendments (CLIA) certification, so it is usually performed by a clinical laboratory, nephrologist, or trained physician or technician.

6.1 Urine Color[1]

Color	Causes	
Cloudy or turbid	Pyuria	Heavy crystalluria
	Bacteriuria	Fecal or vaginal contamination
White	WBCs	Chyle
Red or cola-colored	RBCs (supernatant may be clear)	Cascara
	Free Hgb	Senna
	Myoglobin	Beets
	Porphyria (porphobilin porphyrins)	
	Dye	**Drugs**
	Phenolphthalein	Doxorubicin
		Phenazopyridine
		Phenytoin
Yellow	**Vitamin supplement**	**Dye**
	Riboflavin	Yellow dye
Dark yellow/orange	**Drugs**	
	Sulfasalazine	
	Rifampin	
	Bilirubin	
	Phenazopyrazine	

Color	Causes	
Black/brown	**Drugs**	**Other**
	Methyldopa	Melanin
	Levodopa	**Condition**
	Metronidazole	Homogentisic acid (alkaptonuria)
	Imipenem-cilastatin	
Dull blue/green	**Drugs**	**Drug/dye**
	Triamterene	Methylene blue
	Amitriptyline	**Infection**
	Propofol	Pseudomonas UTI
	Endogenous metabolite: Biliverdin	
Purple	**Seen in the setting of foley bag collection, not in the passed urine[2]**	
	Infection	
	Proteus mirabilis	
	Escherichia coli	
	Pseudomonas aeruginosa	
	Morganella morganii	
	Klebsiella pneumoniae	
	Enterococcus spp.	

Hgb, Hemoglobin; RBCs, red blood cells; UTI, urinary tract infection; WBCs, white blood cells.

6.2 Dipstick Test[3]

Dipstick	Positive	False Positive	False Negative
Blood	Detects RBCs as low as 1–2/hpf, but also reacts to free Hgb (hemolysis) and myoglobin (rhabdomyolysis)	Uncommon contamination with hypochlorite or bacteria with pseudoperoxidase activity	Rare; high concentration of ascorbic acid can mask low-grade hematuria
Proteins	Detects albumin >30 mg/dL (normal is negative; trace- 27% will have microalbuminuria; 1+protein- 47% will have micro- or macroalbuminuria)	Highly buffered alkaline urine, some antiseptics, such as chlorhexidine, ejaculation	Light chains and other immunoglobulins, beta-2-microglobulin, dilute urine with <30 mg/dL of albumin
Nitrites	Denotes Enterobacteriaceae, which convert urinary nitrate to nitrite in UTI	None	Short incubation time in the bladder (<4 hr), pathogen doesn't convert nitrate to nitrite, not enough nitrate or too much ascorbic acid in urine
Glucose	Detects diabetes and renal glucosuria	None	Ascorbic acid or ketones in urine decrease positive tests

Continued on following page

Dipstick	Positive	False Positive	False Negative
Ketones	Detects acetoacetate in diabetic and starvation/alcoholic ketosis	High quantities of levodopa, mesna, tiopronin, captopril, penicillamine, acetyl-cysteine in urine	Doesn't detect acetone or beta-hydroxybutyrate ketone bodies
Leukocyte esterase	Detects pyuria ≥6 WBCs/hpf but may indicate interstitial nephritis or leukemia rather than infection	Contamination with vaginal discharge or saliva	High glucose or specific gravity, some antibiotics, only mononuclear leukocytes in transplant rejection
SG	Measures urine concentration, correlating roughly with osmolarity, normally SG = 1.003–1.030 (see figure below)	High SG >1.030 usually due to radiocontrast; also, glucose or protein will raise SG > osmolarity	Low SG shows dilute urine, but agents affecting urine color cause inaccurate results

Hgb, Hemoglobin; *hpf*, high power field; *RBCs*, red blood cells; *SG*, specific gravity; *UTI*, urinary tract infection.

6.3 Proteinuria

6.3.1 PROTEIN TO CREATININE RATIO AND ALBUMIN TO CREATININE RATIO

6.3.1.1 Estimating the Degree of Proteinuria in a Random or Spot Urine Sample[4,5]

Urine protein to creatinine ratio (PCR) measures all proteins, can be expressed as grams of protein per gram of creatinine (Cr) or a unit-free number, and is calculated as:

$$\frac{U_{protein}\left(mg/dL\right)}{U_{creatinine}\left(mg/dL\right)} = \frac{protein\left(g\right)}{creatinine\left(g\right)}$$

This correlates with grams of protein excreted per day per 1.73 m² body surface area (BSA).

6.3.1.2 Detecting Micro- or Macroalbuminuria (See Below for Definitions) in a Random or Spot Urine Sample

Urine albumin to creatinine ratio (ACR) is expressed as milligrams of albumin per gram of Cr and is calculated as:

$$\frac{U_{albumin}\left(mg/L\right)}{U_{creatinine}\left(g/L\right)} = \frac{albumin\left(mg\right)}{creatinine\left(g\right)}$$

Proteinuria	PCR on Spot Urine	24-Hour Urine Collection
Normal	<0.2 (usually unit-free but can be g/g)	<150 mg/24 hr
Mild proteinuria	0.2–1.0	150 mg–1.0 g/24 hr
Moderate proteinuria	1.0–3.0	1.0–3.0 g/24 hr
Nephrotic range	>3.0	>3.0 g/24 hr

Albuminuria	ACR on Spot Urine	24-Hour Urine Collection
Normal	<30 mg/g is considered normal, but sex-based normals are: <17 mg/g (males) <25 mg/g (females)	<30 mg/24 hr
Microalbuminuria	30–300 mg/g (either sex) or 17–300 mg/g (males) 25–300 mg/g (females)	30–300 mg/24 hr
Macroalbuminuria	>300 mg/g	>300 mg/24 hr

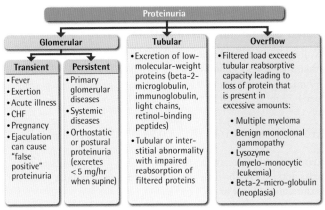

CHF, Congestive heart failure.

6.4 Estimation of Renal Function

6.4.1.1 Measured Creatinine Clearance (CrCl)

Collect timed urine for volume and total Cr excretion (usually 24-hour collection in which total urine volume is 1440 min/24 hr in the formula below):

$$\text{Normal daily Cr excretion: Males: } 15-20 \text{ mg/kg/24 hr*}$$

$$\text{Females: } 10-15 \text{ mg/kg/24 hr*}$$

$$(\text{*assuming normal muscle mass})$$

$$\text{Creatinine clearance mL/min} = \frac{U_{Cr}\left(mg/dL\right) \times U_{Vol}\left(mL/min\right)}{S_{Cr}\left(mg/dL\right)}$$

6.4.1.2 Measured Glomerular Filtration Rate (GFR)

Rarely done except for research studies:
- Inulin clearance
- I^{125} iothalamate clearance

Estimated GFR using cystatin C[6]:
- Biomarker similar to Cr used to estimate GFR
- Is filtered but not secreted
- Avoids confounding factors seen with Cr related to diet and muscle mass
- Typically is a test that is sent out, so results take longer than they do for Cr

6.4.1.3 Cockcroft-Gault Formula[7]

Estimated creatinine clearance calculated from serum creatinine (SCr):

$$eC_{Cr}(ml/min) = \frac{(140 - age)}{S_{Cr}(mg/dL)} \times \frac{Body\ weight(kg)}{72} \times (0.85\ if\ female)$$

Original formula used actual body weight (BW), but to avoid overestimate of eC_{Cr} if weight is >120% of ideal body weight (IBW), it is better to use:

Either IBM or $0.4(BW - IBW) + IBW$ where IBW is calculated as:
- IBW for females $(kg) = 45 + (2.3 \times inches\ over\ 60")$
- IBW for males $(kg) = 50 + (2.3 \times inches\ over\ 60")$

6.4.1.4 Estimated Glomerular Filtration Rate (eGFR) Calculated From SCr[8]

The Chronic Kidney Disease Epidemiology Collaboration (CKD-EPI) equation for eGFR is more accurate than the Modification of Diet in Renal Disease (MDRD) formulae, particularly with GFRs >60 mL/min per 1.73 m². However, many experts favor reporting only that eGFR >60 mL/min per 1.73 m² for "normal" eGFRs due to lack of accuracy in this range.

$$eGFR=$$
$$141 \times min(Scr/\kappa,1)^{\alpha} \times max(Scr/\kappa,1)^{-1.209} \times 0.993^{age} \times 1.018\,[if\ female] \times 1.159\,[if\ black]$$

SCr is standardized serum creatinine (mg/dL), κ is 0.7 for females and 0.9 for males, α is −0.329 for females and −0.411 for males, min indicates the minimum of SCr/κ or 1, and max indicates the maximum of SCr/κ or 1.

However, there have been controversies about the use of race in the estimation of GFR,[9] so the National Kidney Foundation and the American Society of Nephrology established a task force in 2020 that reassessed the inclusion of race in eGFR calculations (see discussion in Chapter 11). While research for new biomarkers takes place, the task force has made the following two recommendations: "(1) …immediate implementation of the CKD-EPI Cr equation refit (CKD-EPIcr_R) without the race variable in all laboratories in the U.S. because it does not include race in the calculation and reporting, and …has acceptable performance characteristics and potential consequences that do not disproportionately affect any one group of individuals; and (2) …increased, routine, and timely use of cystatin C, especially to confirm eGFR in adults who are at risk for or have chronic kidney disease, because combining filtration markers (Cr and cystatin C, i.e., CKD-EPIcr- cys_R) is more accurate and would support better clinical decisions than either one marker alone".[10]

These two non-race-based "refit" formulae are as follows:

$$CKD-EPIcr\_R=$$
$$142 \times min(Scr/\kappa,1)^{\alpha} \times max(Scr/\kappa,1)^{-1.200} \times 0.9938^{age} \times 1.012\,[if\ female]$$

where SCr is serum creatinine in mg/dL, k is 0.7 for females and 0.9 males, α is −0.241 for females and −0.302 for males, age is in years, min indicates the minimum of SCr/k or 1, and max indicates the maximum of SCr/k or 1.[10]

$$CKD-EPIcr-cys\_R=$$
$$135 \times min(Scr/\kappa,1)^{\alpha} \times max(Scr/\kappa,1)^{-0.544}$$
$$\times min(scys/0.8,1)^{-0.323} \times max(Scys/0.8,1)^{-0.778} \times 0.995^{age} \times 0.963\,[if\ female]$$

where SCr is serum creatinine in mg/dL, Scys is serum cystatin C in mg/L, κ is 0.7 for females and 0.9 for males, α is −0.219 for females and −0.144 for males, age is in years, min indicates the minimum of SCr/κ or 1, and max indicates the maximum of SCr/κ or 1.[11]

Currently, it is on a hospital/lab basis as to whether or not eGFR is reported with or without the race coefficient, but increasingly, the race-free formulae have become preferred. We advise the routine use of the non-race-based refit first creatinine-based formula above as more accurate overall for all races than the initial CKD-EPI equation and the use of the second formula with both creatinine and cystatin C for greater accuracy in certain situations. These can be easily utilized with online calculators (https://www.kidney.org/professionals/kdoqi/gfr_calculator).

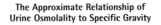

The Approximate Relationship of Urine Osmolality to Specific Gravity

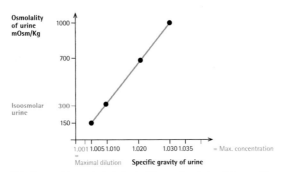

Note: Presence of dense molecules in the urine (glucose, radiocontrast media, heavy proteinuria) can produce large changes in SG with relatively little change in osmolality, so SG should not be used to estimate osmolality in such cases.

6.5 Preparing Urine for Evaluation by Microscopy[12]

How to perform a urinalysis with sediment examination:
1. Pour about 10 to 12 mL of urine into a test tube (preferably a conical test tube).
2. Create a counterweight test tube with an equal amount of water.
3. Place the test tube and water in a centrifuge in opposite slots.
4. Close the centrifuge until it locks.
5. Set a timer for 5 minutes.
6. Dip a test strip into the extra unspun urine.
7. Lay the test strip down to develop for the times specified on the test strip container.
8. Once developed, use the test strip container guide to interpret the results.
9. Once the urine is done spinning, remove the test tube.
10. Pour off the excess fluid, leaving about 0.5 mL.
11. Resuspend the pellet in the remaining fluid using a pipette.
12. Place 1 drop of urine on a slide.
13. Place the slide cover slip over the drop of urine.
14. View the slide under a microscope, starting with a low power objective (10×) and then switching to high power (40×) for identification of cells, casts, bacteria, or crystals.

6.6 Microscope Techniques

6.6.1 LIGHT MICROSCOPY

Uses:
Provides a general overview of all objects. Elements with a low refractive index can be difficult to see if the light source is turned up too high. It can be helpful to turn down the intensity of the light to better see these elements.

6.6.2 PHASE CONTRAST

Uses:
Provides enhanced contrast of object edges and of elements with a low refractive index, including hyaline protein matrix within casts, membranes of RBCs with low Hgb ("ghost cells"), and lipids. Phase contrast is also the best tool for cellular detail, and is especially useful for identifying acanthocytes.

6.6.3 STERNHEIMER-MALBIN (SM) STAIN

Uses:

Facilitates visualization of the various components of cells (e.g., the nucleus vs. cytoplasm) and enhances the identification of WBCs, tubular epithelial cells, and protein matrix of casts.

6.6.4 DARK FIELD OR POLARIZED

Uses:

Elements in the sediment with a high refractive index such as crystals and lipids appear especially "bright" under dark field illumination. Dark field or microscopic visualization through cross-polarized lenses is useful for low-power scanning of a slide to identify casts, lipids, and crystals.

6.7 Urine Sediment Findings

Cells	Casts	Crystals (Chapter 15)
RBCs: Hematuria may be of nonglomerular or glomerular origin, the latter indicated by acanthocytic RBCs or RBC casts	Organic matrix composed primarily of Tamm-Horsfall mucoprotein (also called uromodulin) **Hyaline casts:** Signifies low urinary flow, observed with small volumes of concentrated urine or with diuretic therapy	**Uric acid crystals:** Observed in acid urine from conversion of more soluble urate salt into less soluble uric acid
WBCs: Polymorphs (pyuria in UTI) Eosinophils (need staining to identify) Lymphocytes (in acute transplant rejection or interstitial nephritis) Macrophages (uncertain significance)	**RBC casts:** Diagnostic of glomerulonephritis or vasculitis **WBC casts:** Pyelonephritis, acute glomerulonephritis, tubulointerstitial disease **Renal epithelial cell casts:** ATN, interstitial nephritis, and rarely in acute glomerulonephritis	**Calcium phosphate:** Form in a relatively alkaline urine **Calcium oxalate:** Most common crystal and kidney stone, not dependent upon the urine pH **Cystine crystals:** Seen only in cystinuria
Epithelial cells: Renal tubular cells (ATN, nephrotic syndrome, transplant rejection, interstitial nephritis) Squamous epithelial cells (may signify vaginal or skin contamination) Transitional cells (bladder, ureters, or renal pelvis origin; usually benign but can be malignant)	**Lipid or fatty casts:** Nephrotic-range proteinuria (can see characteristic "Maltese cross" droplets composed of cholesterol esters and cholesterol, which may also be observed as free fat or as oval fat bodies in the urine) **Granular casts:** Observed in numerous disorders, represent degenerating cells or aggregated proteins in casts **Muddy brown casts:** Granular casts containing degenerated cellular pigments; indicate tubular necrosis **Waxy casts:** Represent proteinaceous matrix in the final stage of degeneration of granular casts	**Triple phosphate crystals:** Magnesium ammonium phosphate crystals + calcium carbonate apatite = struvite or "triple phosphate" crystals (occurs only when ammonia production is increased and the urine pH is elevated to decrease the solubility of phosphate in the setting of urease-producing organisms such as *Proteus* or *Klebsiella*) **Drug crystals:** Mainly acyclovir, indinavir, atazanavir, triamterene, methotrexate, and sulfonamide antibiotics
Bacteria, fungi, or parasites	**Broad casts:** May be waxy or granular; form in the enlarged tubules of nephrons that have hypertrophied in advanced renal failure	

ATN, Acute tubular necrosis; *RBC*, red blood cell; *UTI*, urinary tract infection; *WBC*, white blood cell.

6.8 Hematuria[13]

Hematuria is defined (arbitrarily) as the presence of ≥2 to 3 RBCs per hpf in spun urine.

6.8.1 CLASSIFICATION OF HEMATURIA

The amount of blood determines whether the hematuria is visible to the naked eye or requires microscopy for detection:
- Macroscopic (or gross) hematuria
- Microscopic hematuria

6.8.2 CAUSES OF HEMATURIA

Urological Diseases (Nonglomerular and Usually Without Proteinuria)

- Transient hematuria:
  - Most common cause of hematuria is infection (cystitis, prostatitis, or pyelonephritis)
  - Trauma, exercise
  - Menstruation
  - Sexual intercourse
- Persistent hematuria:
  - Neoplasms
  - Nephrolithiasis
  - Hypercalciuria or hyperuricosuria
  - Renal cystic disease
  - Tuberculosis

Hematological Disorders

- Sickle cell trait or disease
- Coagulopathies, particularly high INR
- HUS/TTP

Glomerular Disorders

- Signs of glomerular origin: RBC casts, acanthocytes (dysmorphic RBCs), proteinuria >500 mg/day, cola-colored urine
- Persistent hematuria:
  - Any glomerular disease, but more common in acute nephritic disease
  - IgA nephropathy
  - Hereditary nephritis (Alport syndrome)
  - Thin basement membrane disease
  - Renal vasculitis

Other

- Vascular disease
- Systemic vasculitis
- Renal infarction
- AV malformation, renal angiomas
- Renal AV fistula
- Malignant hypertension
- Papillary necrosis
- Loin pain hematuria syndrome

HUS/TPP, Hemolytic uremic syndrome/thrombotic thrombocytopenic purpura; *INR*, international normalized ratio; *RBC*, red blood cell.

6.8.3 HEMATURIA EVALUATION[13–15]

- Examine urinary sediment for glomerular etiology (i.e., RBC casts, >5% acanthocytes)
- Radiological imaging for renal anatomy (tumor mass, stones, polycystic kidneys, hydronephrosis, AV malformation, medullary sponge kidney, kidney size)
  - Ultrasound—safe, can be used in pregnancy, less expensive
  - Intravenous pyelography (IVP)—no longer routinely used, shows ureters, poor differentiation of solid versus cystic masses

- CT scan—best for stones (without contrast) and masses (with contrast), can show vasculature and detect some bladder tumors
- MRI (without and with gadolinium)—equal to CT for masses and vasculature, less risk of contrast toxicity, but gadolinium to be used in late stage 4 or stage 5 chronic kidney disease (CKD) only if clearly necessary due to risk of gadolinium-induced nephrogenic systemic fibrosis
  - Renal arteriography—if CT suggests infarction or AV malformation
  - Retrograde or percutaneous antegrade pyelography—to evaluate obstruction in hydronephrosis
- Cystoscopy (bladder mass or stone, unresolving cystitis)—indicated in gross hematuria or persistent nonglomerular microscopic hematuria in patients 40 to 50 years of age or with risk factors for transitional cell cancer[15]
- Urine cytology—rarely used, can detect transitional cell cancer with high specificity but low sensitivity, not useful for renal cell cancer[16]
- Renal biopsy low yield unless proteinuria, renal insufficiency, or clinical evidence of glomerular disease[17,18]

6.9 Eosinophiluria[19,20]

6.9.1 DETECT WITH HANSEL'S STAIN OF THE URINARY SEDIMENT*

- Allergic interstitial nephritis
- Acute prostatitis or UTI
- Atheroembolic disease
- Occasionally vasculitis or rapidly progressive glomerulonephritis
- Transplant rejection

*Note: Eosinophiluria is neither sensitive nor specific.

Urine Light Microscopic Sediment Findings

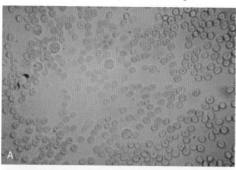

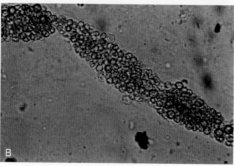

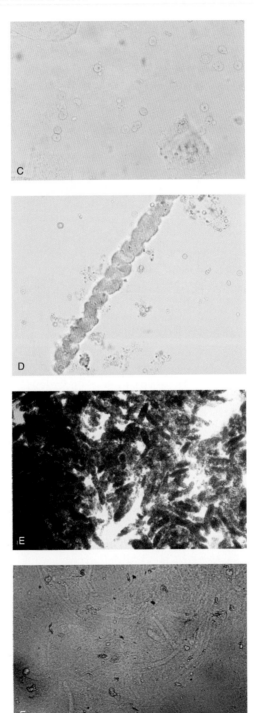

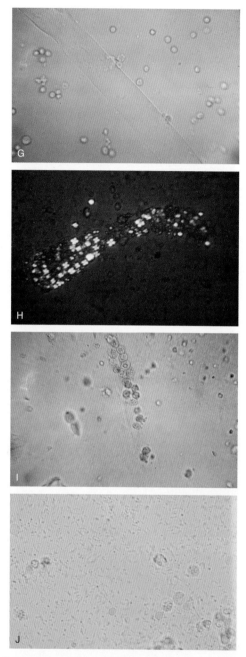

A. Many red blood cells (isomorphic) and several white blood cells. **B.** A red blood cell cast suggesting he-maturia of glomerular origin. **C.** Multiple acanthocytes suggesting RBCs of glomerular origin. **D.** Granular cast, often seen in CKD, but not specific. **E.** Many "muddy brown" casts suggestive of ischemic/toxic acute kidney injury. **F.** Many hyaline casts (note low refraction of casts making it important to keep light low) seen in normal concentrated urine. **G.** Waxy 'broad' cast (and RBCs) seen in chronic kidney disease. **H.** Lipid cast with appearance of "Maltese crosses" under polarized light and free fat droplets in nephrotic syndrome. **I.** Renal tubular cell and WBC cast suggestive of interstitial nephritis. **J.** Many bacterial rods, granulocytic WBCs and RBCs indicative of high grade bacteriuria. (A-B, D-J, Courtesy of the late Dr. Richard Nesson)

6.10 Kidney Biopsy[21,22]

6.10.1 INDICATIONS FOR KIDNEY BIOPSY

- **Acute renal failure:** Rising Cr when cause is unclear or >3 to 4 weeks of supportive treatment without recovery
- **Nephritis of uncertain etiology:** Acute nephritic syndrome, progressive renal insufficiency
- **Proteinuria:** Without evidence of known causative systemic disease—Nephrotic syndrome or >1 to 2 g/day nonnephrotic range proteinuria to determine diagnosis and prognosis
- **Hematuria:** Recurrent gross hematuria or persistent microscopic hematuria of suspected renal etiology or family history of hematuria when diagnosis would help management
- **Systemic disease:** Systemic lupus erythematosus (SLE) or systemic vasculitis with renal findings, undiagnosed systemic disease, monoclonal gammopathy of potential renal significance, or atypical course of diabetic nephropathy
- **Transplant kidney:** Allograft dysfunction to differentiate ATN versus transplant rejection, drug toxicity, viral interstitial nephritis, recurrent or de novo glomerulonephritis, or thrombotic microangiopathy

6.10.2 RELATIVE CONTRAINDICATIONS FOR KIDNEY BIOPSY

- Anatomic abnormalities: for example, solitary, ectopic, cystic, or horseshoe kidney may be more effectively biopsied using CT rather than ultrasound (US) localization
- Uncorrected coagulation disorders and thrombocytopenia
- Uremic platelet dysfunction is a relative contraindication that may be helped by DDAVP (desmopressin) pretreatment
- Severe uncontrolled hypertension (HTN) (goal systolic blood pressure [SBP] is <140–150)
- Hydronephrosis
- Small kidneys (<9 cm) in an adult is usually indicative of chronic irreversible disease; therefore, diagnostic yield is likely very low
- Impaired mental status or uncooperative patient will probably necessitate sedation for safety

6.10.3 ABSOLUTE CONTRAINDICATIONS FOR KIDNEY BIOPSY

- Pyelonephritis, cellulitis at site of biopsy needle entry

6.10.4 COMPLICATIONS OF KIDNEY BIOPSY[23–27]

- Gross hematuria occurs in 3% to 10% of patients and is usually self-limited
- Hematuria or perinephric bleeding that causes hypotension occurs in 1% to 2% of cases
- Bleeding requiring blood transfusion occurs in 1% to 2% of cases
- Infection is rare unless UTI is present prebiopsy
- AV fistula formation is rare but may cause persistent hematuria and a renal bruit
- Death occurs in about 0.06%–0.1% of patients, angiographic intervention in about 0.4%, and nephrectomy in <0.1%
- An observation period of ≤8 hours risks missing 20% to 33% of complications, but most centers sent patients home after observation periods of about 4 hr

References

1. Aycock RD, Kass DA. Abnormal urine color. *South Med J*. 2012;105(1):43–47. doi:10.1097/SMJ.0b013e31823c413e.
2. de Menezes Neves PDM, Coelho Ferreira BM, Mohrbacher S, Renato Chocair P, Cuvello-Neto AL. Purple urine bag syndrome: a colourful complication of urinary tract infection. *Lancet Infect Dis*. 2020;20(10):1215. doi:10.1016/S1473-3099(20)30323-6.

3. Fogazzi GB, Verdesca S, Garigali G. Urinalysis: core curriculum 2008. *Am J Kidney Dis.* 2008;51(6): 1052–1067. doi:10.1053/j.ajkd.2007.11.039.

4. Ginsberg JM, Chang BS, Matarese RA, Garella S. Use of single voided urine samples to estimate quantitative proteinuria. *N Engl J Med.* 1983;309(25):1543–1546. doi:10.1056/nejm198312223092503.

5. Schwab SJ, Christensen RL, Dougherty K, Klahr S. Quantitation of proteinuria by the use of protein-to-creatinine ratios in single urine samples. *Arch Intern Med.* 1987;147(5):943–944. doi:10.1001/archinte. 1987.00370050135022.

6. Ferguson TW, Komenda P, Tangri N. Cystatin C as a biomarker for estimating glomerular filtration rate. *Curr Opin Nephrol Hypertens.* 2015;24(3):295–300. doi:10.1097/MNH.0000000000000115.

7. Cockcroft DW, Gault MH. Prediction of creatinine clearance from serum creatinine. *Nephron.* 1976; 16(1):31–41. doi:10.1159/000180580.

8. Levey AS, Bosch JP, Lewis JB, Greene T, Rogers N, Roth D. A more accurate method to estimate glomerular filtration rate from serum creatinine: a new prediction equation. Modification of Diet in Renal Disease Study Group. *Ann Intern Med.* 1999;130(6):461–70. doi:10.7326/0003-4819-130-6-199903160-00002.

9. Delgado C, Baweja M, Burrows NR, et al. Reassessing the inclusion of race in diagnosing kidney diseases: an interim report from the NKF-ASN task force. *J Am Soc Nephrol.* 2021;32(6):1305–1317. doi:10.1681/ASN.2021010039.

10. Delgado C, Baweja M, Crews D, et al. A unifying approach for GFR estimation: recommendations of the NKF-ASN Task Force on Reassessing the Inclusion of Race in Diagnosing Kidney Disease. *J Am Soc Nephrol.* 2021;32(12):2994–3015. doi:10.1681/asn.2021070988.

11. Inker LA, Eneanya ND, Coresh J, et al. New creatinine- and cystatin C–based equations to estimate GFR without race. *N Engl J Med.* 2021;385(19):1737–1749. doi:10.1056/nejmoa2102953.

12. Cavanaugh C, Perazella MA. Urine sediment examination in the diagnosis and management of kidney disease: core curriculum 2019. *Am J Kidney Dis.* 2019;73(2):258–272. doi:10.1053/j.ajkd.2018.07.012.

13. Cohen RA, Brown RS. Clinical practice. Microscopic hematuria. *N Engl J Med.* 2003;348(23):2330–2338. doi:10.1056/NEJMcp012694.

14. Niemi MA, Cohen RA. Evaluation of microscopic hematuria: a critical review and proposed algorithm. *Adv Chronic Kidney Dis.* 2015;22(4):289–296. doi:10.1053/j.ackd.2015.04.006.

15. Grossfeld GD, Wolf JS, Litwin MS, et al. Asymptomatic microscopic hematuria in adults: summary of the AUA best practice policy recommendations. *Am Fam Physician.* 2001;63(6):1145–1154.

16. Feifer AH, Steinberg J, Tanguay S, Aprikian AG, Brimo F, Kassouf W. Utility of urine cytology in the workup of asymptomatic microscopic hematuria in low-risk patients. *Urology.* 2010;75(6):1278–1282. doi:10.1016/j.urology.2009.09.091.

17. Hall CL, Bradley R, Kerr A, Attoti R, Peat D. Clinical value of renal biopsy in patients with asymptomatic microscopic hematuria with and without low-grade proteinuria. *Clin Nephrol.* 2004;62(4):267–272. doi:10.5414/cnp62267.

18. Mc Gregor DO, Lynn KL, Bailey RR, Robson RA, Gardner J. Clinical audit of the use of renal biopsy in the management of isolated microscopic hematuria. *Clin Nephrol.* 1998;49(6):345–348.

19. Fletcher A. Eosinophiluria and acute interstitial nephritis. *N Engl J Med.* 2008;358(16):1760–1761. doi:10.1056/nejmc0708475.

20. Kaye M, Gagnon RF. Acute allergic interstitial nephritis and eosinophiluria. *Kidney Int.* 2008;73(8):980. doi:10.1038/sj.ki.5002777.

21. Luciano RL, Moeckel GW. Update on the native kidney biopsy: core curriculum 2019. *Am J Kidney Dis.* 2019;73(3):404–415. doi:10.1053/j.ajkd.2018.10.011.

22. Whittier WL, Korbet SM. Renal biopsy: update. *Curr Opin Nephrol Hypertens.* 2004;13(6):661–665. doi:10.1097/00041552-200411000-00013.

23. Atwell TD, Smith RL, Hesley GK, et al. Incidence of bleeding after 15,181 percutaneous biopsies and the role of aspirin. *Am J Roentgenol.* 2010;194(3):784–789. doi:10.2214/AJR.08.2122.

24. Hergesell O, Felten H, Andrassy K, Kühn K, Ritz E. Safety of ultrasound-guided percutaneous renal biopsy-retrospective analysis of 1090 consecutive cases. *Nephrol Dial Transplant.* 1998;13(4):975–977. doi:10.1093/ndt/13.4.975.

25. Marwah DS, Korbet SM. Timing of complications in percutaneous renal biopsy: what is the optimal period of observation? *Am J Kidney Dis.* 1996;28(1):47–52. doi:10.1016/S0272-6386(96)90129-8.

26. Schorr M, Roshanov PS, Weir MA, House AA. Frequency, timing, and prediction of major bleeding complications from percutaneous renal biopsy. *Can J Kidney Health and Dis.* 2020;7:2054358120923527. doi:10.1177/2054358120923527.

27. Koirala A, Jefferson JA. How safe is a native kidney biopsy? *CJASN.* 2020;15(11):1541–1542. doi:10. 2215/CJN.14890920.

CHAPTER 7

Acute Kidney Injury

Robert Stephen Brown ▦ Alexander Goldfarb-Rumyantzev ▦ Nathan H. Raines

7.1 Definition of AKI[1]

- Increase in serum creatinine (SCr) by ≥0.3 mg/dL within 48 hours; or
- Increase in SCr to ≥1.5 times baseline, which is known or presumed to have occurred within the prior 7 days; or
- Urine volume <0.5 mL/kg/hr for 6 hours.

7.2 Epidemiology of AKI

Incidence of acute kidney injury (AKI) can be thought of in three different ways:
1. Contacts with the healthcare system with a primary diagnosis of AKI,
2. AKI arising among hospitalized patients, especially those in the intensive care unit (ICU), or
3. AKI leading to dialysis requirement.

Overall, data suggest an increase in the incidence of AKI across all three categories over the past 3 decades. This increase is thought to be driven by a number of factors[2]:
- Aging population with more comorbidities;
- New medications which have nephrotoxic side effects, and greater degree of polypharmacy (see sections 7.10 and 7.11);
- Increased frequency of procedures that place risk to kidney function; and
- Changing definitions of AKI (see section 7.3);
- Changing diagnostic practices (e.g., urinary biomarkers for AKI).

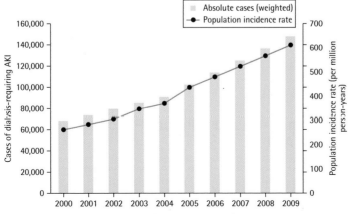

Population Incidence of Dialysis-requiring AKI in United States from 2000 to 2009 (absolute count & incidence rate per million person-years)[4]

From Hsu RK, McCulloch CE, Dudley RA, Lo LJ, Hsu CY. Temporal changes in incidence of dialysis-requiring AKI. *J Am Soc Nephrol.* 2013;24(1):37–42. doi:10.1681/ASN.2012080800.

The diagnosis of AKI, whether requiring dialysis or not, carries with it an increased risk for mortality both in-hospital and post-hospitalization.[3] However, mortality among individuals hospitalized with AKI has trended in the opposite direction of AKI incidence. Among those with AKI requiring dialysis, mortality fell from more than 40% in 1988 to less than 25% in 2009.[4,5] However, no improvement in mortality rates, and even higher death rates in the critically ill, have been reported over the past decade[6]. AKI also increases the subsequent risk for chronic kidney disease (CKD),[7,8] cardiovascular disease,[9] and hypertension (HTN).[10]

Because of these long-term effects, patients who develop AKI should have ongoing monitoring for kidney-related and other sequelae after their hospitalization, even if their creatinine (Cr) returns to baseline.

7.3 Staging of AKI[1]

The KDIGO (Kidney Disease: Improving Global Outcomes) staging system has largely replaced the RIFLE (Risk, Injury, Failure, Loss of kidney function, and End-stage kidney disease) and AKIN (Acute Kidney Injury Network) staging systems as a means of diagnosing and categorizing the severity of AKI. Note the use of SCr rather than estimated glomerular filtration rate (eGFR): remember that formulae designed for calculating eGFR or creatinine clearance (CrCl) from SCr levels must not be used in patients with AKI or in any case in which the SCr level is unstable. Providers often neglect to consider urine output (UO) criteria, which can lead to missed cases and incorrect prognostic evaluation.[11]

Stage	SCr	UO
1	1.5–1.9 times baseline *or* ≥0.3-mg/dL (≥26.5-mmol/L) increase	<0.5 mL/kg/hr for 6–12 hr
2	2.0–2.9 times baseline	<0.5 mL/kg/hr for ≥12 hr
3	3.0 times baseline *or* Increase in SCr to ≥4.0 mg/dL *or* Initiation of renal replacement therapy *or* In patients <18 years, decrease in eGFR to <35 mL/min/1.73 m^2	<0.3 mL/kg/hr for ≥24 hr *or* Anuria for ≥12 hr

eGFR, Estimated glomerular filtration rate; *SCr*, serum creatinine; *UO*, urine output.

Kellum J A, Lameire N, Aspelin P, et al. Kidney Disease: Improving Global Outcomes (KDIGO) acute kidney injury work group. KDIGO clinical practice guideline for acute kidney injury. *Kidney Int Suppl*. 2012;2(1):1–138. doi:10.1038/kisup.2012.1.

7.4 KDIGO Stage-Based Clinical Practice Guideline for AKI

Using the stages of AKI severity listed above, the KDIGO guidelines suggest general evaluation and management strategies as shown in the following algorithms:

Stage-Based Evaluation and Management of AKI

	KDIGO AKI Stage		
High Risk	**1**	**2**	**3**
Discontinue all nephrotoxic agents when possible			
Ensure volume status and perfusion pressure			
Consider functional hemodynamic monitoring			
Monitor SCr and UO			
Avoid hyperglycemia			
Consider alternatives to radiocontrast procedures			
	Noninvasive diagnostic workup (US, serologies)		
	Consider invasive diagnostic workup (kidney biopsy)		
		Check for changes in drug dosing	
		Consider renal replacement therapy	
		Consider ICU admission	
			Avoid subclavian catheters if possible

AKI, Acute kidney injury; *ICU*, intensive care unit; *SCr*, serum creatinine; *UO*, urine output; *US*, ultrasound.

Kellum J A, Lameire N, Aspelin P, et al. Kidney Disease: Improving Global Outcomes (KDIGO) acute kidney injury work group. KDIGO clinical practice guideline for acute kidney injury. *Kidney Int Suppl.* 2012;2(1):1–138. doi:10.1038/kisup.2012.1.

7.5 Diagnostic Steps to Establish the Cause of AKI

7.5.1 DETERMINATION OF AKI VERSUS CKD

The initial step in the diagnostic approach to patients with kidney insufficiency is to determine whether the injury is acute or chronic:

Source of Information	Acute	Chronic
Medical history	Abrupt ↑ in SCr over days	Slow increase in SCr over weeks to months
Symptoms	Recent onset of symptoms (e.g., fever, flank pain, decreased or discolored urine)	No symptoms or slow onset of fatigue, anorexia, weakness, nausea, and/or pruritus
Labs	Further ↑ in SCr after initial evaluation	Relatively stable SCr
Anemia	Less typical or secondary to other than renal causes	More typical although not very specific
Ultrasound	Normal size or enlarged kidneys; can have findings of hydronephrosis or vascular occlusion depending on underlying cause	Small kidneys with increased echogenicity, although may be of normal or enlarged size, particularly with diabetes, amyloidosis, or polycystic kidney disease

SCr, Serum creatinine.

7.5.2 INITIAL DIAGNOSTIC APPROACH

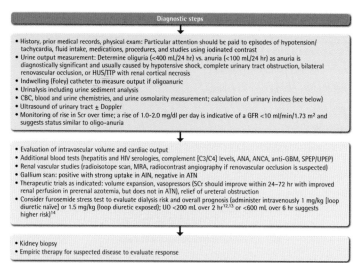

Diagnostic steps

- History, prior medical records, physical exam: Particular attention should be paid to episodes of hypotension/tachycardia, fluid intake, medications, procedures, and studies using iodinated contrast
- Urine output measurement: Determine oliguria (<400 mL/24 hr) vs. anuria (<100 mL/24 hr) as anuria is diagnostically significant and usually caused by hypotensive shock, complete urinary tract obstruction, bilateral renovascular occlusion, or HUS/TTP with renal cortical necrosis
- Indwelling (Foley) catheter to measure output if oligoanuric
- Urinalysis including urine sediment analysis
- CBC, blood and urine chemistries, and urine osmolarity measurement; calculation of urinary indices (see below)
- Ultrasound of urinary tract ± Doppler
- Monitoring of rise in Scr over time; a rise of 1.0–2.0 mg/dl per day is indicative of a GFR <10 ml/min/1.73 m^2 and suggests status similar to oligo-anuria

- Evaluation of intravascular volume and cardiac output
- Additional blood tests (hepatitis and HIV serologies, complement [C3/C4] levels, ANA, ANCA, anti-GBM, SPEP/UPEP)
- Renal vascular studies (radioisotope scan, MRA, radiocontrast angiography if renovascular occlusion is suspected)
- Gallium scan: positive with strong uptake in AIN, negative in ATN
- Therapeutic trials as indicated: volume expansion, vasopressors (SCr should improve within 24–72 hr with improved renal perfusion in prerenal azotemia, but does not in ATN), relief of ureteral obstruction
- Consider furosemide stress test to evaluate dialysis risk and overall prognosis (administer intravenously 1 mg/kg [loop diuretic naïve] or 1.5 mg/kg [loop diuretic exposed]; UO <200 mL over 2 hr[12,13] or <600 mL over 6 hr suggests higher risk)[14]

- Kidney biopsy
- Empiric therapy for suspected disease to evaluate response

AIN, Acute interstitial nephritis; *ANA,* antinuclear antibody; *ANCA,* antoneutrophil cytoplasmic antibodies; *anti-GBM,* antiglomeruler basement antibody; *ATN,* acute tubular necrosis; *CBC,* complete blood count; *HUS/TTP,* hemolytic uremic syndrome/thrombotic thrombocytopenic purpura; *MRA,* magnetic resonance angiography; *SCr,* serum creatinine; *SPEP/UPEP,* serum and urine protein electrophoresis; *UO,* urine output.

7.5.3 DIAGNOSTIC ALGORITHM FOR AKI

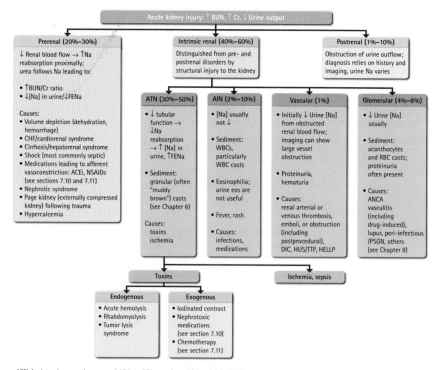

ACEi, Angiotensin converting enzyme inhibitor; *AIN,* acute interstitial nephritis; *ANCA,* antineutrophil cytoplasmic antibody; *ATN,* acute tubular necrosis; *DIC,* disseminated intravascular coagulation; *FENa,* fractional excretion of sodium; *HELLP,* Hemolysis, Elevated Liver enzymes and Low Platelets syndrome; *HUS/TTP,* hemolytic uremic syndrome/thrombotic thrombocytopenic purpura; *[Na],* sodium concentration; *NSAID,* nonsteroidal antiinflammatory drug; *PSGN,* post-streptococcal glomerulonephritis.

7.6 Urinary Indices in AKI

Urinary indices and other signs to differentiate between prerenal azotemia and acute tubular necrosis (ATN) can be diagnostically useful in distinguishing possible causes of AKI (see below). Conceptually, these indices are ways to evaluate whether renal tubular function is intact or compromised: Are the kidneys appropriately able to hold on to Na? Can they concentrate the urine in response to hypovolemia? Does urea follow Na reabsorption appropriately in the proximal tubule?

Lab Test	Prerenal Azotemia	ATN
Urine to plasma Cr ratio	>40	<20
BUN/Cr ratio	>20	<10–12
Urea nitrogen/BUN	>8	<3
UNa (mEq/L)	<20	>40
FENa (%)	<1	>2
FE urea (%); useful when on loop diuretics that alter Na handling	<35	>50
Urinalysis (see Chapter 6)	Hyaline casts or negative sediment	Abnormal: muddy brown granular and epithelial cell casts, free epithelial cells
Specific gravity	>1.020	<1.010–1.015
Uosm (mOsm/kg H_2O)	>500	<350–450

ATN, Acute tubular necrosis; BUN, blood urea nitrogen; Cr, creatinine; FENa, fractional excretion of sodium; mOsm, milliosmoles; UNa, urine sodium concentration; Uosm, urine osmolality.

The above criteria of prerenal disease may not be present in patients with underlying CKD since the tubular function may be impaired at baseline.

7.6.1 FRACTIONAL EXCRETION OF SODIUM (FENa)

FENa is probably the urinary index most commonly used in the workup of AKI.

$$FENa = \frac{Na^+excreted}{Na^+filtered} = \frac{\left(U_{Na} \times S_{Cr} \times 100\right)}{\left(S_{Na} \times U_{Cr}\right)}$$

However, certain conditions can create altered handling of Na in the kidney, diminishing its utility as an assessment of volumetric stress or ↓ renal blood flow.

When FENa Might not Be Helpful	
↑ FENa in Prerenal ARF or Other Non-ATN Azotemia	↓ FENa in ATN or Other Nonprerenal Azotemia
• Diuretics • Osmotic agents: mannitol, glucose, urea, post-radiocontrast • Adrenal insufficiency • Underlying chronic renal insufficiency • Underlying interstitial disease • Acute volume expansion with ↑ Na excretion • Obstructive uropathy	• Early in ATN secondary to sepsis or ischemia ("intermediate" syndrome with features of both ATN and prerenal failure) • Radiocontrast • Hemolysis, rhabdomyolysis • AIN • Acute GN, vasculitis • Renal artery occlusion

AIN, Acute interstitial nephritis; ARF, acute renal failure; ATN, acute tubular necrosis; GN, glomerulonephritis.

7.6.2 BUN/CREATININE RATIO

Another index is the serum BUN/Cr ratio. A normal value for the BUN/Cr ratio is between 10 and 20. However, certain conditions may alter the metabolic production of urea or its handling in the kidneys:

Disproportional BUN/Cr Ratio

↑ BUN/Cr	↓ BUN/Cr
• Prerenal failure	• Hepatic insufficiency
• GI bleeding	• Rhabdomyolysis
• Catabolic states	• Malnutrition
• Antianabolic agents	
• Postrenal obstruction	
• ↓ Cr with ↓ muscle mass in elderly or paralyzed patient	
• Steroids and tetracycline	

BUN, Blood urea nitrogen; *Cr*, creatinine; *GI*, gastrointestinal.

7.7 Red Flags

While most cases of AKI are due to either prerenal conditions or ATN, one should be able to identify "red flags" for other potential etiologies of AKI. In addition, do not miss urinary obstruction—kidney ultrasound (US) should be done in most AKI cases.

Signs and Symptoms	Potential Etiology
Proteinuria and hematuria	Glomerulonephritis, vascular causes
Heavy proteinuria (>3 g/day)	Glomerulonephritis, renal vein thrombosis
Thrombocytopenia	HUS/TTP, HELLP, DIC
Lung infiltrates/nodules, hemoptysis	Pulmonary renal syndromes
Purpura (palpable purpura)	HSP, vasculitis, cryoglobulinemia
Nonpurpuric skin rash	AIN, SLE
Very high blood pressure	Scleroderma crisis, malignant hypertension
Joint pain	SLE, rheumatoid arthritis, HSP

AIN, Acute interstitial nephritis; *DIC*, disseminated intravascular coagulation; *HELLP*, Hemolysis, Elevated Liver enzymes and Low Platelets syndrome; *HSP*, Henoch-Schönlein purpura; *HUS/TTP*, hemolytic uremic syndrome and thrombotic thrombocytopenic purpura; *SLE*, systemic lupus erythematosus.

7.8 Prerenal AKI

Prerenal AKI encompasses a spectrum of conditions that share a common feature: the decline in glomerular filtration rate (GFR) observed in these conditions arises not due to any structural injury to the kidney itself, but to compromise in glomerular blood flow. Prerenal AKI can progress to ATN if prolonged blood flow compromise leads to ischemia.

The most common cause of prerenal AKI is hypovolemia, and administration of isotonic fluids or blood transfusion when history, exam, and laboratory findings are suggestive of hypovolemia or blood loss is both diagnostic and therapeutic. Medications are also a frequent cause and are discussed further in section 7.10 and 7.11. There are two other important variations on prerenal AKI that merit further discussion, since their management is quite different. We discuss these variations in the following subsections:

7.8.1 HEPATORENAL SYNDROME

Patients with portal HTN from cirrhosis or fulminant liver failure are at risk for developing hepatorenal syndrome (HRS), a rise in SCr without an alternative cause.

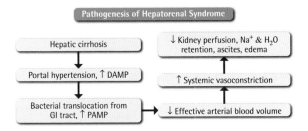

DAMP, danger-associated (or damage-associated) molecular pattern (endogenous molecules released from damaged cells); GI, gastrointestinal; PAMP, pathogen-associated molecular pattern

Adapted from Angeli P, Garcia-Tsao G, Nadim MK, Parikh CR. News in pathophysiology, definition and classification of hepatorenal syndrome: a step beyond the International Club of Ascites (ICA) consensus document. *J Hepatol.* 2019;71(4):811–822. doi:10.1016/j.jhep.2019.07.002.

7.8.1.1 Diagnosis of HRS[15]

HRS was reclassified in 2015 into HRS-AKI and HRS–non-AKI, which in turn is subdivided into HRS-AKD (acute kidney disease) and HRS-CKD. HRS–non-AKI will not be discussed at length here, but entails chronic GFR reduction for <3 months (AKD) or >3 months (CKD) in the absence of other causes.

Features of HRS-AKI	↑ SCr ≥0.3 mg/dL in 48 hr; UO ≤0.5 mL/kg for ≥6 hr *or* ↑ SCr ≥50% No response to 2-day diuretic withdrawal and albumin 1 g/kg of body weight No nephrotoxins or alternative etiologies (shock)
Urinalysis	Bland sediment with no or minimal proteinuria
Urine indices	FENa <1%; urine [Na] <20 mEq/L
Prognosis	Poor without liver transplant

FENa, Fractional excretion of sodium; SCr, serum creatinine; UO, urine output.

7.8.1.2 Management of HRS-AKI[15]

ICU	Non-ICU
Norepinephrine: raise MAP by 10 mmHg	Terlipressin; where terlipressin is not available, midodrine + octreotide
Albumin 25–50 g/d after 1g/kg body weight	
Stop beta-blockers and diuretics, avoid nephrotoxins	
Consider transjugular intrahepatic portosystemic shunt (TIPS) for refractory disease	
Liver transplant	

7.8.2 CARDIORENAL SYNDROME

Cardiorenal syndrome can be divided into five classes. Only Class 1 is a cause of AKI.[16]

Class	Features
1	AKI resulting from acute decompensation of CHF
2	Chronic heart disease leads to CKD
3	AKI leads to acute cardiac complications
4	CKD leads to chronic cardiac complications
5	A systemic disorder leads to both heart and kidney disease

AKI, Acute kidney injury; *CHF*, congestive heart failure; *CKD*, chronic kidney disease.

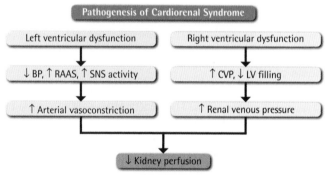

BP, blood pressure; *CVP*, central venous pressure; *LV*, left ventricular; *RAAS*, renal angiotensin aldosterone system; *SNS*, systemic nervous system

7.8.2.1 Diagnosis of Cardiorenal Syndrome

History	↑ SCr in the presence of decompensated CHF; ↑ weight; ↑ diuretic resistance
Exam	Pulmonary and peripheral edema; ↑ JVP
Labs	Elevated BNP; ↑ BUN/Cr
Urine	↓FENa, ↓ urine [Na]; hyaline casts
Imaging	Echocardiogram: ↑ filling pressures; CXR: pulmonary edema

BNP, B-type natriuretic peptide; *BUN*, blood urea nitrogen; *CHF*, congestive heart failure; *Cr*, creatinine; *CXR*, chest X-ray; *JVP*, jugular venous pressure.

7.8.2.2 Management of Cardiorenal Syndrome

Loop diuretics are first-line therapy and may be associated with improved mortality but do not consistently produce improvement in SCr in cardiorenal syndrome.[17] Loop diuretics can be augmented with thiazide-like diuretics if inadequate diuretic response is observed. Inotropes can be beneficial in cardiogenic shock but are otherwise not effective in treating cardiorenal syndrome. Ultrafiltration is not effective in treating AKI arising from cardiorenal syndrome, although it may become necessary when injury progresses to become completely refractory to diuretics.[18]

7.9 Acute Tubular Necrosis[19,20]

ATN is characterized by toxic or ischemic injury to kidney tubular cells, leading to cell damage or cell death. Decline in GFR is observed, not because of direct injury to the glomerulus, but because tubular injury decreases proximal tubular Na reabsorption, leading to increased Na and Cl delivery to the macula densa resulting in afferent arterial vasoconstriction via tubuloglomerular feedback. A decrease in renal blood flow accompanies these changes in AKI. Specific causes of ATN are discussed in this section.

Causes of ATN

Ischemic	Toxicity
• Sepsis, including COVID-19 • Hypovolemia (GI, renal or skin losses, bleeding), hypotension • Decreased renal plasma flow in edematous states (CHF, cirrhosis, hepatorenal syndrome, nephrotic syndrome) • Medications (ACEi, calcineurin inhibitors, NSAIDs, amphotericin, radiocontrast) • Renal vascular disease (renal artery thrombosis, stenosis, or embolization; atheroemboli, HUS, other forms of vasculitis or small vessel injury including transplant rejection, sickle cell anemia, preeclampsia, malignant HTN)	• Gentamicin, vancomycin, amphotericin, other drugs (see 7.10) • Chemotherapy agents (see 7.11) • Iodinated contrast (see 7.9.2) • Hemoglobin (hemolysis) • Myoglobin (rhabdomyolysis) • Other toxins (e.g., heavy metals, ethylene glycol)

ACEi, Angiotensin-converting enzyme inhibitors; *CHF,* congestive heart failure; *GI,* gastrointestinal; *HTN,* hypertension; *HUS,* hemolytic uremic syndrome; *NSAIDs,* nonsteroidal antiinflammatory drugs.

7.9.1 ISCHEMIA/SEPSIS-ASSOCIATED ATN

Ischemia/sepsis-associated ATN is the most common variety of ATN among hospitalized patients, particularly the critically ill. Injury arises from inadequate perfusion of renal tubular epithelial cells, leading to ischemia and cell death. Diagnosis is typically made by history and physical examination (Hx & Px) and microscopic examination of urine:

History/exam	Hypotension (including intraoperative); tachycardia (including arrhythmia); decreased urine output; pressor requirement
Urine	↑ FENa, ↑ urine [Na]; granular/muddy brown casts
Prognosis	Dependent on degree of injury; may recover in 3–5 days to 2–3 weeks, or can lead to long-term dialysis

There is no specific management other than maintenance of renal perfusion, avoidance of additional insults, and provision of dialysis should it become indicated (see 7.16).

7.9.2 RADIOCONTRAST-ASSOCIATED/INDUCED AKI

Contrast-associated AKI (CA-AKI) is AKI by KDIGO guidelines occurring within 48 hours of intravenous radiocontrast administration. If there are no other clear precipitating factors, AKI can be considered contrast-induced AKI (CI-AKI).[21]

7.9.2.1 Incidence of CI-AKI[21]

The overall risk of CA-AKI, which may or may not be caused by the contrast administration, appears to be related to the underlying pre-contrast kidney function whereas the incidence of

CI-AKI likely depends upon more severely decreased GFR and multiple other factors (see Table below).[21]

GFR (mL/min/1.73 m²)	CA-AKI	CI-AKI
>60	5%	0%
45–59	10%	0%
30–44	15%	0%–2%
<30	30%	0%–17%

7.9.2.2 Pathophysiology of CI-AKI[22]

- Hyperosmolarity and increased viscosity of the radiocontrast agent lead to compromised renal blood flow and other hemodynamic changes, which results in medullary ischemia.
- Oxidative stress and direct cellular toxicity lead to:
  - Endothelial cell dysfunction → Alterations in the metabolism of nitric oxide (NO), thromboxane A2, endothelin, angiotensin II, and prostaglandins → compromised renal hemodynamics
  - Tubular epithelial cell toxicity → compromised tubular function, increased tubuloglomerular feedback → compromised renal hemodynamics with decreased GFR

7.9.2.3 Diagnosis of CA/CI-AKI

History	Contrast exposure 24–48 hours prior to initial rise in SCr in an individual with appropriate risk factors (see below)
Urine	↑ Urine specific gravity (close to exposure); ↓ urine [Na]; granular casts
Imaging	Can see contrast stasis in renal cortex on subsequent CT
Prognosis	Usually resolves in 7–10 days

SCr, Serum creatinine.

7.9.2.4 Risk Factors for CA-AKI[21]

- Decreased GFR
- Concurrent exposure to other nephrotoxic agents
- Proteinuria
- Diabetes
- Intraarterial contrast[23]
- Impaired kidney perfusion
- Peripheral vascular disease
- CHF
- Shock
- Volume depletion
- Chronic liver disease

Decreased GFR is the major risk factor for CI-AKI.

7.9.2.5 Management of CA/CI—AKI

- Limit the dose of contrast.
- Use alternative imaging techniques whenever possible.

- Volume expansion with isotonic fluid. Optimal regimen is not known; typically, 1–3 mL/kg/hr are given for at least 1 hour before and 3 hours after contrast exposure, although a longer duration after exposure may be beneficial.[21]
- Use of iso-osmolar contrast compared to low-osmolar contrast has not been shown to reduce risk in a meaningful way though it is likely best to avoid hyper-osmolar contrast.

7.9.3 HEME PIGMENT-INDUCED AKI

Rhabdomyolysis and hemolysis can cause AKI due to toxicity from heme pigment released from myoglobin and hemoglobin, respectively. Heme pigment causes injury through a combination of tubular obstruction, tubular epithelial cell toxicity, and vasoconstriction.[24]

7.9.3.1 Diagnosis of Heme Pigment-Induced AKI

	Rhabdomyolysis	Hemolysis
History	Trauma; prolonged inability to get off floor; strenuous exercise (particularly with NSAIDs); illicit drug use; medications (see 7.10); viral and tick-borne infections; metabolic myopathies	Toxins; medications; infection, particularly malaria; G6PD deficiency; PNH
Exam	Muscle tenderness	
Labs	↑ CK (>20,000 IU/L), ↑ LDH, ↑ AST, ↑ ALT, ↑ K^+; ↓ Ca^{++} initially (often ↑ in recovery phase)	↓ Hemoglobin, ↓ haptoglobin, ↑ K^+, ↑ LDH; abnormal blood smear
Urine	Blood positive on dipstick but no RBCs on microscopy; pigmented granular casts; dark or tea-colored; FENa often ↓	
Prognosis	Most recover if underlying cause of pigment release is addressed	

CK (or CPK), creatine kinase (or creatine phosphokinase); NSAIDs, Nonsteroidal antiinflammatory drugs; PNH, paroxysmal nocturnal hemoglobinuria; RBCs, red blood cells.

7.9.3.2 Management of Heme Pigment-Induced AKI

- Address underlying cause.
- Aggressive fluid administration (as long as not contraindicated):
  - For rhabdomyolysis, can be >1 L/hr initially then 1 L/3-6hr; goal is to have CK decline to <5 k u/L, should check CK every 4 to 6 hours.
- Urine alkalinization in rhabdomyolysis with bicarbonate, as long as alkalemia and hypocalcemia are not present:
  - Goal urine pH >6.5
- Mannitol[25] and loop diuretics[26] are *not* effective.
- Treat hyperkalemia aggressively.
- Treat hypocalcemia judiciously, as hypercalcemia often occurs in the recovery phase.
- Consider allopurinol if uric acid levels are elevated as a complication of cell lysis.
- Dialysis may be implemented for complications of renal failure, but is not effective in removing heme pigment.[27]

7.10 AKI Induced by Medications[28,29]

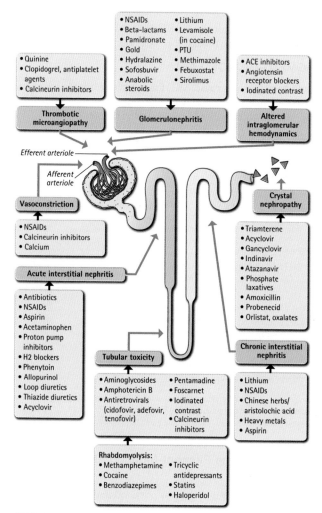

ACEi, Angiotensin-converting enzyme inhibitors; NSAIDs, nonsteroidal antiinflammatory drugs; PTU, propylthiouracil.

7.11 AKI Induced by Cancer/Chemotherapy[28,30,31]

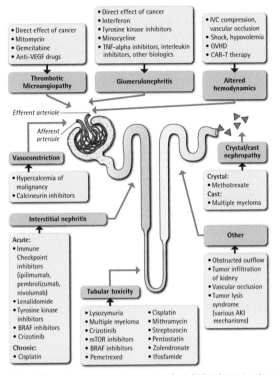

AKI, Acute kidney injury; CAR-T, chimeric antigen receptor T-cell; GVHD, graft versus host disease; IVC, inferior vena cava; mTOR, mammalian target of rapamycin.

7.12 Acute Kidney Injury Due to Glomerular Disease

(See Chapter 8 for further details of glomerular diseases)

Acute Glomerulonephritis Causing AKI	
Primary GN	**Secondary Disease**
• IgA nephropathy	• Poststreptococcal GN
• Membranoproliferative GN	• GN secondary to infection (e.g., endocarditis, HIV, shunt nephritis)
• Idiopathic crescentic GN	• Lupus nephritis
• Collapsing glomerulopathy	• Cryoglobulinemic GN
• C3 glomerulopathy	• Goodpasture's syndrome, anti-GBM GN
	• HSP
	• Vasculitis (e.g., granulomatosis with polyangiitis (formerly Wegener's granulomatosis), ANCA vasculitis, polyarteritis nodosa)

ANCA, anti-neutrophil cytoplasmic antibody; C3, complement component 3; IgA, immunoglobulin A; GBM, glomerular basement membrane; GN, glomerulonephritis; HSP, Henoch-Schönlein purpura.

7.12.1 PULMONARY-RENAL VASCULITIC SYNDROMES[32]

Pulmonary renal syndromes are a subset of diseases causing acute glomerulonephritis and diffuse alveolar hemorrhage. Many cases will be associated with characteristic antibody patterns, although these patterns do not have perfect positive or negative predictive value.

- Microscopic polyangiitis, often associated with perinuclear anti-neutrophil cytoplasmic antibodies/myeloperoxidase antibodies (p-ANCA/MPO antibodies)
- Granulomatosis with polyangiitis (formerly Wegener's granulomatosis), often associated with cytoplasmic anti-neutrophil cytoplasmic antibodies/proteinase 3 antibodies (c-ANCA/PR3 antibodies)
- Churg-Strauss syndrome (also called eosinophilic granulomatosis with polyangiitis), often associated with p-ANCA/MPO antibodies
- Systemic lupus erythematosus with lung involvement, which can be associated with anti-nuclear antibody (ANA), anti-smith, anti-double stranded DNA (anti-dsDNA), and low complement levels
- Goodpasture's syndrome, associated with an anti-GBM antibody
- Behcet's disease, evaluated with a skin pathergy test
- Rheumatoid vasculitis, often associated with ANA, ANCA, and low complement levels

7.13 Acute Interstitial Nephritis[33]

(Also see Chapter 9)

7.13.1 CAUSES OF AIN

- Infection
  - Bacterial (*Corynebacterium diphtheriae*, *Legionella*, *staphylococci*, *streptococci*, *yersinia*)
  - Viral (cytomegalovirus [CMV], Epstein-Barr virus [EBV], hantavirus, HIV, herpes viruses, hepatitis viruses, mumps, BK polyomavirus, SARS-CoV-2 virus [severe acute respiratory syndrome coronavirus 2])[34]
  - Other (Leptospira, mycobacterium, mycoplasma, rickettsia, syphilis, toxoplasmosis)
- Immune diseases (systemic lupus erythematosus [SLE], sarcoid, Sjögren's syndrome, vasculitis, lymphoproliferative disorders, tubulointerstitial nephritis with uveitis syndrome)
- Acute rejection of kidney transplant
- Medications
  - Antivirals
  - Antibiotics (penicillin, cephalosporins other beta-lactam antibiotics, rifampin, ciprofloxacin)
  - Sulfa-based drugs (sulfamethaxozaole/trimethoprim, thiazides, furosemide)
  - Proton pump inhibitors
  - NSAIDs, 5-aminosalicylic acid (5-ASA), others

7.13.2 DIAGNOSIS OF AIN

- Fever, rash on physical exam
- Low level proteinuria (<2 g/day), WBCs in urinary sediment
- Eosinophilia
- Gallium scan positivity of kidneys
- Kidney biopsy

7.13.3 TREATMENT OF AIN

- Removing drug responsible for acute interstitial nephritis (AIN)
- Brief course of corticosteroids (see Chapter 9)

7.14 Postrenal AKI[35-37]

Obstructions throughout the urinary tract can result in AKI. An important element to remember is that, if an individual has normal baseline kidney function and two kidneys, unilateral obstruction *will not* result in AKI.

History	• May report noticing a decrease in UO or pain, but often asymptomatic • Increased risk with history of cancer, prior urinary tract obstruction or instrumentation, or solitary kidney
Urine	Urine indices can vary. Hematuria is often present.
Imaging	Diagnosis is typically made by imaging. Hydronephrosis is the characteristic findings, seen on US, CT, or MRI. A distended bladder is evidence of obstruction lower in the urinary tract (outlet obstruction, neurogenic bladder).
Prognosis	Can resolve as soon as obstruction is relieved. Persistence of injury tends to increase with severity and duration of obstruction

UO, Urine output; *US*, ultrasound.

7.14.1 CAUSES OF POSTRENAL AKI

Kidney calyces/pelvis	Stones/crystals, including drug crystals; tumors; sloughed papillae
Ureter	Stones/crystals; tumors; retroperitoneal fibrosis; blood clots; trauma; prior ureteral instrumentation/stents
Bladder	Tumors; blood clots; neurogenic bladder; posterior urethral valves
Urethra	Prostate enlargement; strictures; stones; urinary catheter dysfunction

7.14.2 MANAGEMENT OF POSTRENAL AKI

Management also varies by location and cause of obstruction. There are three common interventions used to relieve obstruction:

1. Bladder catheterization: Typically, the first-line intervention if the obstruction is at the level of the bladder or urethra; not effective with more proximal obstruction.
2. Percutaneous nephrostomy (PCN) tube placement: Often the most rapid and effective way to relieve an obstruction proximal to the bladder, at institutions where it is available. Can also be used when catheter or stent placement is not possible/desirable. Can include placement of a nephroureteral stent such as a percutaneous nephroureteral (PCNU) tube.
3. Ureteral stenting via cystoscopy: an alternative to PCN for obstruction proximal to the bladder.

Management of post-obstructive diuresis, if it occurs, with half-normal saline intravenous infusion, initially matching urine output and then decreasing progressively.

7.15 AKI Associated With COVID-19

AKI is one of the most frequent extrapulmonary manifestations of COVID-19, with some studies suggesting it arises in up to 50% of hospitalized patients.[38] AKI secondary to COVID-19 may occur through a variety of mechanisms, giving rise to various kidney manifestations as follows[38-40]:

- Prenal failure due to hemodynamic compromise
- Acute tubular necrosis secondary to ischemia (the most common intrinsic kidney lesion)
- Collapsing focal segmental glomerulosclerosis (particularly in African Americans with the high-risk APOL1 genotype)

- Thrombotic microangiopathy which rarely may even lead to kidney infarction
- Acute interstitial nephritis
- ANCA/Anti-GBM glomerulonephritis

The role of direct SARS-COV-2 viral tropism for the kidney in various forms of AKI remains uncertain.[38,39] Not surprisingly, older age, underlying CKD, diabetes, or cardiovascular disease are risk factors for COVID AKI, and AKI is associated with significantly increased mortality.[40-43] In addition, many patients do not recover normal kidney function after AKI[40-43], and a follow-up study of hospitalized COVID patients showed decreased kidney function at 6 months in 35%, even in some with unrecognized kidney involvement during hospitalization.[44] From 5% to 45% of COVID ICU patients required dialysis management, with continuous renal replacement therapy (continuous venovenous hemofiltration, CVVH) being used most commonly.[45]

7.16 General Management Considerations in AKI

7.16.1 TREATMENT OF AKI

- First look for reversible causative factors (e.g., infection, obstruction, nephrotoxins, circulatory failure, hypercalcemia, etc.).
- Provide supportive care with careful fluid balance to maintain euvolemia; for some causes of AKI, implement volume expansion to increase urine volume.
- Correct electrolyte and acid-base disorders.
- Pharmacological manipulations that do not address causative factors (i.e., pressors to maintain MAP >65 or dopamine) have limited effect. Loop diuretics may increase UO, but overall, most drug trials have been ineffective at improving AKI.
- Utilize phosphate binders for hyperphosphatemia ($CaCO_3$ if serum Ca^{++} is low; aluminum hydroxide or carbonate can be used for acute management without aluminum toxicity in short courses of <1 month).
- Provide renal replacement therapy (RRT) when indicated.

7.16.2 INDICATIONS FOR RRT IN AKI

- Symptoms or signs of a uremic syndrome (pericarditis, neuropathy, encephalopathy, seizures, coagulopathy, enteropathy with GI symptoms)
- Severe uncontrolled electrolyte abnormalities (e.g., hyperkalemia)
- Severe uncontrolled acid-base disorder (e.g., metabolic acidosis)
- Severe volume overload threatening to compromise respiratory function, or refractory hypervolemia
- Early initiation of dialysis in critically ill patients *is not* beneficial for survival[46]
- Probability of death is unchanged by intensive versus adequate renal replacement therapy[47]

7.16.3 POTENTIAL NEGATIVE EFFECT OF DIALYSIS IN AKI

- Decreased UO caused by removal of volume and urea by dialysis
- Repeated episodes of hypotension (less common with PD and continuous RRT; i.e., CVVH)
- Complement activation caused by dialyzer membranes (less severe with more biocompatible dialysis membranes)

7.16.4 NUTRITIONAL CONSIDERATIONS IN PATIENTS WITH AKI

- Energy requirements: 35 kcal/kg/day

- Protein requirements: 1.2 g protein/kg/day but >1.25 g/kg/day is not beneficial and will increase rate of BUN rise
- Other nutrients: ratio between glucose and lipids 70/30 to provide calories and minimize muscle protein catabolism
- Usually low Na, low K, low phosphate diet is desirable to control fluid retention, hyperkalemia and hyperphosphatemia
- Avoid catabolic agents that raise the BUN, if possible (e.g., corticosteroids, tetracycline)

7.17 Biomarkers of ATN

Numerous biomarkers that are potentially useful in the diagnosis of ATN have been proposed.[48] Use of these biomarkers largely remains limited to research, with only uncommon clinical application at present. The most commonly used biomarkers are summarized in the following table.

Biomarker	Function
Urine/serum neutrophil gelatinase-associated lipocalin (NGAL)	Growth differentiation factor; also participates in iron trafficking; upregulated in ischemic injury and released into urine
Urine kidney injury molecule-1 (KIM-1)	Membrane glycoprotein; shed into urine during acute Injury; production increases in response to injury
Urine/serum IL-18	Immunomodulation, inflammation; upregulated in ischemic injury and released into urine
Urine/serum cystatin C	Protein produced by nucleated cells, cysteine protease inhibitor; during injury, filtration and proximal tubule metabolism decrease with rise in serum level
Urine liver fatty-acid binding protein (L-FABP)	Fatty acid trafficking protein that translocates from cytosol to tubular lumen during ischemic injury
Plasma IL-6	Immunomodulation, inflammation; production increases and clearance decreases in association with AKI
Urine alpha glutathione S-transferase (GST)	Cytosolic enzymes released into the urine during kidney injury
Urine N-acetyl-beta-glucosaminidase (NAG)	Lysosomal enzyme (glucosidase) expressed in proximal tubules, released into the urine with renal damage

References

1. Kellum J A, Lameire N, Aspelin P, et al. Kidney Disease: Improving Global Outcomes (KDIGO) acute kidney injury work group. KDIGO clinical practice guideline for acute kidney injury. *Kidney Int Suppl.* 2012;2(1):1–138. doi:10.1038/kisup.2012.1.
2. Siew ED, Davenport A. The growth of acute kidney injury: a rising tide or just closer attention to detail? *Kidney Int.* 2015;87(1):46–61. doi:10.1038/ki.2014.293.
3. Coca SG, Peixoto AJ, Garg AX, Krumholz HM, Parikh CR. The prognostic importance of a small acute decrement in kidney function in hospitalized patients: a systematic review and meta-analysis. *Am J Kidney Dis.* 2007;50(5):712–720. doi:10.1053/j.ajkd.2007.07.018.
4. Hsu RK, McCulloch CE, Dudley RA, Lo LJ, Hsu CY. Temporal changes in incidence of dialysis-requiring AKI. *J Am Soc Nephrol.* 2013;24(1):37–42. doi:10.1681/ASN.2012080800.
5. Waikar SS, Curhan GC, Wald R, McCarthy EP, Chertow GM. Declining mortality in patients with acute renal failure, 1988 to 2002. *J Am Soc Nephrol.* 2006;17(4):1143–1150. doi:10.1681/ASN.2005091017.
6. Griffin BR, Liu KD, Teixeira JP. Critical Care Nephrology: Core Curriculum 2020. *Am J Kidney Dis.* 2020;75(3):435–452. doi:10.1053/j.ajkd.2019.10.010.

7. Bucaloiu ID, Kirchner HL, Norfolk ER, Hartle JE 2nd, Perkins RM. Increased risk of death and de novo chronic kidney disease following reversible acute kidney injury. *Kidney Int.* 2012;81(5):477–785. doi:10.1038/ki.2011.405.

8. Hsu C-Y, Chinchilli VM, Coca S, et al. Post-acute kidney injury proteinuria and subsequent kidney disease progression: the Assessment, Serial Evaluation, and Subsequent Sequelae in Acute Kidney Injury (ASSESS-AKI) Study. *JAMA Intern Med.* 2020;180(3):402–410. doi:10.1001/jamainternmed.2019.6390.

9. Wu V-C, Wu C-H, Huang T-M, et al. Long-term risk of coronary events after AKI. *J Am Soc Nephrol.* 2014;25(3):595–605. doi:10.1681/ASN.2013060610.

10. Hsu C-Y, Hsu RK, Yang J, Ordonez JD, Zheng S, Go AS. Elevated BP after AKI. *J Am Soc Nephrol.* 2016;27(3):914–923. doi:10.1681/ASN.2014111114.

11. Kellum JA, Sileanu FE, Murugan R, Lucko N, Shaw AD, Clermont G. Classifying AKI by urine output versus serum creatinine level. *J Am Soc Nephrol.* 2015;26(9):2231–2238. doi:10.1681/ASN.2014070724.

12. Chawla LS, Davison DL, Brasha-Mitchell E, et al. Development and standardization of a furosemide stress test to predict the severity of acute kidney injury. *Crit Care.* 2013;17(5):R207. doi:10.1186/cc13015.

13. Chen JJ, Chang CH, Huang YT, Kuo G. Furosemide stress test as a predictive marker of acute kidney injury progression or renal replacement therapy: a systemic review and meta-analysis. *Crit Care.* 2020;24(1):202. doi:10.1186/s13054-020-02912-8.

14. Sakhuja A, Bandak G, Barreto EF, et al. Role of loop diuretic challenge in stage 3 acute kidney injury. *Mayo Clin Proc.* 2019;94(8):1509–1515. doi:10.1016/j.mayocp.2019.01.040.

15. Angeli P, Garcia-Tsao G, Nadim MK, Parikh CR. News in pathophysiology, definition and classification of hepatorenal syndrome: a step beyond the International Club of Ascites (ICA) consensus document. *J Hepatol.* 2019;71(4):811–822. doi:10.1016/j.jhep.2019.07.002.

16. Ronco C, Haapio M, House AA, Anavekar N, Bellomo R. Cardiorenal syndrome. *J Am Coll Cardiol.* 2008;52(19):1527–1539. doi:10.1016/j.jacc.2008.07.051.

17. Testani JM, Chen J, McCauley BD, Kimmel SE, Shannon RP. Potential effects of aggressive decongestion during the treatment of decompensated heart failure on renal function and survival. *Circulation.* 2010;122(3):265–272. doi:10.1161/CIRCULATIONAHA.109.933275.

18. Bart BA, Goldsmith SR, Lee KL, et al. Ultrafiltration in decompensated heart failure with cardiorenal syndrome. *N Engl J Med.* 2012;367(24):2296–2304. doi:10.1056/NEJMoa1210357.

19. Rosen S, Stillman IE. Acute tubular necrosis is a syndrome of physiologic and pathologic dissociation. *J Am Soc Nephrol.* 2008;19(5):871–875. doi:10.1681/ASN.2007080913.

20. Maremonti F, Meyer C, Linkermann A. Mechanisms and Models of Kidney Tubular Necrosis and Nephron Loss. *J Am Soc Nephrol.* 2022;33(3):472–486. doi: 10.1681/ASN.2021101293.

21. Davenport MS, Perazella MA, Yee J, et al. Use of intravenous iodinated contrast media in patients with kidney disease: consensus statements from the American College of Radiology and the National Kidney Foundation. *Radiology.* 2020;294(3):660–668. doi:10.1148/radiol.2019192094.

22. Faucon AL, Bobrie G, Clément O. Nephrotoxicity of iodinated contrast media: from pathophysiology to prevention strategies. *Eur J Radiol.* 2019;116:231–241. doi:10.1016/j.ejrad.2019.03.008.

23. Andreucci M, Faga T, Serra R, De Sarro G, Michael A. Update on the renal toxicity of iodinated contrast drugs used in clinical medicine. *Drug Healthc Patient Saf.* 2017;9:25–37. doi:0.2147/DHPS.S122207.

24. Zager RA. Rhabdomyolysis and myohemoglobinuric acute renal failure. *Kidney Int.* 1996;49(2):314–326. doi:10.1038/ki.1996.48.

25. Zager RA. Combined mannitol and deferoxamine therapy for myohemoglobinuric renal injury and oxidant tubular stress. Mechanistic and therapeutic implications. *J Clin Invest.* 1992;90(3):711–719. doi:10.1172/JCI115942.

26. Sever MS, Vanholder R, Lameire N. Management of crush-related injuries after disasters. *N Engl J Med.* 2006;354(10):1052–1063. doi:10.1056/NEJMra054329.

27. Mikkelsen TS, Toft P. Prognostic value, kinetics and effect of CVVHDF on serum of the myoglobin and creatine kinase in critically ill patients with rhabdomyolysis. *Acta Anaesthesiol Scand.* 2005;49(6):859–864. doi:10.1111/j.1399-6576.2005.00577.x.

28. Izzedine H, Escudier B, Rouvier P, et al. Acute tubular necrosis associated with mTOR inhibitor therapy: a real entity biopsy-proven. *Ann Oncol.* 2013;24(9):2421–2425. doi:10.1093/annonc/mdt233.

29. Shahrbaf FG, Assadi F. Drug-induced renal disorders. *J Renal Inj Prev.* 2015;4(3):57–60. doi:0.12861/jrip.2015.12.

30. Shirali AC, Perazella MA. Tubulointerstitial injury associated with chemotherapeutic agents. *Adv Chronic Kidney Dis.* 2014;21(1):56–63. doi:10.1053/j.ackd.2013.06.010.

31. Rosner MH, Perazella MA. Acute kidney injury in patients with cancer. *N Engl J Med.* 2017;376(18): 1770–1781. doi:10.1056/NEJMra1613984.

32. McCabe C, Jones Q, Nikolopoulou A, Wathen C, Luqmani R. Pulmonary-renal syndromes: an update for respiratory physicians. *Respir Med.* 2011;105(10):1413–1421. doi:10.1016/j.rmed.2011.05.012.

33. Raghavan R, Eknoyan G. Acute interstitial nephritis - a reappraisal and update. *Clin Nephrol.* 2014; 82(3):149–162. doi:10.5414/cn108386.

34. Masset C, Le Turnier P, Bressollette-Bodin C, Renaudin K, Raffi F, Dantal J. Virus-Associated Nephropathies: A Narrative Review. *Int. J. Mol. Sci.* 2022;23(19):12014. https://doi.org/10.3390/ijms 231912014.

35. Rishor-Olney CR, Hinson MR. Obstructive Uropathy. In: *StatPearls* [Internet]. Treasure Island (FL): StatPearls Publishing; 2022.

36. Tseng TY, Stoller ML. Obstructive uropathy. *Clin Geriatr Med.* 2009;25(3):437–443. doi:10.1016/j.cger. 2009.06.003.

37. Yap E, Salifu M, Ahmad T, Sanusi A, Joseph A, Mallappallil M. Atypical Causes of Urinary Tract Obstruction. *Case Rep Nephrol.* 2019;2019:4903693. doi:10.1155/2019/4903693.

38. Bruchfeld A. The COVID-19 pandemic: consequences for nephrology. *Nat Rev Nephrol.* 2021;17(2): 81–82. doi:10.1038/s41581-020-00381-4.

39. Sharma P, Uppal NN, Wanchoo R, et al. COVID-19-Associated Kidney Injury: A Case Series of Kidney Biopsy Findings. *J Am Soc Nephrol.* 2020;31(9):1948–1958. doi:10.1681/ASN.2020050699.

40. Hirsch JS, Ng JH, Ross DW, Sharma P, Shah HH, Barnett RL, Hazzan AD, Fishbane S, Jhaveri KD; Northwell COVID-19 Research Consortium; Northwell Nephrology COVID-19 Research Consortium. Acute kidney injury in patients hospitalized with COVID-19. *Kidney Int.* 2020 Jul;98(1):209-218. doi: 10.1016/j.kint.2020.05.006.

41. Pei G, Zhang Z, Peng J, et al. Renal Involvement and Early Prognosis in Patients with COVID-19 Pneumonia. *J Am Soc Nephrol.* 2020;31(6):1157-1165. doi:10.1681/ASN.2020030276.

42. Cheng Y, Luo R, Wang K, et al. Kidney disease is associated with in-hospital death of patients with COVID-19. *Kidney Int.* 2020;97(5):829-838. doi:10.1016/j.kint.2020.03.005.

43. Tan BWL, Tan BWQ, Tan ALM, Schriver ER, et al. Long-term kidney function recovery and mortality after COVID-19-associated acute kidney injury: An international multi-centre observational cohort study. *EClinicalMedicine.* 2022;55:101724. doi:10.1016/j.eclinm.2022.101724.

44. Yende S, Parikh CR. Long COVID and kidney disease. Nat Rev Nephrol. 2021;17(12):792-793. doi:10. 1038/s41581-021-00487-3.

45. Gupta S, Coca SG, Chan L, et al. AKI Treated with Renal Replacement Therapy in Critically Ill Patients with COVID-19. *J Am Soc Nephrol.* 2021;32(1):161-176. doi:10.1681/ASN.2020060897.

46. Bagshaw SM, Wald R, Adhikari NKJ, et al. Timing of initiation of renal-replacement therapy in acute kidney injury. *N Engl J Med.* 2020;383(3):240–251. doi:10.1056/NEJMoa2000741.

47. Palevsky PM, Zhang JH, O'Connor TZ, et al. Intensity of renal support in critically ill patients with acute kidney injury. *N Engl J Med.* 2008;359(1):7–20. doi:10.1056/NEJMoa0802639.

48. Desanti De Oliveira B, Xu K, Shen TH, et al. Molecular nephrology: types of acute tubular injury. *Nat Rev Nephrol.* 2019;15(10):599–612. doi:10.1038/s41581-019-0184-x.

CHAPTER 8

Glomerular Diseases

Robert Stephen Brown ■ Alexander Goldfarb-Rumyantzev ■
Subhash Paudel ■ Stewart H. Lecker

8.1 Glomerular Disease Presentation[1-3]

Glomerular disease may present with a nephritic pattern (proliferative, inflammatory histology), a nephrotic pattern (nonproliferative or fibrotic/sclerotic histology), or both. The initial presentation is very helpful in establishing an initial differential diagnosis.

Nephrotic	Nephritic
• Proteinuria $\geq$ 3 g/24 hr/1.73 m² • Lipiduria (free fat, fatty casts, oval fat bodies) • Hypoalbuminemia • Hyperlipidemia • Edema is common • May be complicated by thrombosis, infection, atherosclerosis, malnutrition	• Active urinary sediment with RBCs, WBCs, casts • Proteinuria: minimal, moderate, or heavy • HTN is common • May have azotemia or oliguria • May have edema
Histology	
Nonproliferative (GBM or podocyte disease, sclerosing)	• Proliferative histology: mesangial, epithelial, or endothelial cell proliferation, focal or diffuse • Glomerular inflammation mediated by infiltrating inflammatory cells • May have crescents in Bowman's space with parietal epithelial cell proliferation and fibrosis • May have glomerular vasculitis or thrombotic microangiopathy • May have mesangial, subendothelial, subepithelial, or intramembranous immune deposits or anti-GBM antibody deposition
Differential diagnosis	
• Membranous nephropathy • Minimal change disease • FSGS • Membranoproliferative GN (e.g., hepatitis C, SLE) • Diabetic nephropathy • Amyloidosis	• Poststreptococcal (postinfectious) GN • IgA nephropathy • Membranoproliferative GN (e.g., hepatitis C, SLE) • Crescentic "rapidly progressive" GN (e.g., ANCA-positive pauci-immune GN, granulomatosis with polyangiitis [formerly Wegener's granulomatosis], anti-GBM antibody GN, or Goodpasture's syndrome)

Nephrotic	Nephritic
Less commonly:	• HUS/TTP
• IgA nephropathy	• Vasculitis (e.g., polyarteritis nodosa, cryoglobulinemia)
• Light chain deposition disease	• Hereditary nephritis (e.g., Alport syndrome)
• Fibrillary GN	
• Hereditary nephritis (Alport syndrome)	

ANCA, antineutrophilic cytoplasmic autoantibody; *FSGS*, focal segmental glomerulosclerosis; *GBM*, glomerular basement membrane; *GN*, glomerulonephritis; *HTN*, hypertension; *HUS/TTP*, hemolytic uremic syndrome/thrombotic thrombocytopenic purpura; *RBCs*, red blood cells; *SLE*, systemic lupus erythematosus; *WBCs*, white blood cells.

Initial tests

In patients with suspected glomerulonephritis (nephrotic or nephritic syndromes)
• Complement levels (C3, C4)
• ANA
• ANCA, if rapidly progressive GN or vasculitis is suspected
• Anti-GBM antibody (if rapidly progressive GN)
• Urine and plasma protein electrophoresis to assess source of proteinuria: UPEP (if > 60–70%, is albumin presume due to glomerular proteinuria; if mainly globulins with multiple "polyclonal" peaks presume due to tubular proteinuria; if single "monoclonal" globulin peak signifies prerenal "overflow" proteinuria due to monoclonal gammopathy)
• Renal ultrasound to evaluate kidney size: small kidneys (= chronicity), r/o PKD, obstructive or reflux nephropathy
More specific tests:
• Antistreptococcal antibodies
• Hepatitis B and C serology
• HIV antibody
• Cryoglobulins (must deliver warm blood to laboratory to avoid false-negative result)
• VDRL

ANA, Antinuclear antibody; *ANCA*, antineutrophilic cytoplasmic autoantibody; *GBM*, glomerular basement membrane; *GN*, glomerulonephritis; *PKD*, polycystic kidney disease; *UPEP*, urine protein electrophoresis; *VDRL*, Venereal Disease Research Laboratory.

8.1.1 SERUM COMPLEMENT COMPONENTS C3 AND C4[4]

C3 and C4 are useful initial tests to narrow the differential diagnosis of glomerular disease.

Decreased Serum Complement

• Poststreptococcal GN (complement returns to normal in 2–3 months)
• Periinfectious GN: subacute bacterial endocarditis, infected ventriculoatrial "shunt" nephritis
• Membranoproliferative GN (complement stays low)
• SLE
• Cryoglobulinemia (complement is often low)
• May be seen at times in HUS/TTP, rheumatoid vasculitis, and atheroembolic disease

Continued on following page

Normal Serum Complement

- Minimal change disease
- FSGS
- Membranous nephropathy
- IgA nephropathy, HSP (rarely low)
- Antiglomerular basement membrane disease
- Pauci-immune RPGN (ANCA positive or negative)
- Vasculitis: granulomatosis with polyangiitis (formerly Wegener's), polyarteritis nodosa
- Hereditary nephritis (including Alport syndrome)

ANCA, Antineutrophilic cytoplasmic autoantibody; *FSGS*, focal segmental glomerulosclerosis; *GN*, glomerulo-nephritis; *HSP*, Henoch-Schönlein purpura; *HUS/TTP*, hemolytic uremic syndrome/thrombotic thrombocyto-penic purpura; *RPGN*, rapidly progressive glomerulonephritis; *SLE*, systemic lupus erythematosus.

8.2 Nephrotic Syndrome

Minimal Change	Focal Segmental Glomerular Sclerosis	Membranous Glomerulopathy
Potential Causes		

• Idiopathic most common
• Secondary causes:
  • Drugs (e.g., NSAIDs, lithium, pamidronate)
  • Hodgkin's disease, non-Hodgkin's lymphoma, leukemias
  • Acute variant of IgA nephropathy
	• Idiopathic most common (particularly in Black patients who may have APOL1 high-risk genetic alleles)
	• Secondary causes:
	  • HIV nephropathy
	  • Heroin nephropathy
	  • Ureteral reflux nephropathy
	  • Sickle cell disease
	  • Malignancy (lymphomas)
	  • Transplant rejection
	  • Drugs (e.g., lithium, anabolic steroids, pamidronate, interferon, adriamycin)
	  • Secondary to other glomerulopa-thies (often without the nephrotic syndrome)
	  • Reduced renal mass and glomeru-lomegaly: hyperfiltration due to underlying renal injury or obesity
		• Idiopathic most common; it appears that the majority of idiopathic cases have autoanti-bodies, mainly IgG4, directed against the PLA2R in glomerular podocytes
		• Secondary causes:
		  • SLE
		  • Hepatitis B or C
		  • Malignancy (solid tumors, lymphomas)
		  • Sarcoidosis, rheumatoid arthri-tis, Sjögren syndrome
		  • Syphilis, malaria
		  • Drugs (e.g., penicillamine, gold, NSAIDs, clopidogrel)
		  • Sickle cell disease
		  • HIV

Pathology		
• LM: normal glomeruli, no inter-stitial disease • IF: no immune deposition • EM: diffuse efface-ment or fusion of visceral epithelial foot processes	• LM: focal segmental glomerular sclerosis, mesangial hypercellularity, endocapillary foam cells, tubulointer-stitial disease • IF: either no immune deposition or segmental deposits of IgM and C3 in the area of scarring • EM: effacement or fusion of visceral epithelial foot processes, usually less diffuse in secondary FSGS	• LM: diffusely thickened GBMs • IF: IgG and C3 in fine granular distribution along all GBMs • EM: subepithelial electron-dense deposits in all GBMs

---

EM, Electron microscopy; *FSGS*, focal segmental glomerulosclerosis; *GBMs*, glomerular basement mem-branes; *IF*, immunofluorescent microscopy; *LM*, light microscopy; *NSAIDs*, nonsteroidal antiinflammatory drugs; *PLA2R*, phospholipase A2 receptor; *SLE*, systemic lupus erythematosus.

General Principles of Nephrotic Syndrome Treatment

Treatment of Underlying Disease	Treatment of Complications	Treatment of Proteinuria
• Specific to the type of glomerular disease (see below)	• Edema: sodium restriction, diuretics • Hyperlipidemia: statins, fibrates • Hypercoagulability: heparin followed by warfarin in those with a documented thrombotic or embolic event as long as heavy proteinuria persists; direct oral anticoagulants, while less tested, have also been used[5]	• ACEi or ARB, aliskiren if intolerant to ACEi/ARB • Blood pressure control • Mineralocorticoid receptor antagonists (e.g., spirono-lactone)[6]

ACEi, Angiotensin converting enzyme inhibitor; *ARB*, angiotensin receptor blocker.

8.3 Nephritic Syndrome

Mesangial Proliferative or Focal Proliferative GN	Poststreptococcal GN
IgA nephropathy, HSP, IgM nephropathy (variant of minimal change disease) • IgA nephropathy or HSP may present concomitantly with upper respiratory tract or other infections	• >10 days after infection with group A β-hemolytic *Streptococcus*
Pathology	
• LM: mesangial cell proliferation • IF: glomerular IgA deposits, frequently with C3 and sometimes IgG or IgM deposits • EM: electron-dense deposits in the glomerular mesangium	• LM: enlarged hypercellular glomeruli, endothelial cell proliferation, polymorphs in glomeruli • IF: deposits of IgG, C3, sometimes IgM, and IgA in glomerular capillaries and mesangium • EM: scattered, large, electrodense subepithelial deposits and subendothelial deposits in glomerular capillaries
Membranoproliferative or mesangiocapillary GN	**Crescentic (rapidly progressive) GN**

• **Immune complex deposition:**
  • Hepatitis C (with or without cryoglobulins)
  • SLE
  • Infections (endocarditis, abscess, parasitic diseases)
  • Monoclonal gammopathy (myeloma, CLL, lymphomas)
• **Complement deposition:**
  • Dense deposit disease
  • Disordered complement conditions (C3 glomerulopathy)
• **No immune complex or complement deposition:**
  • Transplant nephropathy
  • Antiphospholipid syndrome
  • HUS/TTP
	• Type 1—anti-GBM antibodies (Goodpasture's syndrome): 20%
	• Type 2—immune complex deposition (SLE, crescentic IgA nephropathy, postinfectious GN, membranous, membranoproliferative GN, HSP): 30%–40%
	• Type 3—no immune deposition; e.g., pauci-immune (granulomatosis with polyangiitis [formerly Wegener's], microscopic polyarteritis, polyarteritis nodosa). 40%–50%

Continued on following page

Membranoproliferative or mesangiocapillary GN	Crescentic (rapidly progressive) GN
Pathology	

• MPGN has several histologies defined by either immune deposition or electron microscopy findings; see chart of MPGN Pathology in section below.	• **LM:** extensive crescent formation (extracapillary proliferation in Bowman's space of the glomeruli)
	• **IF:**
	  • Type 1—linear GBM localization of Ig
	  • Type 2—granular localization of glomerular immune complexes and complement
	  • Type 3—no or scanty glomerular immunoglobulin deposition

CLL, Chronic lymphocytic leukemia; *GBM*, glomerular basement membrane; *GN*, glomerulonephritis; *HSP*, Henoch-Schönlein purpura; *HUS/TTP*, hemolytic uremic syndrome/thrombotic thrombocytopenic purpura; *IF*, immunofluorescent microscopy; *LM*, light microscopy; *MPGN*, membranoproliferative glomerulonephritis; *SLE*, systemic lupus erythematosus.

8.4 IgA Nephropathy[7,8]

IgA nephropathy is the most common form of primary glomerulonephritis, with as many as 40% of patients progressing to end-stage kidney disease (ESKD). Predictors of a poor prognosis, dialysis, or death are as follows: HTN or impaired renal function at presentation, proteinuria ≥ 1 g/24 hr or nephrotic syndrome, older age, or severe pathological lesions such as crescents on biopsy. Blood pressure control and reduction of proteinuria reduce the risk of death or dialysis.

8.4.1 CONDITIONS ASSOCIATED WITH GLOMERULAR IgA DEPOSITS

- **Idiopathic IgA nephropathy is most common**
- **Henoch-Schönlein purpura (IgA vasculitis**
- **Gastrointestinal**
  - Hepatic cirrhosis
  - Celiac disease
  - Inflammatory bowel disease
- **Rheumatological**
  - Behcet's syndrome
  - Rheumatoid arthritis
  - Ankylosing spondylitis
  - Psoriatic arthritis
  - Reiter's syndrome
  - Relapsing polychondritis
- Neoplastic
  - Renal cell carcinoma
  - Non-Hodgkin's lymphoma
  - Bronchogenic carcinoma
  - Mesothelioma
- Infectious
  - Epstein-Barr virus
  - HIV
  - Osteomyelitis

- ■ Mycoplasma pneumoniae
- ■ Tuberculosis, leprosy, brucella
- ■ Dermatological
  - ■ Psoriasis
  - ■ Erythema nodosum
  - ■ Dermatitis herpetiformis
- ■ Ophthalmological
  - ■ Uveitis
  - ■ Scleritis
- ■ Miscellaneous
  - ■ Granulomatosis with polyangiitis (formerly Wegener's)
  - ■ Familial Mediterranean fever
  - ■ Myasthenia gravis
  - ■ Hemochromatosis
  - ■ Sarcoidosis

8.4.2 TREATMENT OF IgA[9–11]

Treatment of IgA Nephropathy or Henoch-Schönlein Purpura

Proteinuria 0.5–1 g/24 hr	Proteinuria >1 g/24 hr	Persistent Proteinuria >1 g/24 hr
• ACEi or ARB if proteinuria is >0.5–1 g/day • BP goal <130/80 if proteinuria is <1 g/day[12–14]	• BP goal <120 mmHg systolic BP if initial proteinuria >1 g/day (and for most CKD patients)[12–14]	• If proteinuria >1 g/day after 3–6 months of optimized supportive care, add 6 months of prednisone (e.g., 1 mg/kg/day for 2 months and then taper) if eGFR >50 mL/min, consider enrolling in a clinical trial or adding immunosuppressive medication

Other therapeutic options for IgA nephropathy or HSP

- • Crescentic IgA nephropathy: pulse corticosteroids/plasmapheresis/immunosuppressives (e.g., cyclophosphamide ± azathioprine)
- • High-dose IV immunoglobulin in severe IgA or HSP
- • Add a sodium/glucose cotransporter 2 (SGLT2) inhibitor[14a]
- • Tonsillectomy with or without pulse corticosteroids[15]
- • Add fish oil[14a]

ACEi, Angiotensin-converting-enzyme inhibitors; *ARB*, angiotensin II receptor blocker; *BP*, blood pressure; *CKD*, chronic kidney disease; *eGFR*, estimated glomerular filtration rate; *HSP*, Henoch-Schönlein purpura.

8.5 Membranous Nephropathy[16]

Membranous nephropathy is the most common form of nephrotic syndrome in adults. In one quarter of cases it is caused by an underlying disease (see chart of Nephrotic Syndrome above for causes). Approximately one-third of patients have a spontaneous remission, one-third remain stable, and one-third progress to ESKD.[17]

8.5.1 HISTOLOGICAL FEATURES THAT HELP TO DIFFERENTIATE PRIMARY (IDIOPATHIC) FROM SECONDARY MEMBRANOUS NEPHROPATHY

- Positive staining for IgG4 in primary nephropathy, while IgG1 and IgG3 may be found in SLE or IgG1 and IgG2 with malignancies.
- Increased staining for PLA2R in glomeruli correlates with antibodies to PLA2R consistent with primary membranous nephropathy.[18]
- Subepithelial and intramembranous deposits characterize primary nephropathy, while mesangial or subendothelial deposits or tubular immune staining may be found in secondary nephropathy. Treatment of membranous nephropathy is discussed below.[19–21]

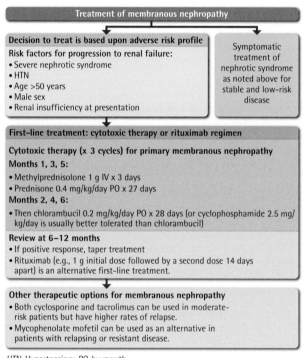

Treatment of membranous nephropathy

Decision to treat is based upon adverse risk profile

Risk factors for progression to renal failure:
- Severe nephrotic syndrome
- HTN
- Age >50 years
- Male sex
- Renal insufficiency at presentation

Symptomatic treatment of nephrotic syndrome as noted above for stable and low-risk disease

First-line treatment: cytotoxic therapy or rituximab regimen

Cytotoxic therapy (x 3 cycles) for primary membranous nephropathy
Months 1, 3, 5:
- Methylprednisolone 1 g IV x 3 days
- Prednisone 0.4 mg/kg/day PO x 27 days
Months 2, 4, 6:
- Then chlorambucil 0.2 mg/kg/day PO x 28 days (or cyclophosphamide 2.5 mg/kg/day is usually better tolerated than chlorambucil)

Review at 6–12 months
- If positive response, taper treatment
- Rituximab (e.g., 1 g initial dose followed by a second dose 14 days apart) is an alternative first-line treatment.

Other therapeutic options for membranous nephropathy
- Both cyclosporine and tacrolimus can be used in moderate-risk patients but have higher rates of relapse.
- Mycophenolate mofetil can be used as an alternative in patients with relapsing or resistant disease.

HTN, Hypertension; *PO*, by mouth.

8.6 Focal Segmental Glomerular Sclerosis[22–24]

Focal segmental glomerular sclerosis (FSGS) may present as a primary (idiopathic) disease or secondary to an underlying disorder with treatment dependent on managing the primary cause.[25]

Negative prognostic indicators:
- ↑ creatinine (Cr) at diagnosis (>1.3 mg/dL)
- Nephrotic range proteinuria
- HTN
- Interstitial fibrosis (≥20%) on biopsy

8.6.1 FEATURES DIFFERENTIATING PRIMARY FROM SECONDARY FSGS

Primary (Idiopathic)	Secondary
Presentation • Characterized by sudden onset, presence of edema, and hypoalbuminemia • High-risk APOL1 genotype is present in 75% of Black patients with FSGS[26,27] **Histological forms** • Cellular, collapsing glomerulopathy, or glomerular tip lesion • Podocytes are uniformly effaced **Treatment** • See below	**Causes** • See chart of *Nephrotic Syndrome* above for causes **Presentation** • Slow onset • Absence of edema and hypoalbuminemia **Histology** • Enlarged glomeruli • Heterogenous effacement of podocytes **Treatment** • ACEi or ARB • BP control • Treatment of underlying cause (e.g., HAART Rx for HIV, weight loss for morbid obesity)

Treatment of primary FSGS

Corticosteroid therapy

- Prednisone 0.5–2 mg/kg/day (remission associated with ≥60 mg/day for 3 months). If positive response ⇒ ↓ to 0.5 mg/kg/day and treat for another 1.5–2 months, then taper over 1–1.5 months. In the elderly (>60 years), 1.0–1.6 mg/kg (up to 100 mg) every other day for 3–5 months.
- Treat for 6 months before defining as steroid resistant.

Mild or moderate disease (proteinuria 0.5–2.0 g/24 hr, stable Cr):

- ACEi or ARB
- BP control
- Sodium restriction and diuretics, if needed
- CVD risk factor management (e.g., statins)

Steroid-resistant cases

- Cyclosporine 5–10 mg/kg/day (to maintain whole blood trough level of 100–200 ng/mL) for 6 months, then reduce by 25% every 2 months for a total of 12 months. Relapses after stopping or reducing the dose are common.
- Cytotoxic therapy (cyclophosphamide, azathioprine, chlorambucil): inconclusive evidence.

Relapse

- If relapse after prolonged remission, repeat a course of steroids
- Frequent relapsers/steroid dependent: steroids (1 mg/kg/day up to 80 mg/day for up to 1 month, then taper over 1 month) + cyclosporine (5–6 mg/kg/day) or cytotoxics (limited to 3-month course)

Other therapeutic options for FSGS

- Calcineurin inhibitors (cyclosporine, tacrolimus) or cytotoxic therapy as above instead of steroids
- Mycophenolate mofetil
- Sirolimus
- Plasmapheresis or protein adsorption for kidney transplant patients with recurrent FSGS

ACEi, Angiotensin-converting-enzyme inhibitors; *ARB*, angiotensin II receptor blocker; *BP*, blood pressure; *CVD*, cardiovascular disease; *FSGS*, focal segmental glomerulosclerosis; *HAART*, highly active antiretroviral therapy.

8.7 Minimal Change Disease[28]

Minimal change disease (MCD) is the most common cause of nephrotic syndrome in children, but is less common in adults (10%–15% of nephrotic syndrome cases). Similar to other nephrotic diseases, MCD can be idiopathic (primary), which is by far the more common, or it can be secondary to underlying disorders (e.g., associated with neoplastic diseases, toxic or allergic reactions to drugs, infections, autoimmune disorders). However, primary and secondary MCD present similarly, and the histological features of effacement of foot processes on electron microscopy, but no changes on light microscopy, are similar. In some cases, particularly in older patients, MCD can present with acute renal failure accompanying the nephrotic syndrome, with reversibility upon successful treatment.

8.7.1 TREATMENT OF MINIMAL CHANGE DISEASE

Treatment of Primary MCD

Corticosteroid therapy

- Prednisone 60 mg/m^2/day (up to 80 mg/day) for 4–6 weeks, or 120 mg/m^2 (up to 150 mg every other day)
- If positive response, taper dose: 40 mg/m^2/day every other day for 4–6 weeks until urine is protein-free, then taper off

Mild disease: Nonspecific treatment of nephrotic syndrome

- ACEi or ARB
- BP control
- Sodium restriction and diuretics, if needed
- CVD risk factor management (e.g., statins)

Relapse

- Prednisone 60 mg/m^2/day (up to 80 mg/day) until urine is protein free, then 40 mg/m^2 on alternate days for 4 weeks

Steroid-resistant cases

- If no response to initial treatment (60 mg/m^2/day for 4–6 weeks) or
- If frequent relapses occur or
- If steroid dependent
- Consider other therapeutic options below

Other therapeutic options for MCD

- Cyclophosphamide 2 mg/kg/day for 8 weeks
- In steroid resistant or dependent cases: cyclosporine 5 mg/kg/day (in children, 6 mg/kg/day) for 6–12 months
- In cases with frequent relapses:
  - Chlorambucil 0.15 mg/kg/day with tapering alternate-day prednisone for 8 weeks
  - Levamisole
  - Long-term alternate-day prednisone
  - Long-term cyclosporine at lowest maintenance dose
- Alternative/newer therapies:
  - Mycophenolate mofetil
  - Rituximab

ACEi, Angiotensin-converting-enzyme inhibitors; *ARB*, angiotensin II receptor blocker; *BP*, blood pressure; *CVD*, cardiovascular disease; *FSGS*, focal segmental glomerulosclerosis; *MCD*, minimal change disease.

8.8 Membranoproliferative Glomerulonephritis[29]

Patients with membranoproliferative glomerulonephritis (MPGN) may have a nephritic and/or nephrotic presentation. Primary MPGN is a group of disorders that have a similar histological pattern on light microscopy with hypercellularity and basement membrane thickening. Traditionally, MPGN has been classified based on electron microscopic pattern. However, recent understanding of the underlying mechanism has led to a change in classification from the former Type I, II, and III.[30] MPGN is classified as immune complex MPGN if Ig and/or C3 deposits are found on IF, and is classified as C3 glomerulopathy if it is predominantly complement staining.[29] C3 glomeru-lopathy is characterized by alternative complement pathway dysregulation resulting in complement C3 deposition in the glomerulus. It is further divided based on electron microscopic findings into C3 complement-mediated glomerulonephritis (C3GN) and dense deposit disease (DDD).

MPGN is caused by genetic mutations (e.g., CFHR5) or antibodies to the complement factors (e.g., C3 nephritic factor) or complement-regulating proteins (e.g., factor H and factor I).[30,31]

A form of MPGN without immune complexes or complement may be seen after endothelial injury and repair in patients with kidney transplant nephropathy, antiphospholipid syndrome, HUS/TTP, malignant hypertension, radiation nephritis, or bone marrow transplantation[30]

8.8.1 MPGN: PATHOPHYSIOLOGY

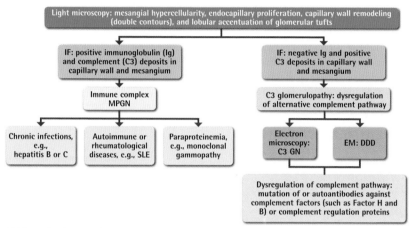

DDD, Dense deposit disease; EM, electron microscopy; GN, glomerulonephritis; IF, immunofluorescent microscopy; MPGN, membranoproliferative glomerulonephritis; SLE, systemic lupus erythematosus.

8.8.2 TREATMENT OF MPGN[11,29-31]

Immune complex GN (ICGN) from underlying disease	Treat the underlying disease, e.g., infection, autoimmune disease, or monoclonal gammopathy
Idiopathic ICGN with normal GFR and non-nephrotic range proteinuria	ACEi or ARB
Idiopathic ICGN with nephrotic syndrome	Limited time trial of prednisone 1 mg/kg/day (≤80 mg/day), tapering over 3 months Consider cyclosporine or tacrolimus trial, if steroid-resistant
Idiopathic ICGN with abnormal kidney function without crescents	Prednisone 1 mg/kg/day (≤80 mg/day), tapering over 3-6 months Alternatively, mycophenolate mofetil ± low-dose prednisone If response is inadequate, consider either oral cyclophosphamide 2mg/kg/day or intravenous rituximab 1 g twice 14 days apart
Idiopathic ICGN with crescents	Pulse IV methylprednisolone followed by oral prednisone and either cyclophosphamide or rituximab as described for Pauci-immune (commonly ANCA-positive) crescentic GN described in 8.10.2 below
C3 Glomerulopathy or Dense Deposit Disease	Initial therapy with oral prednisone plus MMF. If severe disease with inadequate response, consider a trial of intravenous eculizumab (off-label usage)

8.9 Poststreptococcal or Postinfectious GN[32,33]

Most cases of poststreptococcal glomerulonephritis (PSGN) have a relatively benign disease course or are at least reversible. The symptoms should resolve in a few weeks, and C3 should normalize in 6 to 8 weeks (kidney biopsy becomes indicated for persistent disease to rule out MPGN or SLE, etc.). However, some patients develop crescentic disease with a rapid decline in renal function, and rarely, patients develop CKD with persistent hematuria, proteinuria, and a decline in renal function.[34]

Staphylococcus-associated GN is an immune complex–mediated disease that is associated with an ongoing staphylococcus infection. Use of immunosuppression is usually not recommended.[35]

8.9.1 DIAGNOSTIC TESTS

Since the most common pathogen causing postinfectious glomerulonephritis (PIGN) is group A beta-hemolytic *Streptococcus* infection occurring >10 days previously, tests indicating the exposure are helpful in diagnosis:

- Anti-DNase B (antibodies to a product of group A *Strep*)
- Serum ASO (antibodies against streptolysin O)
- **Nonspecific tests to help diagnostically:**
- Serum complement levels: expect low C3 and C4
- Kidney biopsy: pathology as noted in *Nephritic Syndrome* chart (Section 8.2)

8.9.2 TREATMENT OF PIGN

Nonspecific Therapy	Immunosuppressive Therapy
• Blood pressure control • Treat fluid overload and edema (e.g., sodium restriction, diuretics) • Provide supportive treatment with temporary dialysis, if needed • Treat infection (if still present)	• Corticosteroids for crescentic disease

8.10 Crescentic GN[36,37]

Crescent formation indicates severe injury of the glomerular capillary wall with a fibrin leak into Bowman's space, parietal epithelial cell proliferation, and phagocyte migration, leading to crescent formation.

Clinically, crescentic GN usually presents with a rapid progression of acute or subacute renal failure (rapidly progressive GN). Many forms of glomerular disease may present with crescent formation, necrotizing glomerular lesions, and rapid progression (see below).

8.10.1 CRESCENTIC GN

Type 1	Type 2	Type 3
Caused by antibodies against the GBM: anti-GBM nephritis or Goodpasture's syndrome if lung hemorrhage is present (linear deposition along the GBM)	Caused by glomerular deposition of immune complexes, frequently RPGN superimposed on a primary glomerular disease: crescentic IgA nephropathy, HSP, MPGN, hepatitis B or C nephropathy, cryoglobulinemia, SLE, PSGN or PIGN, amyloidosis, multiple myeloma	Pauci-immune—no or scant immune complex deposition: ANCA-associated vasculitides, granulomatosis with polyangiitis (formerly Wegener's), microscopic polyarteritis, Churg-Strauss syndrome (also called eosinophilic granulomatosis with polyangiitis), medication associated (propylthiouracil, allopurinol, penicillamine, hydralazine, others), ANCA-negative RPGN, polyarteritis nodosa

ANCA, Antineutrophilic cytoplasmic autoantibody; *GBM*, glomerular basement membrane; *GN*, glomerulonephritis; *HSP*, Henoch-Schönlein purpura; *PIGN*, postinfectious glomerulonephritis; *PSGN*, poststreptococcal glomerulonephritis; *RPGN*, rapidly progressive glomerulonephritis; *SLE*, systemic lupus erythematosus.

8.10.2 TREATMENT OF CRESCENTIC GN

Anti-GBM Ab: linear IgG staining on IF

SCr <6 mg/dL (<~600 µmol/L), <85% crescents on biopsy
- TPE: daily 40-50 ml/kg plasma exchange for 7 days, then daily or alternate day for 7–14 days or until anti-GBM Ab titer is low or negative
- Pulse methylprednisolone + prednisone: methyprednisolone 500–1000 mg/day for 3 days, then prednisone 60 mg/day, tapered off by 6 months[4,38].
- Cyclophosphamide: for age <55 years, 3 mg/kg/day (down to nearest 50 mg) for 8–12 weeks; for age >55 years, 2 mg/kg/day for 8–12 weeks
- Prolonged Rx if anti-GBM Ab remains detectable

Anti-GBM Ab: linear staining on IF

SCr >6 mg/dL (>~600 µmol/L), dialysis-dependence or >85% crescents on biopsy
- Prognosis for renal recovery is ~5%, so risk–benefit assessment of aggressive Rx is warranted
- Supportive therapy including dialysis when needed may be best
- For pulmonary hemorrhage, TPE ± immune-suppressive Rx as described above

Immune complex deposition: granular localization

- Treatment based on specific glomerular disorder

Pauci-immune (commonly ANCA-positive)[39-41]

- Induction treatment for pauci-immune GN: combination of corticosteroid with cyclophosphamide or rituximab
- Pulse methylprednisolone 500–1000 mg/day for 3 days, then prednisone 1 mg/kg/day for 1 month, gradually tapered over 6–12 months
- Cyclophosphamide IV or PO can be used. IV dose 15 mg/kg every 2 weeks x 3 doses, and then every 3 weeks for 3–6 weeks. PO dose 2 mg/kg/day until stable remission (usually 3–6 months). There is less cumulative dose and leukopenia with IV than with oral route.
- Rituximab can be given instead of cyclophosphamide as 1 g IV at weeks 0 and 2 or 375 mg/m^2/week for 4 weeks.
- Cyclophosphamide may be preferable to rituximab in more severe disease with alveolar hemorrhage and severe renal disease.
- Role of TPE is unclear but is usually reserved for pulmonary hemorrhage.

GBM, Glomerular basement membrane; *GN*, glomerulonephritis; *IF*, immunofluorescent microscopy; *IV*, intravenous; *PO*, by mouth; *SCr*, serum creatinine; *TPE*, therapeutic plasma exchange.

References

1. Madaio MP, Harrington JT. The diagnosis of glomerular diseases. *Arch Intern Med.* 2001;161(1): 25–34. doi:10.1001/archinte.161.1.25.
2. Kodner C. Diagnosis and management of nephrotic syndrome in adults. *Am Fam Physician.* 2016; 93(6):479–485.
3. Floege J, Amann K. Primary glomerulonephritides. *Lancet.* 2016;387(10032):2036–2048. doi:10.1016/S0140-6736(16)00272-5.
4. Rovin BH, Adler SG, Barratt J, et al. Executive summary of the KDIGO 2021 guideline for the management of glomerular Diseases. *Kidney Int.* 2021;100(4):753–779. doi:10.1016/j.kint.2021.05.015.
5. Sexton DJ, de Freitas DG, Little MA, et al. Direct-acting oral anticoagulants as prophylaxis against thromboembolism in the nephrotic syndrome. *Kidney Int Reports.* 2018;3(4):784–793. doi:10.1016/j.ekir.2018.02.010.
6. Alexandrou ME, Papagianni A, Tsapas A, et al. Effects of mineralocorticoid receptor antagonists in proteinuric kidney disease: a systematic review and meta-analysis of randomized controlled trials. *J Hypertens.* 2019;37(12):2307–2324. doi:10.1097/HJH.0000000000002187.

7. Hassler JR. IgA nephropathy: a brief review. *Semin Diagn Pathol.* 2020;37(3):143–147. doi:10.1053/J. SEMDP.2020.03.001.
8. Lai KN. Pathogenesis of IgA nephropathy. *Nat Rev Nephrol.* 2012;8(5):275–283. doi:10.1038/nrneph.2012.58.
9. Wyatt RJ, Julian BA. Medical progress IgA nephropathy. *N Engl J Med.* 2013;368(25):2402–2416. doi:10.1056/NEJMra1206793.
10. Zhang YM, Zhang H. Update on treatment of immunoglobulin A nephropathy. *Nephrology (Carlton).* 2018;23(suppl 4):62–67. doi:10.1111/nep.13453.
11. KDIGO. *KDIGO Clinical Practice Guideline for Glomerulonephritis.* Vol 2, Issue 2, 2012. http://www.kidney-international.org. Accessed August 11, 2021.
12. Kidney Disease: Improving Global Outcomes (KDIGO) Blood Pressure Work Group. KDIGO 2021 clinical practice guideline for the management of blood pressure in chronic kidney disease. *Kidney Int.* 2021;99(3S):S1–S87. doi:10.1016/j.kint.2020.11.003.
13. Foti KE, Wang D, Chang AR, et al. Potential implications of the 2021 KDIGO blood pressure guideline for adults with chronic kidney disease in the United States. *Kidney Int.* 2021;99(3):686–695. doi:10.1016/J.KINT.2020.12.019.
14. Zhuo M, Yang D, Goldfarb-Rumyantzev A, Brown RS. The association of SBP with mortality in patients with stage 1–4 chronic kidney disease. *J Hypertens.* 2021;39(11):2250–2257. doi:10.1097/HJH.0000000000002927.
14a. Pattrapornpisut P, Avila-Casado C, Reich HN. IgA Nephropathy: Core Curriculum 2021. *Am J Kidney Dis.* 2021;78(3):429–441. doi:10.1053/j.ajkd.2021.01.024.
15. Nakagawa N, Kabara M, Matsuki M, et al. Retrospective comparison of the efficacy of tonsillectomy with and without steroid-pulse therapy in IgA nephropathy patients. *Intern Med.* 2012;51(11):1323–1328. doi:10.2169/INTERNALMEDICINE.51.7238.
16. Alsharhan L, Beck LH. Membranous nephropathy: core curriculum 2021. *Am J Kidney Dis.* 2021;77(3):440–453. doi:10.1053/J.AJKD.2020.10.009.
17. Couser WG. Primary membranous nephropathy. *Clin J Am Soc Nephrol.* 2017;12(6):983–997. doi:10.2215/CJN.11761116.
18. Beck LH, Bonegio RGB, Lambeau G, et al. M-type phospholipase A2 receptor as target antigen in idiopathic membranous nephropathy. *N Engl J Med.* 2009;361(1):11–21. doi:10.1056/nejmoa0810457.
19. Ruggenenti P, Fervenza FC, Remuzzi G. Treatment of membranous nephropathy: time for a paradigm shift. *Nat Rev Nephrol.* 2017;13(9):563–579. doi:10.1038/nrneph.2017.92.
20. Fervenza FC, Appel GB, Barbour SJ, et al. Rituximab or cyclosporine in the treatment of membranous nephropathy. *N Engl J Med.* 2019;381(1):36–46. doi:10.1056/nejmoa1814427.
21. Scolari F, Delbarba E, Santoro D, et al. Rituximab or cyclophosphamide in the treatment of membranous nephropathy: the RI-CYCLO Randomized Trial. *J Am Soc Nephrol.* 2021;32(4):972–982. doi:10.1681/ASN.2020071091.
22. Ahn W, Bomback AS. Approach to diagnosis and management of primary glomerular diseases due to podocytopathies in adults: core curriculum 2020. *Am J Kidney Dis.* 2020;75(6):955–964. doi:10.1053/j.ajkd.2019.12.019.
23. De Vriese AS, Sethi S, Nath KA, Glassock RJ, Fervenza FC. Differentiating primary, genetic, and secondary FSGS in adults: a clinicopathologic approach. *J Am Soc Nephrol.* 2018;29(3):759–774. doi:10.1681/ASN.2017090958.
24. Forster BM, Nee R, Little DJ, et al. Focal segmental glomerulosclerosis, risk factors for end stage kidney disease, and response to immunosuppression. *Kidney360.* 2021;2(1):105–113. doi:10.34067/kid.0006172020.
25. Rosenberg AZ, Kopp JB. Focal segmental glomerulosclerosis. *Clin J Am Soc Nephrol.* 2017;12(3):502–517. doi:10.2215/CJN.05960616.
26. Friedman DJ, Pollak MR. APOL1 nephropathy: from genetics to clinical applications. *Clin J Am Soc Nephrol.* 2021;16(2):294–303. doi:10.2215/CJN.15161219.
27. Genovese G, Tonna SJ, Knob AU, et al. A risk allele for focal segmental glomerulosclerosis in African Americans is located within a region containing APOL1 and MYH9. *Kidney Int.* 2010;78(7):698–704. doi:10.1038/ki.2010.251.
28. Vivarelli M, Massella L, Ruggiero B, Emma F. Minimal change disease. *Clin J Am Soc Nephrol.* 2017;12(2):332–345. doi:10.2215/CJN.05000516.

29. Rovin BH, Caster DJ, Cattran DC, et al. Management and treatment of glomerular diseases (part 2): conclusions from a Kidney Disease: Improving Global Outcomes (KDIGO) Controversies Conference. *Kidney Int.* 2019;95(2):281–295. doi:10.1016/j.kint.2018.11.008.
30. Sethi S, Fervenza FC. Membranoproliferative glomerulonephritis—a new look at an old entity. *N Engl J Med.* 2012;366(12):1119–1131. doi:10.1056/nejmra1108178.
31. Smith RJH, Appel GB, Blom AM, et al. C3 glomerulopathy—understanding a rare complement-driven renal disease. *Nat Rev Nephrol.* 2019;15(3):129–143. doi:10.1038/s41581-018-0107-2.
32. Rawla P, Padala SA, Ludhwani D. Poststreptococcal glomerulonephritis. In: *StatPearls [Internet]*. Treasure Island, FL: StatPearls Publishing; 2021. https://www.ncbi.nlm.nih.gov/books/NBK538255.
33. Noris M, Remuzzi G. Challenges in understanding acute postinfectious glomerulonephritis: are antifactor B autoantibodies the answer? *J Am Soc Nephrol.* 2020;31(4):670–672. doi:10.1681/ASN.2020020168.
34. Nast CC. Infection-related glomerulonephritis: changing demographics and outcomes. *Adv Chronic Kidney Dis.* 2012;19(2):68–75. doi:10.1053/j.ackd.2012.02.014.
35. Glassock RJ, Alvarado A, Prosek J, et al. Staphylococcus-related glomerulonephritis and poststreptococcal glomerulonephritis: why defining "post" is important in understanding and treating infection-related glomerulonephritis. *Am J Kidney Dis.* 2015;65(6):826–832. doi:10.1053/j.ajkd.2015.01.023.
36. Parmar MS, Bashir K. Crescentric glomerulonephritis. In: *StatPearls [Internet]*. Treasure Island, FL: StatPearls Publishing; 2021. https://www.ncbi.nlm.nih.gov/books/NBK430727.
37. Naik RH, Shawar SH. Rapidly progressive glomerulonephritis. In: *StatPearls [Internet]*. Treasure Island, FL: StatPearls Publishing; 2021. https://www.ncbi.nlm.nih.gov/books/NBK557430.
38. Benchimol C. Anti-glomerular basement membrane disease. In: Trachtman H, Herlitz L, Lerma E, Hogan J, eds. *Glomerulonephritis.* 2019;12:359–366. Springer, Cham. doi:10.1007/978-3-319-49379-4_19.
39. Kitching AR, Anders HJ, Basu N, et al. ANCA-associated vasculitis. *Nat Rev Dis Prim.* 2020;6(1)71. doi:10.1038/s41572-020-0204-y.
40. Stone JH, Merkel PA, Spiera R, et al. Rituximab versus cyclophosphamide for ANCA-associated vasculitis. *N Engl J Med.* 2010;363(3):221–232. doi:10.1056/NEJMoa0909905.
41. Huizinga T, Nigrovic P, Ruderman E, Schulze-Koops H. Rituximab versus cyclophosphamide in ANCA-associated renal vasculitis: commentary. *Int J Adv Rheumatol.* 2010;8(4):148–149.

CHAPTER 9

Various Kidney Diseases: Interstitial, Cystic, Obstructive, and Infectious Diseases

Robert Stephen Brown ■ Alexander Goldfarb-Rumyantzev ■
Parvathy Geetha ■ Stewart H. Lecker

9.1 Acute Interstitial Nephritis

The histopathology of acute interstitial nephritis (AIN) includes edema and infiltration of the renal interstitium with inflammatory cells (mononuclear cells, T lymphocytes, plasma cells, and eosinophils), while the glomeruli and blood vessels are usually spared. AIN can eventually lead to interstitial fibrosis (chronic interstitial nephritis).

9.1.1 CAUSES OF AIN

- **Drug Induced: 70% to 75%[1,2]**
  Not dose dependent, can recur/exacerbate with a second exposure to the same or a related drug[3]
  - Proton pump inhibitors
  - Nonsteroidal antiinflammatory drugs (NSAIDs); may be accompanied by nephrotic syndrome[4]
  - COX-2 inhibitors
  - Antibiotics (e.g., beta-lactams, rifampin, sulfa, ciprofloxacin)
  - Diuretics
  - Allopurinol
  - Mesalamine
  - Cimetidine
  - Immune checkpoint inhibitors[5]
- **Systemic Diseases**
  - Systemic lupus erythematosus (SLE)
  - Sarcoidosis
  - Sjögren's syndrome
  - IgG4-related disease
  - Tubulointerstitial nephritis with uveitis (TINU)
- **Infections**
  - Acute bacterial pyelonephritis (polymorphonuclear leukocytes predominate)
  - Leptospirosis
  - Legionella
  - Granuloma formation: mycobacterium, fungi, spirochetes, parasites
  - Streptococcus, beta-hemolysis (Councilman's nephritis)
  - Viral: cytomegalovirus, Epstein-Barr virus (EBV), BK (polyoma) virus, HIV

9.1.2 CLINICAL PRESENTATION OF AIN

- **"Full-blown" presentation:** Fever, rash, arthralgias, oliguria, renal insufficiency (acute kidney injury [AKI], acute renal failure [ARF]), but typically not all features are present.
- **Urinalysis:** White blood cells (WBCs), red blood cells (RBCs), WBC casts, eosinophiluria (rarely).
- **Proteinuria:** 0 to >1 g/day; nephrotic range proteinuria can be seen with NSAIDs due to concurrent minimal change disease (MCD).
- **Blood count:** Eosinophilia and anemia may be present.

9.1.3 DIAGNOSIS OF AIN

- Kidney biopsy is the gold standard: Interstitial edema and a marked interstitial infiltrate consisting primarily of T lymphocytes and monocytes.
- Positron emission test (PET) scan[6] or gallium-67 renal scan[7] uptake in AIN may distinguish it from acute tubular necrosis (ATN) when biopsy is undesirable or contraindicated.
- Response to discontinuation of the suspected offending agent and a therapeutic trial of corticosteroids over 1 to 2 weeks may be used to make a presumptive diagnosis.

9.1.4 TREATMENT OF AIN

- Treatment aimed at identifying and discontinuing specific offending agents above, if possible.
- Supportive care of ARF (manage volume status and electrolytes).
- If renal function does not improve within 3 to 7 days or if patient needs hemodialysis (HD), perform biopsy and start steroid therapy.[8]
- Prednisone 1 mg/kg/day. Start taper in 2 to 4 weeks based on response.[9]
- If AIN fails to respond to steroids or cannot tolerate steroids, can try mycophenolate mofetil (MMF) 1 to 2 g orally daily.[10]

9.2 Chronic Interstitial Nephritis

Chronic interstitial nephritis is a large and heterogeneous category of diseases leading primarily to interstitial fibrosis and tubular atrophy. Since progressive, sclerosing kidney diseases of all types are associated with eventual interstitial fibrosis and tubular atrophy, it is useful to define chronic interstitial nephritis as those conditions that cause interstitial and tubular damage initially while leaving glomeruli and vasculature intact.

9.2.1 CAUSES OF CHRONIC INTERSTITIAL NEPHRITIS[11,12]

- **Infection**
  - Pyelonephritis
  - HIV
  - Tuberculosis (TB)
  - EBV (Epstein Barr virus)
  - BK (polyoma) virus
- **Anatomic diseases**
  - Obstructive uropathy
  - Nephronophthisis (a renal ciliopathy)
  - Congenital disorders

- **Drug/chemical induced**
  - Lithium nephropathy
  - Analgesic nephropathy (>2–3 kg total intake)
  - Calcineurin inhibitors
  - Chemotherapy (cisplatin, ifosfamide, nitrosoureas)[13]
  - Cocaine and heroin
  - Lead, cadmium, mercury
  - Balkan nephropathy
  - Chinese herbal (aristolochic acid) nephropathy
  - Agricultural toxins ("Mesoamerican nephropathy")[14,15]
- **Immunological diseases[16]**
  - SLE
  - Sarcoidosis
  - Sjögren's syndrome
  - Rheumatoid arthritis
  - IgG4-associated AIN
  - TINU
- **Metabolic disorders**
  - Nephrocalcinosis
  - Oxalosis
  - Gouty nephropathy
  - Hypokalemic nephropathy
- **Other**
  - Consequence of unresolved AIN or ATN
  - Radiation nephritis
  - Myeloma kidney, lymphoma
  - Sickle cell disease
  - Mitochondrial cytopathies

9.3 Interstitial Fibrosis[17]

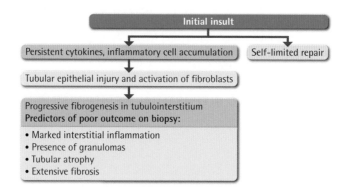

9.4 Role of NSAIDs in Kidney Disease

NSAIDs are probably one of the most commonly used medications as they are available over the counter. NSAIDs can affect the kidneys in several ways.[18]

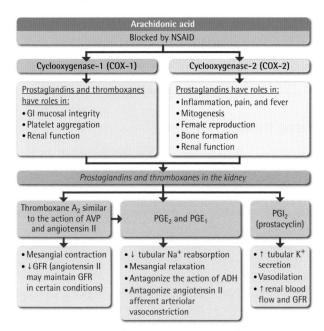

ADH, Antidiuretic hormone; GFR, glomerular filtration rate; GI, gastrointestinal; NSAID, nonsteroidal antiinflammatory drug.

Renal Effects of NSAIDs

Decreased PGE$_2$ Can Cause:	Decreased PGI$_2$ (prostacyclin) Can Cause:
• Sodium retention	• Hyperkalemia
• Peripheral edema	• ↓ Renal blood flow and GFR (may lead to ARF)
• ↑ BP	• Hyporeninemic hypoaldosteronism
• CHF (rarely)	

ARF, Acute renal failure; BP, blood pressure; CHF, congestive heart failure; GFR, glomerular filtration rate.

Renal Insufficiency Mechanisms of NSAIDs

Acute	Chronic
• AIN	• Nephrotic syndrome: MCD
• ATN	• Chronic tubulointerstitial disease
• Hemodynamic compromise	• Papillary necrosis

AIN, Acute interstitial nephritis; ATN, acute tubular necrosis; MCD, minimal change disease; NSAIDs, nonsteroidal antiinflammatory drugs.

9.5 PKD and Other Hereditary Cystic Kidney Diseases[19]

9.5.1 TYPES OF CYSTIC KIDNEY DISEASES

- Autosomal dominant polycystic kidney disease (ADPKD)
- Autosomal recessive polycystic kidney disease (ARPKD)

- Nephronophthisis: Medullary cystic kidney disease (MCKD) complex
- Bardet-Biedl syndrome
- Oral-facial-digital syndrome (OFDS)
- Miscellaneous hereditary polycystic kidney disease (PKD) syndromes:
    - ADPKD associated with tuberous sclerosis
    - ADPKD associated with von Hippel-Lindau disease

9.5.2 POLYCYSTIC KIDNEY DISEASE[20]

PKD is relatively common (1 in every 400–1000 live births, accounts for 5%–10% of ESKD). Most patients with PKD also have liver cysts, but only a fraction of patients develop massive polycystic liver disease.

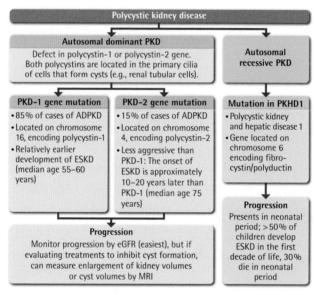

ADPKD, Autosomal dominant polycystic kidney disease; eGFR, estimated glomerular filtration rate; ESKD, end stage kidney disease; PKD, polycystic kidney disease.

Height adjusted kidney volume enlargement along with age helps predict future GFR decline[21]

9.5.2.1 Diagnosis of PKD

Family history, but no family history in 10%–25% of cases
Radiological (US, CT, MRI)[22]
US criteria (based on age) in at-risk (family history) patients:
- 15–39 years: Total of 3 cysts
- 40–59 years: At least 2 cysts in each kidney
- >60 years: 4 or more cysts in each kidney
In patients with no known family history, >10 cysts in each kidney or concomitant liver cysts suggest PKD.

Molecular[23]
- Genetic testing can identify only 70% of all PKD1 and PKD2 mutations.
- Genetic testing by Sanger sequencing of the PKD1 and PKD2 genes followed by multiplex-dependent probe amplification in cases with negative sequencing results.

PKD, Polycystic kidney disease; US, ultrasound.

9.5.2.2 Treatment of PKD

Treatments to Slow Progression of PKD	Potential Therapies
• HTN develops in most patients and is associated with progressive disease: ACEi or ARB drugs of choice for BP control, goal <110/75 mmHg • Dietary sodium restriction, <2 g/day • Increase fluid intake, >3 L/day	• V2 vasopressin receptor antagonist: Tolvaptan • Other potential agents such as mTOR inhibitors, somatostatin analogs, amiloride, and paclitaxel have not demonstrated clear benefits.

ACEi, Angiotensin-converting-enzyme inhibitor; *ARB*, angiotensin II receptor blocker; *BP*, blood pressure; *HTN*, hypertension; *mTOR*, mammalian target of rapamycin.

9.5.3 AUTOSOMAL DOMINANT TUBULOINTERSTITIAL KIDNEY DISEASE/MEDULLARY CYSTIC KIDNEY DISEASE[24,25]

- Suspected when both parent and child have CKD with absent/minimal proteinuria and bland sediment
- Autosomal dominant

ADTKD With UMOD Mutation/MCKD2	ADTKD Due to REN Mutation	ADTKD Due to MUC1 Mutation/MCKD1
• Mutation in gene encoding uromodulin/Tamm-Horsfall mucoprotein • Mutant uromodulin accumulating intracellularly in thick ascending limb leading to tubular cell death • Hyperuricemia from reduced urate excretion[26] • Diagnosis: Strong family history of CKD and gout; confirmation with genetic testing Kidney biopsy nondiagnostic, shows interstitial fibrosis • Treatment: Of gout and to prevent urate CKD progression	• Mutation in REN gene encoding renin • Low plasma renin levels leading to low BP, mild elevation in serum potassium • Progressive CKD, hyperuricemia, anemia • Diagnosis: Genetic testing • Treatment: Fludrocortisone, high-sodium diet, kidney transplantation	• Mutation in gene encoding mucin 1 • Progressive CKD • Hyperuricemia and gout are late manifestations • Renal cysts • Diagnosis: Genetic testing • Treatment: Prevention of gout and urate CKD progression, kidney transplantation

ADTKD, Autosomal dominant tubulointerstitial kidney disease; *BP*, blood pressure; *CKD*, chronic kidney disease.

9.6 Obstructive Uropathy[27,28]

OBSTRUCTIVE UROPATHY (OBSTRUCTION TO URINE FLOW) CAN CAUSE:

- Hydronephrosis (dilatation of the renal pelvis)
- Hydroureter(s)
- Bladder distention and dysfunction
- Nephropathy (renal damage from obstruction):
  - ARF: 5% to 10% caused by high-grade obstruction

- CKD: small percentage caused by long-lasting obstruction
- HTN
- Hyperkalemic distal renal tubular acidosis[29]

9.6.1.2 Causes of Obstructive Uropathy

- Upper urinary tract obstruction:
  - Congenital ureteropelvic junction obstruction or horseshoe kidney
  - Kidney stones, blood clots, or sloughed renal papillae
  - Transitional cell carcinoma obstructing the renal pelvis or ureter
  - Ureteral stricture: Secondary to inflammation, radiation, trauma, surgery, etc.[30]
  - Retroperitoneal malignancy
  - Retroperitoneal fibrosis
- Lower urinary tract obstruction:
  - Benign prostatic hypertrophy or prostate cancer
  - Bladder cancer obstructing the bladder neck or ureter(s): Bladder stones, blood clots, or fungal ball(s)
  - Neurogenic bladder
  - Urethral stricture or valves
  - Malpositioned Foley catheter
- Vesicoureteral reflux in children and young adults: Not a true obstructive uropathy, but high-grade reflux can cause hydronephrosis and reflux nephropathy, a leading to secondary focal segmental glomerulosclerosis (FSGS) manifested by proteinuria and CKD.[31]

9.6.2 DIAGNOSTIC TESTS TO EVALUATE OR RULE OUT OBSTRUCTIVE UROPATHY

- Bladder catheterization
- US (positive predictive value of 70% in patients with a clinical suspicion and negative predictive value of 98%)[32]
- Noncontrast CT if there is suspicion of stone or in patients with ADPKD where stone and hydronephrosis are difficult to differentiate by US
- MRI with/without gadolinium but poor visualization of stones
- Intravenous pyelography (IVP; requires radiocontrast)
- Retrograde or antegrade pyelography
- Radioisotope renography using Tc-99m DTPA (diethylenetriaminepentaacetic acid)
- For evaluation of suspected vesicoureteral reflux, voiding cystourethrogram, radionuclide cystogram, or contrast-enhanced voiding urosonography can be used

9.6.3 TREATMENT OF OBSTRUCTIVE UROPATHY

- For lower urinary tract obstruction: Bladder drainage (straight or Foley catheter or percutaneous suprapubic catheter placement)
- For upper urinary tract obstruction: Percutaneous nephrostomy or retrograde ureteral stent placement
- Eliminate the cause of obstruction, if possible (e.g., remove kidney stones or bladder stones)
- Treat urinary tract infection (UTI) if present

9.7 URINARY TRACT INFECTION[33,34]

Asymptomatic bacteriuria needs to be treated only in:
- Pregnant women,[35]
- Patients undergoing urological interventions, and
- Renal transplant recipients in the first few months after transplant.

9.7.1 TYPES AND TREATMENT OF UTI[36]

Uncomplicated UTI/Cystitis

• **Symptoms:** Dysuria, urinary urgency, frequency, lower abdominal pain • **Findings:** Hematuria or cloudy urine, positive leukocyte esterase and nitrites on dipstick, WBCs (>10/μL in women), and bacteria in sediment microscopy	• **Common Pathogens:** *Escherichia coli* (75%–95%) • Other gram-negatives such as klebsiella, proteus • *Staphylococcus saprophyticus* • Pseudomonas, Enterococcus, and Staphylococcus in healthcare exposure	• **Common Treatment Choices:** Nitrofurantoin 100 mg twice daily for 5 days • Trimethoprim/Sulfamethoxazole double-strength 160/800 mg twice daily for 3 days • Fosfomycin 3-g powder mixed in water as single dose • Beta-lactams (amoxicillin-clavulanate 500 mg twice daily/cefpodoxime 100 mg twice daily) for 5–7 days • Fluoroquinolone (ciprofloxacin 250 mg twice daily or levofloxacin 250 mg daily) for 3 days • In pregnancy: Cefpodoxime, amoxicillin-clavulanate, or fosfomycin; nitrofurantoin can be used in second and third trimesters • In elderly, prescribe for 3–7 days

Acute complicated UTI (Pyelonephritis)

Includes UTI that has extended beyond bladder (UTI with fever or systemic symptoms, pyelonephritis, sepsis, or bacteremia) • **Symptoms:** Fever, chills, flank pain, nausea/vomiting, CVA tenderness, pelvic or perineal pain in men which can suggest prostatitis • **Findings:** CVA tenderness, >100,000 organisms/mL on culture, imaging suggestive of pyelonephritis	• **Common Pathogens:** *E. coli* • Other Gram-negatives • *S. saprophyticus* • Enterococcus • Staphylococcus • Pseudomonas in healthcare patients or instrumentation • Candida species	• **Common Treatment Choices:** Fluoroquinolone for 7–10 days (ciprofloxacin 500 twice daily or levofloxacin 750 daily) If concern for fluroquinolone resistance/MDR, can use ceftriaxone/ertapenem/gentamicin single dose followed by Trimethoprim/Sulfamethoxazole/amoxicillin clavulanate[37] • Inpatient prescription: Ceftriaxone/piperacillin tazobactam/fluroquinolones Concern for MDR: Piperacillin tazobactam/carbapenems • Critically ill/urinary obstruction: Vancomycin + carbapenems • Treatment then guided by culture sensitivity for 7–10 days

CVA, Costovertebral angle; *MDR*, Multi-drug resistence; *UTI*, urinary tract infection; *WBCs*, white blood cells.

References

1. Moledina DG, Perazella MA. Drug-induced acute interstitial nephritis. *Clin J Am Soc Nephrol.* 2017;12(12):2046–2049. doi:10.2215/CJN.07630717.
2. Praga M, González E. Acute interstitial nephritis. *Kidney Int.* 2010;77(11):956–961. doi:10.1038/ki.2010.89.

114   9—VARIOUS KIDNEY DISEASES

3. Schubert C, Bates WD, Moosa MR. Acute tubulointerstitial nephritis related to antituberculous drug therapy. *Clin Nephrol.* 2010;73(6):413–419. doi:10.5414/cnp73413.

4. Bensman A. Non-steroidal anti-inflammatory drugs (NSAIDs) systemic use: the risk of renal failure. *Front Pediatr.* 2020;7:517. doi:10.3389/fped.2019.00517.

5. Draibe JB, García-Carro C, Martinez-Valenzuela L, et al. Acute tubulointerstitial nephritis induced by checkpoint inhibitors versus classical acute tubulointerstitial nephritis: are they the same disease? *Clin Kidney J.* 2020;14(3):884–890. doi:10.1093/ckj/sfaa027.

6. Krishnan N, Perazella MA. The role of PET scanning in the evaluation of patients with kidney disease. *Adv Chronic Kidney Dis.* 2017;24(3):154–161. doi:10.1053/j.ackd.2017.01.002.

7. Love C, Palestro CJ. Radionuclide imaging of inflammation and infection in the acute care setting. *Semin Nucl Med.* 2013;43(2):102–113. doi:10.1053/j.semnuclmed.2012.11.003.

8. González E, Gutiérrez E, Galeano C, et al. Early steroid treatment improves the recovery of renal function in patients with drug-induced acute interstitial nephritis. *Kidney Int.* 2008;73(8):940–946. doi:10.1038/sj.ki.5002776.

9. Fernandez-Juarez G, Perez JV, Caravaca-Fontán F, et al. Duration of treatment with corticosteroids and recovery of kidney function in acute interstitial nephritis. *Clin J Am Soc Nephrol.* 2018;13(12):1851–1858. doi:10.2215/CJN.01390118.

10. Preddie DC, Markowitz GS, Radhakrishnan J, et al. Mycophenolate mofetil for the treatment of interstitial nephritis. *Clin J Am Soc Nephrol.* 2006;1(4):718–722. doi:10.2215/CJN.01711105.

11. Gifford FJ, Gifford RM, Eddleston M, Dhaun N. Endemic nephropathy around the world. *Kidney Int Rep.* 2017;2(2):282–292. doi:10.1016/j.ekir.2016.11.003.

12. Schwarz A, Krause PH, Kunzendorf U, Keller F, Distler A. The outcome of acute interstitial nephritis: risk factors for the transition from acute to chronic interstitial nephritis. *Clin Nephrol.* 2000;54(3):179–190.

13. Shirali AC, Perazella MA. Tubulointerstitial injury associated with chemotherapeutic agents. *Adv Chronic Kidney Dis.* 2014;21(1):56–63. doi:10.1053/j.ackd.2013.06.010.

14. Orantes-Navarro CM, Herrera-Valdés R, Almaguer-López M, et al. Toward a comprehensive hypothesis of chronic interstitial nephritis in agricultural communities. *Adv Chronic Kidney Dis.* 2017;24(2):101–106. doi:10.1053/j.ackd.2017.01.001.

15. Vervaet BA, Nast CC, Jayasumana C, et al. Chronic interstitial nephritis in agricultural communities is a toxin-induced proximal tubular nephropathy. *Kidney Int.* 2020;97(2):350–369. doi:10.1016/j.kint.2019.11.009.

16. Oliva-Damaso N, Oliva-Damaso E, Payan J. Acute and chronic tubulointerstitial nephritis of rheumatic causes. *Rheum Dis Clin North Am.* 2018;44(4):619–633. doi:10.1016/j.rdc.2018.06.009.

17. Zeisberg M, Neilson EG. Mechanisms of tubulointerstitial fibrosis. *J Am Soc Nephrol.* 2010;21(11):1819–1834. doi:10.1681/ASN.2010080793.

18. Huerta C, Castellsague J, Varas-Lorenzo C, Rodríguez LAG. Nonsteroidal anti-inflammatory drugs and risk of ARF in the general population. *Am J Kidney Dis.* 2005;45(3):531–539. doi:10.1053/j.ajkd.2004.12.005.

19. Rohatgi R. Clinical manifestations of hereditary cystic kidney disease. *Front Biosci.* 2008;13:4175–4197. doi:10.2741/2999.

20. Chebib FT, Torres VE. Autosomal dominant polycystic kidney disease: core curriculum 2016. *Am J Kidney Dis.* 2016;67(5):792–810. doi:10.1053/j.ajkd.2015.07.037.

21. Schrier RW, Brosnahan G, Cadnapaphornchai MA, et al. Predictors of autosomal dominant polycystic kidney disease progression. *J Am Soc Nephrol.* 2014;25(11):2399–2418. doi:10.1681/ASN.2013111184.

22. Pei Y, Obaji J, Dupuis A, et al. Unified criteria for ultrasonographic diagnosis of ADPKD. *J Am Soc Nephrol.* 2009;20(1):205–212. doi:10.1681/ASN.2008050507.

23. Song X, Haghighi A, Iliuta I-A, Pei Y. Molecular diagnosis of autosomal dominant polycystic kidney disease. *Expert Rev Mol Diagn.* 2017;17(10):885–895. doi:10.1080/14737159.2017.1358088.

24. Eckardt K-U, Alper SL, Antignac C, et al. Outcomes, autosomal dominant tubulointerstitial kidney disease: diagnosis, classification, and management—a KDIGO consensus report. *Kidney Int.* 2015;88(4):676–683. doi:10.1038/ki.2015.28.

25. Yu SM-W, Bleyer AJ, Anis K, et al. Autosomal dominant tubulointerstitial kidney disease due to MUC1 mutation. *Am J Kidney Dis.* 2018;71(4):495–500. doi:10.1053/j.ajkd.2017.08.024.

26. Dahan K, Devuyst O, Smaers M, et al. A cluster of mutations in the UMOD gene causes familial juvenile hyperuricemic nephropathy with abnormal expression of uromodulin. *J Am Soc Nephrol.* 2003;14(11): 2883–2893. doi:10.1097/01.asn.0000092147.83480.b5.

27. Chávez-Íñiguez JS, Navarro-Gallardo GJ, Medina-González R, Alcantar-Vallin L, García-García G. Acute kidney injury caused by obstructive nephropathy. *Int J Nephrol.* 2020;2020:8846622. doi:10.1155/2020/8846622.

28. Tseng TY, Stoller ML. Obstructive uropathy. *Clin Geriatr Med.* 2009;25(3):437–443. doi:10.1016/j. cger.2009.06.003.

29. Batlle DC, Arruda JAL, Kurtzman NA. Hyperkalemic distal renal tubular acidosis associated with obstructive uropathy. *N Engl J Med.* 1981;304(7):373–380. doi:10.1056/NEJM198102123040701.

30. Washino S, Hosohata K, Miyagawa T. Roles played by biomarkers of kidney injury in patients with upper urinary tract obstruction. *Int J Mol Sci.* 2020;21(15):5490. doi:10.3390/ijms21155490.

31. Matsuo T, Kobayashi Y, Nemoto N, Sano T, Kamata K, Shigematsu H. A nephrotic case of vesicoureteral reflux representing focal segmental glomerulosclerosis associated with podocytic infolding lesions. *Clin Exp Nephrol.* 2008;12(6):494–500. doi:10.1007/s10157-008-0086-x.

32. Ellenbogen P, Scheible F, Talner L, Leopold G. Sensitivity of gray scale ultrasound in detecting urinary tract obstruction. *AJR Am J Roentgenol.* 1978;130(4):731–733. doi:10.2214/ajr.130.4.731.

33. Foxman B. Urinary tract infection syndromes occurrence, recurrence, bacteriology, risk factors, and disease burden. *Infect Dis Clin North Am.* 2014;28(1):1–13. doi:10.1016/j.idc.2013.09.003.

34. McLellan LK, Hunstad DA. Urinary tract infection: pathogenesis and outlook. *Trends Mol Med.* 2016;22(11):946–957. doi:10.1016/j.molmed.2016.09.003.

35. Nicolle LE, Gupta K, Bradley SF, et al. Clinical practice guideline for the management of asymptomatic bacteriuria: 2019 update by the Infectious Diseases Society of America. *Clin Infect Dis.* 2019;68(10): e83–e110. doi:10.1093/cid/ciy1121.

36. Kolman KB. Cystitis and pyelonephritis diagnosis, treatment, and prevention. *Prim Care.* 2019;46(2): 191–202. doi:10.1016/j.pop.2019.01.001.

37. Walker E, Lyman A, Gupta K, Mahoney MV, Snyder GM, Hirsch EB. Clinical management of an increasing threat: outpatient urinary tract infections due to multidrug-resistant uropathogens. *Clin Infect Dis.* 2016;63(7):960–965. doi:10.1093/cid/ciw396..

CHAPTER 10

Kidney Disorders in Other Diseases

Robert Stephen Brown ▦ Alexander Goldfarb-Rumyantzev ▦
Periklis Kyriazis ▦ Stewart H. Lecker

10.1 Diabetic Kidney Disease

Diabetic kidney disease (DKD) is a clinical diagnosis characterized by albuminuria, decreased estimated glomerular filtration rate (eGFR), or both in patients with diabetes, and is the leading cause of chronic kidney disease (CKD) and end-stage kidney disease (ESKD) in the United States and worldwide. Even though DKD is responsible for 30% to 50% of ESKD in the United States, only 20% to 40% of patients with diabetes develop DKD. In DKD, all-cause and cardiovascular mortality is 20 to 30 times higher compared to mortality in the general population. Increased albuminuria and low eGFR are independent risk factors for cardiovascular and renal events among patients with type 2 diabetes, emphasizing the importance of kidney disease as a predictor of clinical outcomes.[1–6]

10.1.1 Stages of Diabetic Nephropathy

Stage of Diabetic Nephropathy	GFR	Albuminuria	Pathology
No nephropathy	Normal	None	Normal
Early diabetic changes: CKD stage 1 (eGFR >90 mL/min/1.73 m²)	Normal or increased (may have hyper-filtration[7])	None (<30 mg/day or mg/g) or microalbuminuria (30–300 mg/day or mg/g)	Glomerular hypertrophy
Initial diabetic nephropathy: Stage 2 (eGFR 60–89 mL/min/1.73 m²) or early stage 3 (eGFR 45–59 mL/min/1.73 m²)	Mildly or moderately decreased	Microalbuminuria (30–300 mg/day or mg/g) or macroalbuminuria (>300 mg/day or mg/g)	Thickening of the GBM, mesangial expansion, change in vascular cells, accumulation of advanced glycosylation end products
Advanced (overt) nephropathy: Late stage 3 (eGFR 30–44 mL/min/1.73 m²) or stage 4 (eGFR 15–29 mL/min/1.73 m²)	eGFR declines by about 10 mL/year in untreated patients	Macroalbuminuria (>300 mg/day or mg/g), and may have nephrotic syndrome (>3 g/day or g/g)	Kimmelstiel-Wilson nodules, increased GBM width, diffuse mesangial sclerosis, hyalinosis, microaneurysms, hyaline arteriosclerosis, tubular and interstitial changes with fibrosis

Stage of Diabetic Nephropathy	GFR	Albuminuria	Pathology
ESKD: Stage 5 (eGFR <15 mL/min/1.73 m²)	Very low	Heavy proteinuria	Advanced changes, including interstitial fibrosis and tubular atrophy

CKD, Chronic kidney disease; *eGFR*, estimated glomerular filtration rate; *ESKD*, end stage kidney disease; *GBM*, glomerular basement membrane; *GFR*, glomerular filtration rate.

10.1.2 Risk Factors[8,9]

Risk Factors for Developing Diabetic Nephropathy	Risk Factors for Progression of Diabetic Nephropathy	Risk Factors for CV Events
• Inadequate glycemic control • HTN • Smoking • Hypercholesterolemia • Advanced age • Insulin resistance • Male gender • Black, Hispanic, Asian, or Native American descent • Obesity • Family history of CV events • Genetic factors (e.g., *VEGF* gene for retinopathy, *ELMO1* gene for nephropathy, and *ADIPOQ* gene for coronary artery disease)	• HTN • Albuminuria • Inadequate glycemic control • Smoking	• Older age • Male gender • Longer duration of diabetes • CV disease history • Degree of albuminuria[10,11] • HTN • Hypercholesterolemia

CV, Cardiovascular; *HTN*, hypertension.

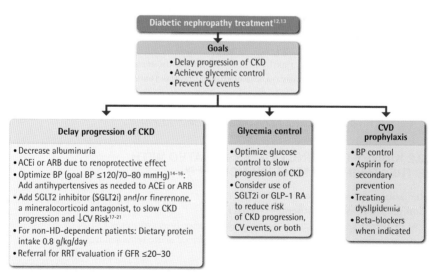

ACEi, Angiotensin-converting-enzyme inhibitors; *ARB*, angiotensin II receptor blocker; *BP*, blood pressure; *CKD*, chronic kidney disease; *CV*, cardiovascular; *CVD*, cardiovascular disease; *GFR*, glomerular filtration rate; *GLP-1 RA*, glucagon-like peptide-1 receptor agonist; *HD*, hemodialysis; *RRT*, renal replacement therapy; *SGLT2*, sodium-glucose cotransporter-2.

10.1.3 Management of Diabetic Nephropathy with CKD[12,13]

- General management as in Chapter 11, with added attention to optimal BP control with ACEi or ARB, nutrition, hypercholesterolemia, sodium balance for better BP control, and avoidance of hyperkalemia (diabetic nephropathy is a common cause of type 4 renal tubular acidosis [RTA] with hyperkalemia).
- SGLT2 inhibitors in patients with CKD delay CKD progression independently of the presence of diabetes.
- SGLT2 inhibitors also significantly decrease risk of death from renal or cardiovascular causes.[22,23]
- Finerenone has been shown to decrease progression of CKD, decrease serious cardiovascular events, and decrease hospitalizations for heart failure even when on RAS blockers and SGLT2 inhibitors but with an increase in hyperkalemia[17-21].
- Control of general complications of CKD: anemia, hyperphosphatemia, hyperparathyroidism, and bone disease.

10.2 Kidney Injury Associated With Malignancies

10.2.1 KIDNEY DYSFUNCTION[24,25]

Mechanical:
- Extrarenal obstruction: Prostate, bladder, retroperitoneal, or pelvic cancers
- Intrarenal tubular obstruction: Acute uric acid nephropathy, myeloma kidney (cast nephropathy)
- Tumor infiltration: Lymphoma or leukemia most commonly
- Renal ischemia: Renal vein occlusion from renal cell carcinoma

Hemodynamic alterations:
- Hypovolemia
- Cardiac toxicity

Glomerular diseases:
- Membranous glomerulopathy (solid tumors)
- Minimal change nephropathy/focal segmental glomerulosclerosis (FSGS) (lymphomas and leukemias)
- Amyloidosis (myeloma, lymphoma; rarely leukemia or renal cell carcinoma)
- Membranoproliferative or rapidly progressive glomerulonephritis (solid tumors, lymphoma)
- Thrombotic microangiopathy: Some adenocarcinomas (pancreas, gastric)

Tubulointerstitial diseases:
- Hypercalcemia: Acute renal failure, nephrogenic diabetes insipidus
- Multiple myeloma: Tubular dysfunction (see below 10.2.4)

10.2.2 KIDNEY DYSFUNCTION ASSOCIATED WITH THE TREATMENT OF MALIGNANCIES[26-29]

Radiation nephropathy or cystitis
Complications of chemotherapy—renal failure
- Hyperuricemia with urate nephropathy: Tumor lysis syndrome (TLS)
- Cisplatin-, carboplatin-, and ifosfamide-induced acute renal failure
- Interferon-induced acute renal failure
- Hemolytic uremic syndrome/thrombotic thrombocytopenic purpura (HUS/TTP) or thrombotic microangiopathy: Anti-tumor therapy (e.g., mitomycin, bleomycin, cisplatin, gemcitabine, radiation +cyclophosphamide (CYC), vascular endothelial growth factor inhibitors)
- High-dose methotrexate nephrotoxicity
- High-dose bisphosphonate-induced acute renal failure or collapsing glomerulopathy

Complications of chemotherapy—tubular disorders, bladder dysfunction
- Tubular dysfunction: Hypokalemia, metabolic acidosis from drug-induced renal tubular acidosis (RTA)—ifosfamide, cisplatin
- Hypomagnesemia: Cisplatin
- Hemorrhagic cystitis: Cyclophosphamide, ifosfamide
- Urinary retention: Vincristine

Complications of cancer immunotherapies
- Interleukin-2: Proteinuria from FSGS/minimal change disease (MCD), cytokine release syndrome (24–48 hr)
- Immune checkpoint inhibitors: Acute tubulointerstitial nephritis, glomerulonephritis[30,31]

10.2.3 ELECTROLYTE ABNORMALITIES ASSOCIATED WITH MALIGNANCIES[31]

- Vomiting and diarrhea: Hypokalemia, hyponatremia, metabolic acidosis or alkalosis
- Hyponatremia/syndrome of inappropriate antidiuretic hormone secretion (SIADH): Tumor secretion of antidiuretic hormone (ADH), high-dose cyclophosphamide, vincristine, vinblastine
- Hypercalcemia: Tumor secretion of parathyroid hormone-related peptide (PTH-RP), bone metastases, overproduction of 1,25-dihydroxyvitamin D, cytokines
- Hyperphosphatemia, hyperkalemia, hypocalcemia with TLS and acute renal failure (ARF)
- Hypokalemia: Lysozymuria with some leukemias causing renal potassium wasting
- Hypophosphatemia and tumor-induced osteomalacia: A rare syndrome characterized by urinary phosphate wasting, reduced 1,25-dihydroxyvitamin D concentrations, and osteomalacia caused by an increased production of fibroblast growth factor 23 (FGF23) by a mesenchymal tumor[31].

10.2.4 KIDNEY DISEASE IN MULTIPLE MYELOMA[32,33]

- Light chain toxicity:
  - Myeloma kidney (AKI or CKD due to glomerular filtration of toxic light chains with tubular injury and obstruction—"cast nephropathy")
  - Renal tubular dysfunction (accumulation of light chains in proximal cells causing type 2 RTA or Fanconi syndrome—kappa chains more commonly)
- Amyloidosis: Proteinuria or nephrotic syndrome, CKD (lambda chains more commonly)
- Cryoglobulinemia type 1: Membranoproliferative glomerular pattern—deposition of monoclonal immunoglobulin, usually IgG or IgM
- Hypercalcemia
- Hyperuricemia
- Increased risk for nonsteroidal antiinflammatory drug (NSAID) or radiocontrast nephrotoxicity
- Plasma cell renal infiltration

10.2.5 MONOCLONAL GAMMOPATHY OF RENAL SIGNIFICANCE[34,35]

- Monoclonal gammopathy of renal significance (MGRS) is a B cell or plasma cell premalignant lymphoproliferative disorder defined by the presence of serum monoclonal immunoglobulin <30 g/L with deposition in the kidney that may cause kidney disease and <10% monoclonal bone marrow plasma cells.
- Three distinct clinical types: Non-IgM, IgM, and light chain monoclonal gammopathy.
- Small risk of progression to a malignant plasma cell dyscrasia.
- In general, no specific treatment is required, but in those with kidney damage, treatment to protect renal function by reducing toxic monoclonal proteins is recommended. When untreated, clinical evaluation for "red flags" and laboratory evaluation with serum protein electrophoresis (SPEP), free light chains, complete blood count (CBC), creatinine (Cr), and serum calcium every 3 to 6 months is necessary.[34]

10.3 Kidney Disease in Hepatitis C[36,37]

Hepatitis C is the most common blood-borne infection in the world and is associated with glomerular disease. Recognized patterns of kidney disease include mixed cryoglobulinemia, membranoproliferative glomerulonephritis, and membranous nephropathy. The prevalence of hepatitis C virus (HCV) in CKD and ESKD patients is higher compared to the general population. Overall, among prevalent hemodialysis patients, HCV prevalence is nearly 10%. However, the advent of direct-acting antivirals (DAAs) has made viral eradication possible in 90% to 100% of cases. All HCV genotypes are now curable with 8- to 24-week courses of DAAs, which are extremely well tolerated. Reliable response to DAAs has also helped increase transplant rates by allowing allocation of HCV renal grafts to HCV-negative recipients.[38,39]

10.3.1.1 Screening and Diagnosis of Hepatitis C

- Initial screening test serological assay that detects HCV antibody.
- Confirmation with nucleic acid test (NAT) for HCV ribonucleic acid and viral load.
- For immunocompromised patients, NAT is the appropriate initial test due to concern for delayed seroconversion in acute HCV infection.
- HCV screening is recommended for all patients who start in-center HD or who transfer from another facility.

10.3.1.2 Treatment of Hepatitis C–Associated Renal Disease[40]

- DAAs are now the first-line therapy in patients with CKD with sustained virological response (SVR) of 90% to 100%. Regimen selection varies by genotype, eGFR, and other patient factors.
- Systemic steroids plus rituximab for moderate to severe mixed cryoglobulinemia syndrome.
- Plasmapheresis ± cytotoxic drugs for cryoglobulinemic membranoproliferative glomerulonephritis (MPGN).

Cryoglobulinemia (may present with vasculitis/palpable purpura, arthralgias, lymphadenopathy, neuropathy, hepatosplenomegaly, hypocomplementemia, or cryoglobulinemic nephropathy)

Type 1: Monoclonal immunoglobulin: (multiple myeloma or Waldenström macroglobulinemia)

Type 2: Essential mixed cryoglobulinemia: Polyclonal immunoglobulins and a monoclonal IgM or IgG rheumatoid factor (infection with HCV or Epstein-Barr virus [EBV] commonly)

Type 3: Mixed cryoglobulinemia: Polyclonal immunoglobulins and polyclonal IgMs (chronic inflammatory and autoimmune disorders such as systemic lupus erythematosus [SLE], other connective tissue diseases, lymphoproliferative malignancies, or HCV)

10.4 HIV Infection

HIV infection can cause multiple renal injuries, including glomerular, interstitial, and/or tubular diseases. Furthermore, antiviral medications used in the treatment of HIV infection have possible adverse effects on the kidneys.[41,42]

10.4.1 KIDNEY DISEASE IN HIV PATIENTS

Glomerular disease:
- An immune complex glomerulonephritis with IgA deposits (IgA Ab against HIV)
- Membranoproliferative glomerulonephritis (associated with hepatitis C or mixed cryoglobulinemia due to HCV or HIV itself)
- FSGS (collapsing glomerulopathy with severe tubulointerstitial injury)

- Postinfectious glomerulonephritis
- Membranous nephropathy, due to concurrent infection with hepatitis B or C virus or syphilis
- Other immune complex kidney diseases (fibrillary glomerulonephritis [GN], immunotactoid GN)
- Thrombotic microangiopathy (HUS/TTP)
- Crescentic GN: Lupus-like GN
- *Pneumocystis jirovecii* or *Cryptococcus neoformans* infection: Clumps of organisms obstructing glomerular and intertubular capillaries

Interstitial disease:

- Viral: EBV, cytomegalovirus (CMV), BK virus, direct infection by HIV, immune restoration inflammatory syndrome after initiation of highly active antiretroviral therapy (HAART)
- Acute interstitial nephritis: beta-lactam antibiotics, quinolones, trimethoprim-sulfamethoxazole (TMP/SMX) rifampin
- Indinavir crystalluria

Acute tubular necrosis (ATN):

- Nephrotoxic medications: Pentamidine, foscarnet, cidofovir, adefovir, amphotericin B, aminoglycosides, TMP/SMX
- Intratubular obstruction (IV high-dose acyclovir or sulfadiazine)
- Infection/sepsis
- Hypotension
- Rhabdomyolysis (mainly medication toxicity)

10.4.2 ANTI-HIV MEDICATIONS AND DRUG-INDUCED KIDNEY DISORDERS

- ATN (pentamidine, foscarnet, cidofovir, adefovir, amphotericin B, aminoglycosides, vancomycin, tenofovir, indinavir)
- Interstitial nephritis (TMP/SMX, NSAIDs, rifampin, beta-lactam antibiotics, ciprofloxacin and other quinolones, tenofovir, indinavir)
- Rhabdomyolysis (pentamidine, TMP/SMX, zidovudine, statins, tenofovir)
- Elevated Cr (trimethoprim-decreased tubular secretion of Cr)
- Hyperkalemia (trimethoprim- or pentamidine-decreased tubular secretion of potassium)
- Hypokalemia (amphotericin B, didanosine, tenofovir)
- Hypocalcemia (pentamidine, foscarnet, didanosine)
- Hypomagnesemia (pentamidine, amphotericin B)
- Acidosis (amphotericin B, tenofovir)
- Diabetes insipidus, nephrogenic (foscarnet, tenofovir)
- Fanconi syndrome (tenofovir; tenofovir disoproxil fumarate [TDF] has fewer side effects compared to tenofovir alafenamide [TAF])
- Renal stones and nephropathy due to indinavir crystalluria

10.4.2.1 Risk Factors for Acute Renal Failure

Risk Factors Specific to HIV	Traditional Risk Factors
• Male sex	• Older age
• Black race	• Diabetes mellitus
• G1/G2 high-risk alleles for APOL1[42,43]	• Chronic kidney disease
• High viral load >400 copies/mL	• Liver failure
• CD4 cell count <200/μL	
• Having ever received HAART	
• Hepatitis C coinfection	

The estimated lifetime risk associated with carrying 2 APOL1 risk alleles is 4% for FSGS in the absence of HIV infection, and as high as 50% for HIV-associated nephropathy.

10.5 Systemic Lupus Erythematosus[44,45]

SLE is an autoimmune disease involving loss of immune tolerance of endogenous nuclear material leading to chronic inflammation and multiorgan damage. Kidney involvement occurs in 25% to 50% of patients with SLE, and 5% to 20% of patients with lupus nephritis develop ESKD within 10 years from the initial diagnosis. The pathological presentations of SLE nephritis are summarized in the International Society of Nephrology/Renal Pathology Society (ISN/RPS) 2003 classification of lupus nephritis.[46]

10.5.1.1 International Society of Nephrology/Renal Pathology Society 2003 Classification of Lupus Nephritis

Class	Definition	Clinical Findings	Treatment
I	Minimal mesangial LN	LM: Normal glomeruli IF: Mesangial deposits	Supportive therapy
II	Mesangial proliferative LN	LM: Mesangial hypercellularity or matrix expansion IF/EM: Few subepithelial or subendothelial deposits Mild hematuria and proteinuria	Supportive therapy
III	Focal LN	Active or inactive focal, segmental, or global endocapillary or extracapillary GN involving <50% of glomeruli Mild hematuria and proteinuria	Glucocorticoids ± CYC or MMF or CNI or MMF and CNI
IV	Diffuse LN	Active or inactive focal, segmental, or global endocapillary or extracapillary GN involving >50% of glomeruli Most common and most severe: AKI/CKD, active lupus serology, active urinary sediment	Glucocorticoids ± CYC or MMF or CNI or MMF and CNI
V	Membranous LN	Global or segmental subepithelial immune deposits or their morphological sequelae by LM and by IF or EM, with or without mesangial alterations. May occur in combination with class III or IV, in which case both classes are diagnosed. May show advanced sclerosis.	Glucocorticoids ± either CNI or MMF or CYC or AZA
VI	Advanced sclerotic LN	≥90% of glomeruli globally sclerosed without residual activity	RAAS blockade
	Tubulointerstitial lesions	Normal renal function, microhematuria, proteinuria hyperkalemia in some	Glucocorticoids
	Vascular disease	Arteriolosclerosis, TMA	Plasma exchange/eculizumab

Class	Definition	Clinical Findings	Treatment
	Podocytopathy[47]	LM: Normal glomeruli, FSGS or mesangial expansion EM: Diffuse and severe foot process effacement on EM Nephrotic-range proteinuria or nephrotic syndrome	Glucocorticoids or CNIs or MMF or CYC or rituximab

AKI, Acute kidney injury; *AZA*, azathioprine; *CKD*, chronic kidney disease; *CNI*, calcineurin inhibitors; *CYC*, cyclophosphamide; *EM*, electron microscopy; *FSGS*, focal segmental glomerulosclerosis; *GN*, glomerulonephritis; *IF*, immunofluorescent microscopy; *LM*, light microscopy; *LN*, lupus nephritis; *MMF*, mycophenolate mofetil; *RAAS*, renin-angiotensin-aldosterone system; *TMA*, thrombotic microangiopathy.

Management of SLE[48-50]:

- Patients with SLE should be on an antimalarial drug (hydroxychloroquine) unless contraindicated.
- Start renin-angiotensin-aldosterone system (RAAS) blockade in patients with proteinuria.
- For class IV and V LN, immunosuppression as described above is indicated to induce remission. Induction phase lasts 3 to 6 months followed by maintenance phase of a prolonged but less intensive treatment.
- In pregnancy, hydroxychloroquine, aspirin, and immunosuppressive drugs such as azathioprine, cyclosporine, or tacrolimus can be continued while methotrexate, MMF, RAAS inhibitors, warfarin, and cyclophosphamide are contraindicated.
- For nonresponders, repeat biopsy is recommended after 6 months from the start of immunosuppression to look for potential progression to a different class and dose adjustment.

10.6 Thrombotic Microangiopathy

10.6.1 TYPES OF TMA[51-53]

- Primary TMA (hereditary or acquired HUS/TTP and atypical TTP)
- Secondary TMA (associated with another underlying disease or drug, e.g., SLE, gemcitabine)
- Infection-related TMA (a form of secondary TMA, e.g., caused by Shiga toxin)

10.6.2 CAUSES OF TMA

Thrombotic microangiopathy is caused by:
- Underlying predisposing factors (e.g., decreased C3 levels, decreased factor H, abnormal von Willebrand factor [VWF] cleaving protease activity or *VWF* gene mutation); and
- Triggering events (e.g., viruses, bacterial Shiga toxin/endotoxins, drugs, antibodies and immune complexes). A combination of the above 2 factors leads to loss of endothelial thromboresistance, leukocyte adhesion, vascular shear stress, consumption of complement, and abnormal VWF fragmentation.[54]

10.6.3 TREATMENT OF TMA[55]

Plasma Therapy	Medications
• Plasma exchange (1–2 plasma volumes/day) • Plasma infusion (FFP) • Plasma cryopheresis (for resistant forms) • Plasma exchange with solvent/detergent-treated plasma (for resistant forms, may limit the risk of viral contamination)	• Prednisone (commonly used) • Eculizumab for complement-mediated TMA **For poor responses:** • Rituximab • IV gammaglobulin • Vincristine • Antithrombotic (heparin, tPA) and antiplatelet (aspirin) agents • Caplacizumab for TTP

FFP, fresh frozen plasma; *TMA*, Thrombotic microangiopathy; *tPA*, tissue plasminogen activator.

10.7 Systemic Sclerosis

The pathogenesis of systemic sclerosis (SSc or scleroderma) includes vascular, immunological, and fibrotic processes. It is characterized by fibrosis of the skin and visceral organs, and it has the highest mortality among connective tissue diseases (55% 10-year survival).[56–58]

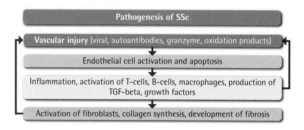

10.7.1 TYPES OF SSc

Limited Cutaneous SSc	Diffuse Cutaneous SSc

• Raynaud phenomenon
• May have CREST syndrome (Calcinosis cutis, Raynaud's, Esophageal motility disorder, Sclerodactyly, Telangiectasia)
• May have other organ involvement, but less likely
	• Raynaud phenomenon
	• Extracutaneous organ involvement more likely:
	  • Interstitial lung disease (earliest changes in the posterior lower lobes)
	  • PAH
	  • Kidney injury and scleroderma renal crisis
	  • GI involvement
	  • Cardiac disease
	  • Arthralgias, myalgias, contractures
	  • Sexual dysfunction

GI, Gastrointestinal; *PAH*, pulmonary arterial hypertension; *SSc*, systemic sclerosis.

10.7.2 PREDICTORS OF INCREASED MORTALITY

- Truncal skin involvement
- Abnormal electrocardiogram (ECG)
- Reduced lung diffusing capacity
- Elevated erythrocyte sedimentation rate (ESR)
- Presence of antibody to topoisomerase I (uncertain)

10.7.3 SCLERODERMA RENAL CRISIS

Scleroderma renal crisis occurs in 5% to 10% of SSc patients (15% of those with diffuse cutaneous SSc), is caused by injury to medium-size arteries in the kidneys, and is a medical emergency.[59]

Presentation:

- Malignant hypertension (HTN) with retinopathy
- Encephalopathy and seizures
- Hyperreninemia
- Acute renal failure/rapidly progressive glomerulonephritis (RPGN)
- Proteinuria
- Pulmonary edema
- Headaches, fevers, malaise
- Normotensive scleroderma renal crisis is associated with a worse outcome

Patients at greatest risk for severe consequences:

- Diffuse cutaneous or rapidly progressive forms of SSc
- Large joint contractures and tendon friction rubs
- Anemia
- New cardiac events
- Recent treatment with high-dose corticosteroids ($\geq$15 mg prednisone/day)
- Positive antinuclear antibody (ANA) with speckled pattern
- Antibodies to RNA polymerase III
- Absence of anticentromere antibodies

Laboratory tests:

- Elevated Cr, proteinuria/glomerulonephritis, microangiopathic hemolytic anemia, thrombocytopenia, hyperreninemia

Treatment:

- Angiotensin-converting-enzyme inhibitors (ACEi, particularly captopril)
- Add dihydropyridine calcium channel blocker to control BP, if necessary
- Role of angiotensin II receptor blocker (ARB) is unknown (use only if ACEi intolerant)
- Endothelin might be a potential target for endothelin receptor blockade
- 40% may require dialysis

10.8 Pregnancy

Consulting on pregnant patients may be an important part of some nephrology practices. Three common issues that trigger consultations are diminished renal function, proteinuria, and HTN as signs of either a non-pregnancy–related condition or preeclampsia. When measuring kidney function, it is important to realize that formulae used to estimate GFR (i.e., CKD-EPI, Modification of Diet in Renal Disease [MDRD] formula) are inaccurate, and a measured creatinine clearance (CrCl) based on a timed urine collection (usually 24 hr) remains the most practical. Similarly, to quantitate proteinuria, the protein to creatinine ratio can be used to monitor changes in the amount of proteinuria over time, but to determine the absolute value of proteinuria over 24 hours, it is best to measure in a 24-hour collection.

10.8.1 Causes of High Blood Pressure in Pregnancy

- Chronic essential HTN
- Secondary HTN
- Preeclampsia
- Preeclampsia superimposed on chronic HTN
- Gestational HTN (BP >140/90 mm Hg after normal BP <20 weeks and no proteinuria)

10.8.2 Proteinuria in Pregnancy[60–64]

Normal	Kidney Disease	Preeclampsia
• <200–300 of protein/24 hr (secondary to ↑ GFR, ↑ basement membrane permeability)	• Pregnancy may: • Unmask kidney disease • Worsen preexisting kidney disease • Be a time in which de novo kidney disease develops	Diagnostic criteria: Gestational HTN (BP >140/90, onset >20 weeks' gestation) + new onset of one of the following: • Proteinuria (300 mg/24 hr) • Cr >1.1 mg/dL or ↑ 2x baseline • Thrombocytopenia • Elevated AST/ALT • Pulmonary edema • Cerebral/visual symptoms

ALT, Alanine aminotransferase; *AST*, aspartate aminotransferase; *Cr*, creatinine; *GFR*, glomerular filtration rate; *HTN*, hypertension.

10.8.3 CAUSES OF ARF IN PREGNANCY

Prerenal (hemodynamic disturbances):
- Hemorrhage, e.g., abruptio placentae or uterine
- Heart failure
- Hyperemesis gravidarum

Intrarenal:
- ATN
- Preeclampsia endotheliosis
- Acute interstitial nephritis (AIN)
- Thrombotic microangiopathies (preeclampsia, HELLP syndrome [Hemolysis, Elevated Liver enzymes, Low Platelet count], acute fatty liver of pregnancy [AFLP], TTP[65])
- Amniotic fluid embolism
- Lupus nephritis exacerbation
- Puerperal sepsis

Postrenal:
- Hydronephrosis due to uterine compression/obstruction at bladder outlet
- Nephrolithiasis
- Iatrogenic (e.g., injury to ureters or bladder during C-section)

10.8.4 TREATMENT OF PREECLAMPSIA

In preeclampsia with severe features/HELLP syndrome,[66] AFLP, renal failure:
- Delivery of the fetus (after corticosteroids for fetal lung maturity, if necessary)
- IV magnesium (MgSO$_4$)—serum therapeutic level 4 to 6 mg/dL (follow hyperreflexia) to prevent seizures (eclampsia)
- BP control as described below

In women with a preterm fetus and gestational HTN or preeclampsia without severe features, there are no randomized controlled trials, but retrospective data suggest that without severe features, the balance should be in favor of continued monitoring until delivery at 37 weeks of gestation.

10.8.5 TREATMENT OF HYPERTENSION IN PREGNANCY

- If BP <140/90 and protein <500 mg/24 hr: mild disease → close follow-up, reduced activity, fetal assessments
- If BP ≥140/95, decreased renal function, increased uric acid, and proteinuria >500 mg/ 24 hr: hospitalization and delivery if >32 to 34 weeks' gestation. If possible, lower BP to 140/90 before delivery with antihypertensives tolerated in pregnancy (e.g., calcium channel blockers, beta-blockers, hydralazine, methyldopa). If <32 weeks, close observation with maternal and fetal monitoring, BP control, seizure (eclampsia) prevention (IV $MgSO_4$), and corticosteroids for fetal lung maturation in an attempt to keep the patient stable to improve fetal viability, but if symptoms/signs worsen, delivery may become necessary.
- If BP >160/100—parenteral Rx (labetalol, hydralazine, nicardipine) → urgent delivery if seizure (eclampsia), severe renal failure, or HELLP syndrome develops.

10.9 Important Inherited Disorders[67-69]

Inherited Disorders	Extrarenal Manifestations	Renal Manifestations
Hereditary nephritis (Alport syndrome[70,71])	Hearing loss, ocular disease, HTN, leiomyomatosis	Microhematuria, proteinuria, progressive CKD, renal pathology of split or laminated GBM on EM and absence of anti-GBM Ab staining on immunofluorescence due to genetic defects in type IV collagen
ADTKD,[72,73] medullary cystic disease (see Chapter 9)	Early onset hyperuricemia and gout; 1 of 3 mutations explain most cases of ADTKD	Low fractional urate excretion, progressive CKD with tubulointerstitial fibrosis and tubular cysts, may develop urinary sodium wasting
von Hippel-Lindau disease[74,75]	Retinal lesions (angiomas), cerebral hemangioma, pheochromocytoma, pancreatic cystadenomas, neuroendocrine tumors	Renal hemangioblastomas, renal cell carcinomas (up to 70%)
Tuberous sclerosis[76]	Seizures, multiorgan tumors, cardiac rhabdomyomas, retinal hamartomas/angiofibromas, pulmonary LAM	Renal angiomyolipomas, multiple cysts, renal hemorrhages, renal cell carcinomas (1%–2%); may benefit from eculizumab treatment
Beckwith-Wiedemann syndrome[77]	Visceromegaly, macroglossia, abdominal wall defect, prenatal and postnatal overgrowth, neonatal hypoglycemia, abdominal organ neoplasms	Wilms' tumor, medullary dysplasia, hypercalciuria, nephrolithiasis
NPHP, a renal ciliopathy associated with several autosomal recessive diseases[78,79]	Retinitis pigmentosa, skeletal, liver, neurological and cardiac disorders	Nephronophthisis (small hyperechoic kidneys with smooth outline cysts), chronic tubulointerstitial disease, renal sodium wasting, CKD

Continued on following page

Inherited Disorders	Extrarenal Manifestations	Renal Manifestations
Fabry disease[80–82]	Neuropathic pain, deafness, heat intolerance, left ventricular hypertrophy, corneal and lenticular opacities, hypertension	Albuminuria, proteinuria, impaired ability to concentrate urine, CKD

ADTKD, Autosomal dominant tubulointerstitial kidney disease; *CKD*, chronic kidney disease; *EM*, electron microscopy; *GBM*, glomerular basement membrane; *HTN*, hypertension; *LAM*, lymphangioleiomyomatosis; *NPHP*, nephronophthisis.
Note: Polycystic kidney disease is included in Chapter 9.

References

1. Zelnick LR, Weiss NS, Kestenbaum BR, et al. Diabetes and CKD in the United States population, 2009–2014. *Clin J Am Soc Nephrol*. 2017;12(12):1984–1990. doi:10.2215/CJN.03700417.
2. Tong L, Adler SG. Diabetic kidney disease. *Clin J Am Soc Nephrol*. 2018;13(2):335–338. doi:10.2215/CJN.04650417.
3. Umanath K, Lewis JB. Update on diabetic nephropathy: core curriculum 2018. *Am J Kidney Dis*. 2018;71(6):884–895. doi:10.1053/j.ajkd.2017.10.026.
4. Hahr AJ, Molitch ME. Management of diabetes mellitus in patients with CKD: core curriculum 2022. *Am J Kidney Dis*. 2022;79(5):728–736. doi:10.1053/j.ajkd.2021.05.023.
5. Fox CS, Matsushita K, Woodward M, et al. Associations of kidney disease measures with mortality and end-stage renal disease in individuals with and without diabetes: a meta-analysis. *Lancet*. 2012;380(9854):1662–1673. doi:10.1016/S0140-6736(12)61350-6.
6. Ninomiya T, Perkovic V, de Galan BE, et al. Albuminuria and kidney function independently predict cardiovascular and renal outcomes in diabetes. *J Am Soc Nephrol*. 2009;20(8):1813–1821. doi:10.1681/ASN.2008121270.
7. Molitch ME, Gao X, Bebu I, et al. Early glomerular hyperfiltration and long-term kidney outcomes in type 1 diabetes: the DCCT/EDIC experience. *Clin J Am Soc Nephrol*. 2019;14(6):854–861. doi:10.2215/CJN.14831218.
8. Radcliffe NJ, Seah J-M, Clarke M, MacIsaac RJ, Jerums G, Ekinci EI. Clinical predictive factors in diabetic kidney disease progression. *J Diabetes Investig*. 2017;8(1):6–18. doi:10.1111/jdi.12533.
9. Maqbool M, Cooper ME, Jandeleit-Dahm KAM. Cardiovascular disease and diabetic kidney disease. *Semin Nephrol*. 2018;38(3):217–232. doi:10.1016/j.semnephrol.2018.02.003.
10. Anyanwagu U, Donnelly R, Idris I. Albuminuria regression and all-cause mortality among insulin-treated patients with type 2 diabetes: analysis of a large UK primary care cohort. *Am J Nephrol*. 2019;49(2):146–155. doi:10.1159/000496276.
11. Fangel MV, Nielsen PB, Kristensen JK, et al. Albuminuria and risk of cardiovascular events and mortality in a general population of patients with type 2 diabetes without cardiovascular disease: a Danish cohort study. *Am J Med*. 2020;133(6):e269–e279. doi:10.1016/j.amjmed.2019.10.042.
12. Barrera-Chimal J, Lima-Posada I, Bakris GL, Jaisser F. Mineralocorticoid receptor antagonists in diabetic kidney disease—mechanistic and therapeutic effects. *Nat Rev Nephrol*. 2022;18(1):56–70. doi:10.1038/s41581-021-00490-8.
13. Sugahara M, Pak WLW, Tanaka T, Tang SCW, Nangaku M. Update on diagnosis, pathophysiology, and management of diabetic kidney disease. *Nephrology (Carlton)*. 2021;26(6):491–500. doi:10.1111/nep.13860.
14. Kidney Disease: Improving Global Outcomes (KDIGO) Blood Pressure Work Group. KDIGO 2021 clinical practice guideline for the management of blood pressure in chronic kidney disease. *Kidney Int*. 2021;99(3S):S1–S87. doi:10.1016/j.kint.2020.11.003.
15. Zhuo M, Yang D, Goldfarb-Rumyantzev A, Brown RS. The association of SBP with mortality in patients with stage 1–4 chronic kidney disease. *J Hypertens*. 2021;39(11):2250–2257. doi:10.1097/HJH.0000000000002927.

16. Li J, Somers VK, Gao X, et al. Evaluation of optimal diastolic blood pressure range among adults with treated systolic blood pressure less than 130 mm Hg. *JAMA Netw Open.* 2021;4(2):e2037554. doi:10.1001/jamanetworkopen.2020.37554.

17. Fioretto P, Pontremoli R. Expanding the therapy options for diabetic kidney disease. *Nat Rev Nephrol.* 2022;18(2):78–79. doi:10.1038/s41581-021-00522-3.

18. Tuttle KR, Brosius FC, Cavender MA, et al. SGLT2 inhibition for CKD and cardiovascular disease in type 2 diabetes: report of a scientific workshop sponsored by the National Kidney Foundation. *Am J Kidney Dis.* 2021;77(1):94–109. doi:10.1053/j.ajkd.2020.08.003.

19. Brown E, Heerspink HJL, Cuthbertson DJ, Wilding JPH. SGLT2 inhibitors and GLP-1 receptor agonists: established and emerging indications. *Lancet.* 2021;398(10296):262–276. doi:10.1016/S0140-6736(21)00536-5.

20. Bakris GL, Agarwal R, Anker SD, et al. Effect of finerenone on chronic kidney disease outcomes in type 2 diabetes. *N Engl J Med.* 2020;383(23):2219–2229. doi:10.1056/NEJMoa2025845.

21. Barrera-Chimal J, Lima-Posada I, Bakris GL, Jaisser F. Mineralocorticoid receptor antagonists in diabetic kidney disease—mechanistic and therapeutic effects. *Nat Rev Nephrol.* 2022;18(1):56–70. doi:10.1038/s41581-021-00490-8.

22. Heerspink HJL, Stefánsson BV, Correa-Rotter R, et al. Dapagliflozin in patients with chronic kidney disease. *N Engl J Med.* 2020;383(15):1436–1446. doi:10.1056/NEJMoa2024816.

23. Li J, Albajrami O, Zhuo M, Hawley CE, Paik JM. Decision algorithm for prescribing SGLT2 inhibitors and GLP-1 receptor agonists for diabetic kidney disease. *Clin J Am Soc Nephrol.* 2020;15(11):1678–1688. doi:10.2215/CJN.02690320.

24. Cosmai L, Porta C, Foramitti M, Rizzo M, Gallieni M. The basics of onco-nephrology in the renal clinic. *J Nephrol.* 2020;33(6):1143–1149. doi:10.1007/s40620-020-00922-x.

25. Porta C, Bamias A, Danesh FR, et al. KDIGO Controversies Conference on onco-nephrology: understanding kidney impairment and solid-organ malignancies, and managing kidney cancer. *Kidney Int.* 2020;98(5):1108–1119. doi:10.1016/j.kint.2020.06.046.

26. Schanz M, Schricker S, Pfister F, Alscher MD, Kimmel M. Renal complications of cancer therapies. *Drugs Today (Barc).* 2018;54(9):561–575. doi:10.1358/dot.2018.54.9.2874064.

27. Piscitani L, Sirolli V, Di Liberato L, Morroni M, Bonomini M. Nephrotoxicity associated with novel anticancer agents (aflibercept, dasatinib, nivolumab): case series and nephrological considerations. *Int J Mol Sci.* 2020;21(14):4878. doi:10.3390/ijms21144878.

28. Wanchoo R, Karam S, Uppal NN, et al. Adverse renal effects of immune checkpoint inhibitors: a narrative review. *Am J Nephrol.* 2017;45(2):160–169. doi:10.1159/000455014.

29. Majeed H, Gupta V. Adverse effects of radiation therapy. In: *StatPearls* [Internet]. Treasure Island (FL): StatPearls Publishing; 2022.

30. Gupta S, Cortazar FB, Riella LV, Leaf DE. Immune checkpoint inhibitor nephrotoxicity: update 2020. *Kidney360.* 2020;1(2):130–140. doi:10.34067/KID.0000852019.

31. Rosner MH, Jhaveri KD, McMahon BA, Perazella MA. Onconephrology: the intersections between the kidney and cancer. *CA Cancer J Clin.* 2021;71(1):47–77. doi:10.3322/caac.21636.

32. Dimopoulos MA, Sonneveld P, Leung N, et al. International Myeloma Working Group recommendations for the diagnosis and management of myeloma-related renal impairment. *J Clin Oncol.* 2016;34(13):1544–1557. doi:10.1200/JCO.2015.65.0044.

33. Vakiti A, Padala SA, Mewawalla P. Myeloma kidney. In: *StatPearls* [Internet]. Treasure Island (FL): StatPearls Publishing; 2022.

34. Leung N, Bridoux F, Nasr SH. Monoclonal gammopathy of renal significance. *N Engl J Med.* 2021;384(20):1931–1941. doi:10.1056/NEJMra1810907

35. Jain A, Haynes R, Kothari J, Khera A, Soares M, Ramasamy K. Pathophysiology and management of monoclonal gammopathy of renal significance. *Blood Adv.* 2019;3(15):2409–2423. doi:10.1182/bloodadvances.2019031914.

36. Awan AA, Jadoul M, Martin P. Hepatitis C in chronic kidney disease: an overview of the KDIGO guideline. *Clin Gastroenterol Hepatol.* 2020;18(10):2158–2167. doi:10.1016/j.cgh.2019.07.050.

37. Sise ME. Hepatitis C virus infection and the kidney. *Nephrol Dial Transplant.* 2018;34(3):415–418. doi:10.1093/ndt/gfy230.

38. Jalota A, Lindner BK, Thomas B, Lerma EV. Hepatitis C and treatment in patients with chronic kidney disease. *Dis Mon.* 2021;67(2):101017. doi:10.1016/j.disamonth.2020.101017.

39. Weinfurtner K, Reddy KR. Hepatitis C viraemic organs in solid organ transplantation. *J Hepatol.* 2021;74(3):716–733. doi:10.1016/j.jhep.2020.11.014.

40. Almeida PH, Matielo CEL, Curvelo LA, et al. Update on the management and treatment of viral hepatitis. *World J Gastroenterol.* 2021;27(23):3249–3261. doi:10.3748/wjg.v27.i23.3249.

41. Palau L, Menez S, Rodriguez-Sanchez J, et al. HIV-associated nephropathy: links, risks and management. *HIV AIDS (Auckl).* 2018;10:73–81. doi:10.2147/HIV.S141978.

42. Kopp JB, Nelson GW, Sampath K, et al. APOL1 genetic variants in focal segmental glomerulosclerosis and HIV-associated nephropathy. *J Am Soc Nephrol.* 2011;22(11):2129–2137. doi:10.1681/ASN.2011040388.

43. Friedman DJ, Pollak MR. APOL1 nephropathy: from genetics to clinical applications. *Clin J Am Soc Nephrol.* 2021;16(2):294–303. doi:10.2215/CJN.15161219.

44. Parikh SV, Almaani S, Brodsky S, Rovin BH. Update on lupus nephritis: core curriculum 2020. *Am J Kidney Dis.* 2020;76(2):265–281. doi:10.1053/j.ajkd.2019.10.017.

45. Tsokos GC. Systemic lupus erythematosus. *N Engl J Med.* 2011;365(22):2110–2121. doi:10.1056/NEJMra1100359.

46. Anders H-J, Saxena R, Zhao M-H, Parodis I, Salmon JE, Mohan C. Lupus nephritis. *Nat Rev Dis Primers.* 2020;6(1):7. doi:10.1038/s41572-019-0141-9.

47. Oliva-Damaso N, Payan J, Oliva-Damaso E, Pereda T, Bomback AS. Lupus podocytopathy: an overview. *Adv Chronic Kidney Dis.* 2019;26(5):369–375. doi:10.1053/j.ackd.2019.08.011.

48. Basta F, Fasola F, Triantafyllias K, Schwarting A. Systemic lupus erythematosus (SLE) therapy: the old and the new. *Rheumatol Ther.* 2020;7(3):433–446. doi:10.1007/s40744-020-00212-9.

49. Tunnicliffe DJ, Palmer SC, Henderson L, et al. Immunosuppressive treatment for proliferative lupus nephritis. *Cochrane Database Syst Rev.* 2018;6(6):CD002922. doi:10.1002/14651858.CD002922.pub4.

50. Fanouriakis A, Kostopoulou M, Cheema K, et al. 2019 Update of the Joint European League Against Rheumatism and European Renal Association–European Dialysis and Transplant Association (EULAR/ERA-EDTA) recommendations for the management of lupus nephritis. *Ann Rheum Dis.* 2020;79(6):713–723. doi:10.1136/annrheumdis-2020-216924.

51. Bayer G, von Tokarski F, Thoreau B, et al. Etiology and outcomes of thrombotic microangiopathies. *Clin J Am Soc Nephrol.* 2019;14(4):557–566. doi:10.2215/CJN.11470918.

52. Raina R, Grewal MK, Radhakrishnan Y, et al. Optimal management of atypical hemolytic uremic disease: challenges and solutions. *Int J Nephrol Renovasc Dis.* 2019;12:183–204. doi:10.2147/IJNRD.S215370.

53. Joly BS, Coppo P, Veyradier A. An update on pathogenesis and diagnosis of thrombotic thrombocytopenic purpura. *Expert Rev Hematol.* 2019;12(6):383–395. doi:10.1080/17474086.2019.1611423.

54. Brocklebank V, Wood KM, Kavanagh D. Thrombotic microangiopathy and the kidney. *Clin J Am Soc Nephrol.* 2018;13(2):300–317. doi:10.2215/CJN.00620117.

55. Fox LC, Cohney SJ, Kausman JY, et al. Consensus opinion on diagnosis and management of thrombotic microangiopathy in Australia and New Zealand. *Intern Med J.* 2018;48(6):624–636. doi:10.1111/imj.13804.

56. Chrabaszcz M, Małyszko J, Sikora M, et al. Renal involvement in systemic sclerosis: an update. *Kidney Blood Press Res.* 2020;45(4):532–548. doi:10.1159/000507886.

57. Hughes M, Herrick AL. Systemic sclerosis. *Br J Hosp Med (Lond).* 2019;80(9):530–536. doi:10.12968/hmed.2019.80.9.530.

58. Denton CP. Advances in pathogenesis and treatment of systemic sclerosis. *Clin Med (Lond).* 2015;15 Suppl 6:s58–s63. doi:10.7861/clinmedicine.15-6-s58.

59. Nagaraja V. Management of scleroderma renal crisis. *Curr Opin Rheumatol.* 2019;31(3):223–230. doi:10.1097/BOR.0000000000000604.

60. Chappell LC, Cluver CA, Kingdom J, Tong S. Pre-eclampsia. *Lancet.* 2021;398(10297):341–354. doi:10.1016/S0140-6736(20)32335-7.

61. Rana S, Lemoine E, Granger JP, Karumanchi SA. Preeclampsia: pathophysiology, challenges, and perspectives. *Circ Res.* 2019;124(7):1094–1112. doi:10.1161/CIRCRESAHA.118.313276.

62. Tomimatsu T, Mimura K, Matsuzaki S, Endo M, Kumasawa K, Kimura T. Preeclampsia: maternal systemic vascular disorder caused by generalized endothelial dysfunction due to placental antiangiogenic factors. *Int J Mol Sci.* 2019;20(17):4246. doi:10.3390/ijms20174246.

63. Gestational hypertension and preeclampsia: ACOG Practice Bulletin, Number 222. *Obstet Gynecol.* 2020;135(6):e237–e260. doi:10.1097/AOG.0000000000003891.

64. Phipps EA, Thadhani R, Benzing T, Karumanchi SA. Pre-eclampsia: pathogenesis, novel diagnostics and therapies. *Nat Rev Nephrol.* 2019;15(5):275–289. doi:10.1038/s41581-019-0119-6.
65. Gupta M, Feinberg BB, Burwick RM. Thrombotic microangiopathies of pregnancy: differential diagnosis. *Pregnancy Hypertens.* 2018;12:29–34. doi:10.1016/j.preghy.2018.02.007.
66. Fakhouri F, Scully M, Provôt F, et al. Management of thrombotic microangiopathy in pregnancy and postpartum: report from an international working group. *Blood.* 2020;136(19):2103–2117. doi:10.1182/blood.2020005221.
67. Leung JC. Inherited renal diseases. *Curr Pediatr Rev.* 2014;10(2):95–100. doi:10.2174/157339631002140513101755.
68. Cramer MT, Guay-Woodford LM. Cystic kidney disease: a primer. *Adv Chronic Kidney Dis.* 2015;22(4):297–305. doi:10.1053/j.ackd.2015.04.001.
69. Mehta L, Jim B. Hereditary renal diseases. *Semin Nephrol.* 2017;37(4):354–361. doi:10.1016/j.semnephrol.2017.05.007.
70. Kashtan CE. Alport syndrome: achieving early diagnosis and treatment. *Am J Kidney Dis.* 2021;77(2):272–279. doi:10.1053/j.ajkd.2020.03.026.
71. Warady BA, Agarwal R, Bangalore S, et al. Alport syndrome classification and management. *Kidney Med.* 2020;2(5):639–649. doi:10.1016/j.xkme.2020.05.014.
72. Eckardt K-U, Alper SL, Antignac C, et al. Autosomal dominant tubulointerstitial kidney disease: diagnosis, classification, and management—a KDIGO consensus report. *Kidney Int.* 2015;88(4):676–683. doi:10.1038/ki.2015.28.
73. Olinger E, Hofmann P, Kidd K, et al. Clinical and genetic spectra of autosomal dominant tubulointerstitial kidney disease due to mutations in UMOD and MUC1. *Kidney Int.* 2020;98(3):717–731. doi:10.1016/j.kint.2020.04.038.
74. Aronow ME, Wiley HE, Gaudric A, et al. Von Hippel-Lindau disease: update on pathogenesis and systemic aspects. *Retina.* 2019;39(12):2243–2253. doi:10.1097/IAE.0000000000002555.
75. Adamiok-Ostrowska A, Piekiełko-Witkowska A. Ciliary genes in renal cystic diseases. *Cells.* 2020;9(4):907. doi:10.3390/cells9040907.
76. Nair N, Chakraborty R, Mahajan Z, Sharma A, Sethi SK, Raina R. Renal manifestations of tuberous sclerosis complex. *J Kidney Cancer VHL.* 2020;7(3):5–19. doi:10.15586/jkcvhl.2020.131.
77. Wang KH, Kupa J, Duffy KA, Kalish JM. Diagnosis and management of Beckwith-Wiedemann syndrome. *Front Pediatr.* 2020;7:562. doi:10.3389/fped.2019.00562.
78. Srivastava S, Molinari E, Raman S, Sayer JA. Many genes—one disease? Genetics of hephronophthisis (NPHP) and NPHP-associated disorders. *Front Pediatr.* 2018;5:287. doi:10.3389/fped.2017.00287.
79. McConnachie DJ, Stow JL, Mallett AJ. Ciliopathies and the kidney: a review. *Am J Kidney Dis.* 2021;77(3):410–419. doi:10.1053/j.ajkd.2020.08.012.
80. Michaud M, Mauhin W, Belmatoug N, et al. When and how to diagnose Fabry disease in clinical practice. *Am J Med Sci.* 2020;360(6):641–649. doi:10.1016/j.amjms.2020.07.011.
81. Miller JJ, Kanack AJ, Dahms NM. Progress in the understanding and treatment of Fabry disease. *Biochim Biophys Acta Gen Subj.* 2020;1864(1):129437. doi:10.1016/j.bbagen.2019.129437.
82. van der Veen SJ, Hollak CEM, van Kuilenburg ABP, Langeveld M. Developments in the treatment of Fabry disease. *J Inherit Metab Dis.* 2020;43(5):908–921. doi:10.1002/jimd.12228.

CHAPTER 11

Chronic Kidney Disease

Robert Stephen Brown ■ Alexander Goldfarb-Rumyantzev ■ Jeffrey H. William

11.1 KDIGO Stages of Chronic Kidney Disease[1]

The 2012 Kidney Disease: Improving Global Outcomes (KDIGO) guidelines provide significant updates from the original 2002 Kidney Disease Outcomes Quality Initiative (KDOQI) guidelines[2] in order to add the recognized risk of albuminuria to estimated glomerular filtration rate (eGFR) in staging the severity of chronic kidney disease (CKD).

11.1.1 CURRENT CKD NOMENCLATURE USED BY KDIGO

"CKD is defined as abnormalities of kidney structure or function, present for >3 months, with implications for health, and CKD is classified based on cause, GFR category, and albuminuria category" as shown below.

Prognosis of CKD by GFR and albuminuria categories: KDIGO 2012			Persistent albuminuria categories Description and range		
			A1	A2	A3
			Normal to mildly increased	Moderately increased	Severely increased
			<30 mg/g <3 mg/mmol	30–300 mg/g 3–30 mg/mmol	>300 mg/g >3 mg/mmol
GFR categories (mL/min/1.73m²)	G1	Normal or high	≥90		
	G2	Mildly decreased	60–89		
	G3a	Mildly to moderately decreased	45–59		
	G3b	Moderately to severely decreased	30–44		
	G4	Severely decreased	15–29		
	G5	Kidney failure	<15		

Green: low risk (if no other markers of kidney disease, no CKD); Yellow: moderately increased risk; Orange: high risk; Red: very high risk.

KDIGO 2012 Clinical Practice Guideline for the Evaluation and Management of Chronic Kidney Disease.

KDIGO "recommends referral to specialist kidney care services for people with CKD" in the following circumstances:
- Acute kidney injury (AKI) or abrupt sustained fall in glomerular filtration rate (GFR)
- GFR <30 mL/min/1.73 m² or GFR categories G4 to G5
- A consistent finding of significant albuminuria (albumin to creatinine ratio [ACR] > 300 mg/g [>30 mg/mmol] or albumin excretion rate [AER] > 300 mg/24 hours, approximately equivalent to protein to creatinine ratio [PCR] >500 mg/g [>50 mg/mmol] or protein excretion rate [PER] >500 mg/24 hr)

- Progression of CKD, defined based on one or both of the following:
  - A drop in GFR category (e.g., from G1 to G2) accompanied by a 25% or greater drop in eGFR from baseline
  - A sustained decline in eGFR of more than 5 mL/min/1.73 m²
- Urinary red cell casts, RBC >20/hpf sustained and not readily explained
- CKD and hypertension (HTN) refractory to treatment with four or more antihypertensive agents
- Persistent abnormalities of serum potassium
- Recurrent or extensive nephrolithiasis
- Hereditary kidney disease

KDIGO "recommends timely referral for planning renal replacement therapy (RRT) in people with progressive CKD in whom the risk of kidney failure within 1 year is 10% to 20% or higher, as determined by validated risk prediction tools" as shown below.

		Referral to Specialist Services		Persistent albuminuria categories Description and range		
				A1	A2	A3
				Normal to mildly increased	Moderately increased	Severely increased
				<30 mg/g <3 mg/mmol	30–300 mg/g 3–30 mg/mmol	>300 mg/g >3 mg/mmol
GFR categories (mL/min/1.73m²) Description and range	G1	Normal or high	≥ 90		Monitor	Refer*
	G2	Mildly decreased	60–89		Monitor	Refer*
	G3a	Mildly to moderately decreased	45–59	Monitor	Monitor	Refer*
	G3b	Moderately to severely decreased	30–44	Monitor	Monitor	Refer*
	G4	Severely decreased	15–29	Refer*	Refer*	Refer*
	G5	Kidney failure	<15	Refer*	Refer*	Refer*

Referral decision-making by GFR and albuminuria. *Referring clinicians may wish to discuss with their nephrology service depending on local arrangements regarding monitoring or referring.

11.2 Equations to Calculate eGFR Based on Serum Creatinine[3,4]

For over 50 years, the Cockcroft-Gault equation was used to estimate creatinine clearance (CrCl) as a surrogate for GFR.

Cockcroft-Gault equation (to calculate estimated creatinine clearance)[5]:

$$\mathbf{eC_{Cr}\,(mL\,/\,min)} = \frac{(140 - \text{age})}{\text{Scr}\,(\text{mg}\,/\,\text{dL})} \times \frac{\text{Body weight}\,(\text{kg})}{72} \times (0.85\,\text{if female})$$

where age is expressed in years, SCr in mg/dL, and weight in kg. The original formula used actual weight. Today, ideal body weight (IBW) is usually used because of erroneously high results in obese persons.

The Cockcroft-Gault equation is still used for some pharmacological dosing purposes, but has been largely replaced by one of the Modification of Diet in Renal Disease (MDRD) eGFR equations or its updated form, the CKD-EPI equation, which is more accurate and doesn't require body weight.

MDRD eGFR equation[6]:

$$\mathbf{eGFR} = 175 \times (\text{SCr})^{-1.154} \times \text{age}^{-0.203} \times (0.742,\,\text{if female}) \times (1.212\,\text{if Black})$$

where age is expressed in years, SCr in mg/dL, and weight in kg.

The MDRD GFR is an estimate of the GFR using serum creatinine (SCr) and demographic factors. It has not been studied extensively in populations that are not White or Black, while relying on a stable Cr. This estimate may be less accurate for GFR values above 60.

Chronic Kidney Disease Epidemiology Collaboration (CKD-EPI) equation[7]:

$$\textbf{eGFR} = 141 \times \min\left(SCr/\kappa, 1\right)^{\alpha} \times \max\left(SCr/\kappa, 1\right)^{-1.209} \times 0.993^{Age} \times 1.018$$
$$\left[\text{if female}\right] \times 1.159 \left[\text{if Black}\right]$$

where SCr is serum creatinine, κ is 0.7 for females and 0.9 for males, α is −0.329 for females and −0.411 for males, min indicates the minimum of SCr/κ or 1, and max indicates the maximum of SCr/κ or 1.

11.3 Additional Equations to Calculate eGFR (Based on Serum Cystatin C Alone or Creatinine + Cystatin C)[8]

Since studies indicate that serum levels of cystatin C may offer a better estimate of eGFR and of adverse outcomes than Cr, a CKD-EPI-cystatin C formula was developed and is as follows:

$$\textbf{eGFR} = 133 \times \min\left(Scys/0.8, 1\right)^{-0.499} \times \max\left(Scys/0.8, 1\right)^{-1.328} \times 0.996^{age}$$
$$\left[\times 0.932 \text{ if female}\right]$$

where Scys is serum cystatin C, min indicates the minimum of SCr/0.8 or 1, and max indicates the maximum of Scys/0.8 or 1.

Combining both serum markers, Cr and cystatin C, into a single CKD-EPI creatinine-cystatin C equation as shown below, appears to offer still better accuracy:

$$\textbf{eGFR} = 135 \times \min\left(SCr/\kappa, 1\right)^{\alpha} \times \max\left(SCr/\kappa, 1\right)^{-0.601} \times \min\left(Scys/0.8, 1\right)^{-0.375}$$
$$\times \max\left(Scys/0.8, 1\right)^{-0.711} \times 0.995^{age} \left[\times 0.969 \text{ if female}\right] \left[\times 1.08 \text{ if Black}\right]$$

where SCr is serum creatinine, Scys is serum cystatin C, κ is 0.7 for females and 0.9 for males, α is −0.248 for females and −0.207 for males, min indicates the minimum of SCr/κ or 1, and max indicates the maximum of SCr/κ or 1.

NB: Since the formulae shown above aren't easy to use in practice, calculators are available online (e.g., https://www.kidney.org/professionals/kdoqi/gfr_calculator) and in the form of mobile devices. Furthermore, recent practice has often eliminated the use of the "Black race correction factor" and the authors advise using the updated "retrofit"equations without the race variable as described below in "11.6 Controversies about the use of 'race' in the estimation of GFR".

11.4 Problems With Using eGFR

1. Creatinine, a product of the metabolism of creatine and phosphocreatine in skeletal muscle, is not specific to kidney function. Serum creatinine will be increased due to higher production in younger individuals with more muscle mass, and in males compared to females, and will depend on dietary intake (e.g., lower in vegetarians).
2. In addition to glomerular filtration, creatinine has some renal tubular secretion. Certain medications can decrease tubular secretion and increase serum creatinine (e.g., trimethoprim, cimetidine). Some other medications may increase creatinine measurement (e.g.,

flucytosine, cephalosporins, and perhaps tenofovir), while others may decrease it (e.g., methyldopa, ethamsylate).

3. Creatinine assay is not consistent between various laboratories and needs to be calibrated.
4. The estimating equations perform poorly in numerous patient populations, including the very old and very young, normal renal function and very low renal function, very large and very small individuals, and many kidney transplant recipients.

11.5 Comparison of Methods to Measure or Estimate GFR

	Advantages	Problems/Disadvantages
Creatinine clearance based on 24-hour urine collection	Easy to do, as creatinine is an endogenous product	Inaccurate collection by patient may underestimate or overestimate GFR Clearance is often overestimated because of tubular secretion of creatinine
Mean of urea and creatinine clearance based on 24-hour urine collection	Might be more accurate than creatinine clearance, especially in advanced renal insufficiency	Same problem as above
Cystatin C (serum measurement)	A protein from all nucleated cells which undergoes glomerular filtration with reabsorption and catabolism by renal tubular cells	High variability of serum level between patients; is increased in malignancy, HIV, and steroid therapy
Inulin clearance	Gold standard (a 5200-dalton polymer of fructose)	Inulin is difficult to measure and a time-consuming, expensive method
Radioisotopic methods[9] (e.g., 99mTc-labeled diethylenetriaminepentaacetic acid [DTPA], 51Cr-EDTA, 125I-iothalamate)	Accurate and easy to perform	Not readily available and requires infusion of the radionuclide and radioactive precautions; material is expensive, cannot be used in pregnancy, and is less accurate in advanced renal failure
Radiocontrast agents (e.g., iothalamate, diatrizoate, iohexol)	Accurate and easy to perform	Requires infusion of the contrast agent

11.6 Controversies About the Use of Race in the Estimation of GFR[10]

While the field of nephrology has utilized these estimating equations for GFR over the past few decades, the use of the "Black race correction factor" in these formulae has come under increasing scrutiny. A specially convened task force was formed in 2020 by representatives from the National Kidney Foundation and the American Society of Nephrology to address the mounting evidence of disparities in health and healthcare delivery within Black communities. Many have advocated for the removal of this correction factor as it may adversely affect access to care and kidney transplantation in these communities. Large hospital systems across the country have eliminated it from their laboratory reports, but this practice has not been consistent or standardized across all U.S. laboratories.

While research for new biomarkers takes place, the task force has made the following two recommendations: "1) …immediate implementation of the CKD-EPI creatinine equation refit (CKD-EPIcr_R) without the race variable in all laboratories in the United States because it does not include race in the calculation and reporting, and …has acceptable performance characteristics and potential consequences that do not disproportionately affect any one group of individuals. 2) increased, routine, and timely use of cystatin C, especially to confirm eGFR in adults who are at risk for or have chronic kidney disease, because combining filtration markers (creatinine and cystatin C, i.e., CKD-EPIcr- cys_R) is more accurate and would support better clinical decisions than either one marker alone."[11]

These two non–race-based "refit" formulae are as follows:

1. **CKD - EPIcr_R** $= 142 \times \min \left(SCr/\kappa, 1\right)^{\alpha} \times \max \left(SCr/\kappa, 1\right)^{-1.200} \times 0.9938^{age} \times 1.012 \left[\text{if female}\right]$
    where SCr is serum creatinine in mg/dL, κ is 0.7 for females and 0.9 for males, age is in years, α is −0.241 for females and −0.302 for males, age is in years, min indicates the minimum of SCr/κ or 1, and max indicates the maximum of SCr/κ or 1[11]

2. **CKD - EPIcr - cys_R** $= 135 \times \min \left(SCr/\kappa, 1\right)^{\alpha} \times \max \left(SCr/\kappa, 1\right)^{-0.544} \times \min \left(Scys/0.8, 1\right)^{-0.323}$
    $$\times \max \left(Scys/0.8, 1\right)^{-0.788} \times 0.995^{age} \times 0.963 \left[\text{if female}\right],$$

where SCr is serum creatinine in mg/dL, Scys is serum cystatin C in mg/L, κ is 0.7 for females and 0.9 for males, α is −0.219 for females and −0.144 for males, age is in years, min indicates the minimum of SCr/κ or 1, and max indicates the maximum of SCr/κ or 1[12]

We advise the routine use of formula 1 above, as it is more accurate overall for all races than the initial CKD-EPI equation, and the use of formula 2 with both Cr and cystatin C for greater accuracy in certain situations. These can be easily utilized with online calculators (https://www.kidney.org/professionals/kdoqi/gfr_calculator)

11.7 Aging Kidney[13–19]

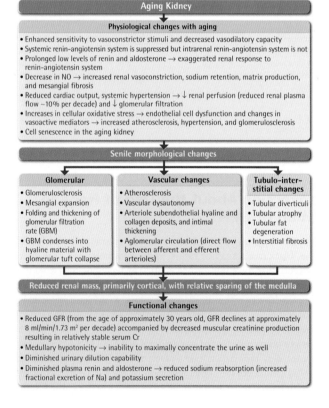

11.7.1 DIFFERENCES BETWEEN A KIDNEY AGING NORMALLY AND A KIDNEY WITH CKD

Based on age-related eGFR below 60 mL/min/1.73 m^2 using an eGFR formula, many healthy elderly are diagnosed with CKD, but actually have normal aging of their kidneys and would not be expected to reach end-stage kidney disease (ESKD) over their lifetime.[17-19] Following are notable factors to suggest that this group of older adults have normal kidney function:

- Proximal tubular function is preserved;
- Serum erythropoietin and hemoglobin levels are normal;
- Urea reabsorption is decreased and serum urea level is normal, whereas it is increased in CKD;
- Calcium, magnesium, phosphate, parathyroid hormone (PTH), and vitamin D levels are normal;
- Urinalysis is normal (no hematuria or proteinuria, however ↓ urinary Cr excretion in the elderly leads to an elevated urine ACR); and
- Preserved renal reserve (the capacity of the kidney to increase its basal GFR by at least 20% after an adequate stimulus such as a protein load), although the magnitude is decreased.

11.8 Management of Patients With CKD/ESKD

- Treat the underlying disease (i.e., control of diabetes, immunosuppression of systemic lupus erythematosus [SLE]).
- Control hypertension (HTN). Targets are controversial in CKD/ESKD, as a subgroup in a SPRINT trial did not show as much benefit with blood pressure (BP) <120/80. However, current evidence and KDIGO advise that an office-measured systolic BP goal is <120 mmHg.[20,21]
- Use renin-angiotensin-aldosterone inhibition or angiotensin receptor blockers for individuals with proteinuria (see Chapter 14).
- Use sodium-glucose co-transporter-2 inhibitors (SGLT-2i), which have been shown to decrease proteinuria, slow the progression of CKD, and lower the risk of ESKD and death from renal causes in patients with or without type 2 diabetes (this could be considered first-line treatment in patients with diabetic nephropathy and type 2 diabetes).[22,23]
- Treat patients with CKD and type 2 diabetes with finerenone (a nonsteroidal selective mineralocorticoid receptor antagonist). Such treatment has resulted in lower risks of CKD progression and cardiovascular events.[24]
- In patients with anemia, address the need for erythropoiesis (EPO) stimulating agents such as epoetin, iron, and additional workup.
- Treat metabolic bone disease with control of calcium, phosphate, PTH, and vitamin D levels. In the future, measurements of FGF-23 and Klotho may become clinically pertinent also.
- Assess nutrition (albumin, prealbumin, vitamins). Consider protein restriction of 0.8 mg/kg/day.
- Measure volume status: sodium restriction ± diuretic use to avoid hypervolemia.[25]
- Assess acid-base state (i.e., bicarbonate supplementation for metabolic acidosis).
- Restrict potassium as needed to avoid hyperkalemia.
- Control lipids to prevent increased risk of CV disease.
- Adjust medications for decreased GFR (e.g., consider stopping metformin) and avoid potential nephrotoxins (e.g., nonsteroidal antiinflammatory drugs [NSAIDs]).

- Monitor potential for preemptive transplantation. Refer when GFR is <20 mL/min/1.73 m^2.
- Provide options counseling for renal replacement modality (i.e., home-based modalities vs. in-center hemodialysis).
- Offer vascular access when hemodialysis is elected. Establish access when GFR <20 mL/min/1.73 m^2, or serum Cr >4 mg/dL, or dialysis is anticipated within 6 months.

Dialysis and renal transplant management are discussed in Chapters 12 and 13.

11.9 Anemia in Chronic Kidney Disease[26,27]

11.9.1 WORKUP

Initiate anemia workup:
- Hemoglobin (Hb) <11 g/dL or hematocrit (Hct) <33% in premenopausal women and prepubertal patients
- Hb <12 g/dL or Hct <37% in adult men and postmenopausal women

Initial workup of anemia in CKD:
- Hb/Hct.
- Red blood cell (RBC) indices, particularly mean corpuscular volume (MCV).
- Reticulocyte count and corrected reticulocytes (i.e., what reticulocyte % would be if patient was not anemic) = (Hct ÷ 45) × %reticulocyte count.
- Iron studies:
  - Serum iron (reflects iron immediately available for Hb synthesis); measured serum iron = iron bound to transferrin
  - Transferrin = total iron binding capacity (TIBC), either of which can be measured directly or calculated from the other
  - Percent transferrin saturation (TSAT; reflects iron immediately available for Hb synthesis)
- Calculate TSAT = (Iron/TIBC) × 100. TSAT indicates how many transferrin binding sites are occupied by iron. TSAT <20% suggests iron deficiency:
  - Serum ferritin (reflects iron stores: normal is 40–200 ng/mL; <15 ng/mL makes iron deficiency most likely; a rise to >100 ng/mL is suggestive of a response to iron supplementation)
  - Hepcidin (not measured clinically) is increased in inflammatory states such as CKD, interferes with intestinal iron uptake and utilization
- Stool for occult blood.
- Vitamin B_{12} and folate.
- If no other cause for anemia is found and SCr is >2 mg/dL, anemia is more likely to be secondary to CKD and relative EPO deficiency.

11.9.2 CAUSES OF ANEMIA

The following diagram shows potential causes of anemia. It is applicable not only to patients with CKD, but to patients with normal kidney function as well. It is important to remember that CKD patients may have anemia due to factors unrelated to CKD itself, such as blood loss or hemolysis (as mentioned above). Although EPO deficiency is a primary cause of anemia in patients with ESKD, a lot of other physiological factors can interfere with EPO, such as iron deficiency, inflammation and infection, elevated hepcidin levels, vitamin deficiency, protein malnutrition, hyperparathyroidism, malignancies, and hematological disorders.

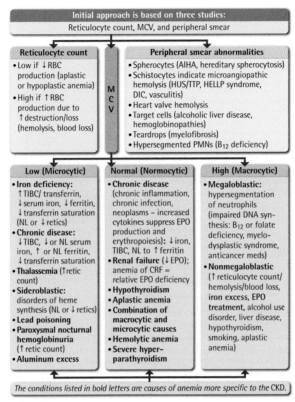

Initial approach is based on three studies:
Reticulocyte count, MCV, and peripheral smear

Reticulocyte count
- Low if ↓RBC production (aplastic or hypoplastic anemia)
- High if ↑RBC production due to ↑destruction/loss (hemolysis, blood loss)

MCV

Peripheral smear abnormalities
- Spherocytes (AIHA, hereditary spherocytosis)
- Schistocytes indicate microangiopathic hemolysis (HUS/TTP, HELLP syndrome, DIC, vasculitis)
- Heart valve hemolysis
- Target cells (alcoholic liver disease, hemoglobinopathies)
- Teardrops (myelofibrosis)
- Hypersegmented PMNs (B$_{12}$ deficiency)

Low (Microcytic)
- **Iron deficiency:** ↑TIBC/ transferrin, ↓serum iron, ↓ferritin, ↓transferrin saturation (NL or ↓retics)
- **Chronic disease:** ↓TIBC, ↓or NL serum iron, ↑ or NL ferritin, ↓transferrin saturation
- **Thalassemia** (↑retic count)
- **Sideroblastic:** disorders of heme synthesis (NL or ↓retics)
- **Lead poisoning**
- **Paroxysmal nocturnal hemoglobinuria** (↑retic count)
- **Aluminum excess**

Normal (Normocytic)
- **Chronic disease** (chronic inflammation, chronic infection, neoplasms – increased cytokines suppress EPO production and erythropoiesis): ↓iron, TIBC, NL to ↑ferritin
- **Renal failure** (↓EPO); anemia of CRF = relative EPO deficiency
- **Hypothyroidism**
- **Aplastic anemia**
- **Combination of macrocytic and microcytic causes**
- **Hemolytic anemia**
- **Severe hyper-parathyroidism**

High (Macrocytic)
- **Megaloblastic:** hypersegmentation of neutrophils (impaired DNA synthesis: B$_{12}$ or folate deficiency, myelodysplastic syndrome, anticancer meds)
- **Nonmegaloblastic** (↑reticulocyte count/ hemolysis/blood loss, iron excess, EPO treatment, alcohol use disorder, liver disease, hypothyroidism, smoking, aplastic anemia)

The conditions listed in bold letters are causes of anemia more specific to the CKD.

AIHA, Autoimmune hemolytic anemia; *CRF*, chronic renal failure; *DIC*, disseminated intravascular coagulation; *EPO*, erythropoietin; *HELLP*, hemolysis elevated liver enzymes and low platelets; *HUS/TTP*, hemolytic uremic syndrome/thrombotic thrombocytopenic purpura; *MCV*, mean corpuscular volume; *NL*, normal; *PMNs*, polymorphonuclear neutrophils; *RBC*, red blood cell; *TIBC*, total iron-binding capacity.

11.9.3 DIFFERENTIAL DIAGNOSIS OF CAUSES OF ANEMIA

Differential diagnosis of common causes of anemia in CKD includes iron deficiency, EPO deficiency, and anemia of chronic disease based on iron studies.

	Iron Deficiency	Anemia of CKD	Anemia of Chronic Disease
Iron and TSAT	↓	NL	↓ or NL
TIBC	↑	NL	↓ or NL
Ferritin and bone marrow iron storages	↓	NL	↑ or NL
Treatment	Iron supplement (may require IV iron, if oral is unsuccessful)	EPO	Treat the cause; if untreatable (e.g., HIV/AIDS), administer EPO unless its effect to increase cancer growth is a contraindication

EPO, Erythropoietin; *NL*, normal; *TIBC*, total iron-binding capacity; *TSAT*, transferrin saturation.

11.9.4 TREATMENT OF ANEMIA OF CKD[28–31]

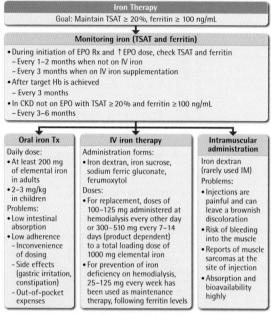

CKD, Chronic kidney disease; *EPO*, erythropoietin; *Hb*, hemoglobin; *IM*, intramuscularly; *IV*, intravenous; *TSAT*, transferrin saturation.

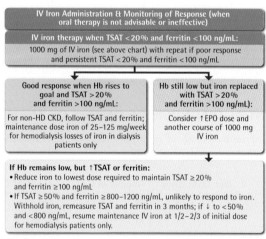

CKD, Chronic kidney disease; *EPO*, erythropoietin; *Hb*, hemoglobin; *HD*, hemodialysis; *TSAT*, transferrin saturation.

11.9.5 ERYTHROPOIESIS STIMULATING AGENTS (ESAs) AND OTHER THERAPIES[29,30]

11.9.5.1 Indications for ESAs (i.e., EPO therapy)

- Anemia associated with CKD with no other cause found and when iron deficiency has been corrected with iron Rx

- Also for treatment of anemia in patients treated with zidovudine for HIV infection and those who are scheduled to undergo elective surgery to reduce the need for blood transfusion

Patients with cancer on chemotherapy require a risk–benefit assessment in the use of EPO due to findings of increased death in those with cancer.

11.9.5.2 Types of ESAs

- Short-acting:
  - EPO
  - Epoetin alfa
  - Epoetin beta
  - Epoetin zeta
- Long-acting:
  - Darbepoetin alfa
  - Methoxy polyethylene glycol-epoetin beta
- Hypoxia- inducible factor prolyl hydroxylase inhibitors (HIF-PHIs)

11.9.5.3 Route of ESA Administration

- Subcutaneous (SC) for predialysis and peritoneal dialysis/home hemodialysis (PD/HHD) patients
- IV for HD patients for comfort (or SC for better dose response)
- Oral for HIF-PHIs (see Section 11.9.5.7 below)

11.9.5.4 If Switching From IV to SC Administration in HD Patients

- If Hb target not yet achieved: SC dose = IV dose
- If at Hb target: SC dose = 2/3 IV dose
- If switching to IV dose = 1.5 SC dose

11.9.5.5 ESA Dosing

- Epoetin (alfa in the United States) SC in adults 80 to 120 U/kg/week (~6000 U/week) in 2–3 doses
- Epoetin (alfa in the United States) IV in HD 120 to 180 U/kg/week (~9000 U/week) in 3 doses
- If failed to ↑Hb by 0.5 to 1.0 g/dL over 2 to 4 weeks, increase EPO dose by 50%.
- If Hb ↑ by >1.5 g/dL per month or if Hb exceeds target, reduce weekly dose by 25% (if rapid responder, stop and restart 1–2 weeks later at 75% of original dose).
- Aim to achieve a target Hb within 2 to 4 months.

11.9.5.6 ESA Controversy[31–34]

- No benefit (CREATE study) and possible cardiovascular harm (CHOIR study) of Hb target >12 g/dL (outcome: composite death and cardiovascular events)
- No event-free survival benefit to having an Hb level of 12.5 g/dL over 10.6 g/dL, but more strokes and more cancer deaths in a subset of patients with previous malignancy, and more venous and arterial thromboses (TREAT study)
- Risk for mortality is the same for an Hb level of 10.0 g/dL up to 12.0 g/dL (DOPPS study)

11.9.5.7 HIF-PHIs: A Novel Therapy for Anemia of CKD[35–37]

Hypoxic inducible factor-prolyl hydroxylase inhibitors (HIF-PHIs) are the newest oral agents studied in both the CKD and dialysis populations for treating anemia of CKD. The awardees of the 2019 Nobel Prize in Physiology or Medicine demonstrated the biological underpinnings of the hypoxia inducible factor pathway (HIF-1), which is responsible for gene regulation in response to low circulating oxygen levels. HIF-PHIs stabilize HIF, which then stimulates endogenous erythropoietin production, increasing hemoglobin levels in patients with CKD. Given the controversies with ESA therapies described above, the HIF-PHI candidates have gained more attention as a potential alternative therapy for anemia in CKD.

Roxadustat and vadadustat have garnered the most attention due to the publication of the most recent studies, meeting prespecified noninferiority criteria for hemoglobin concentration increases (compared to placebo or darbepoetin), with favorable changes in iron profiles and hepcidin levels. Their cardiovascular safety profiles will require further study, as there has been some signal of harm. While multiple HIF-PHIs have gained regulatory approval in Europe and Japan, daprodustat is the only HIF-PHI to achieve United States Food and Drug Administration (FDA) approval, though at this time only for use in the dialysis-dependent patients.[37A,37B,37C]

11.10 Mineral and Bone Disease in CKD[38]

Mineral and bone disease in CKD usually refers to the complex multisystem disorder that involves imbalance of calcium and phosphate, metabolic acidosis, parathyroid dysfunction, vitamin D deficiency, renal osteodystrophy, and vascular calcification. Here, we focus on three aspects that receive most of the attention in clinical practice of nephrology and largely overlap: controlling hyperphosphatemia, hyperparathyroidism, and renal osteodystrophy.

11.10.1 CELLULAR COMPONENTS OF THE BONE AND THEIR REGULATION

Osteoblasts

Function

Derived from mesenchymal stem cells, osteoblasts produce collagen and noncollagen proteins on the bone surface to create a structure for mineralization (matrix). Some of the osteoblasts are buried in the matrix and become osteocytes, and some become lining cells that line most trabecular bone surfaces and separate the bone from marrow space.

Regulation

Osteoblast receptors: For PTH, calcitriol (1,25-dihydroxyvitamin D), glucocorticoids, sex hormones, growth hormone (GH) and thyroid hormone, IL-1, tumor necrosis factor (TNF)-alpha, prostaglandins, insulin-like growth factors (IGFs), transforming growth factor (TGF)-beta, bone morphogenic proteins, fibroblast growth factors, and platelet-derived growth factor. Factors produced by osteoblasts that probably act locally include prostaglandins, IL-6, IGFs and their binding proteins (IGF-BPs), TGF-beta, bone morphogenic proteins, fibroblast growth factors, platelet-derived growth factor, and vascular-endothelial growth factor.

Osteoclasts

Function

- Related to monocyte/macrophage cells, osteoclasts resorb bone by dissolving mineral and degrading matrix
- Excessive osteoclastic resorption occurs in osteoporosis, Paget's disease hyperparathyroidism, and inflammatory bone loss
- Inadequate resorption causes osteopetrosis

Regulation

- Many hormones and local factors can also act on osteoblasts to promote or inhibit osteoclastogenesis
- Stimulators: Calcitriol, PTH, TNF-alpha, prostaglandin E2, IL-1, IL-11, and IL-6
- Inhibitors are IL-4, IL-13, interferon (IFN)-gamma, and denosumab, a human IgG2 monoclonal antibody medication that attaches to and blocks the receptor activator of NF-κβ ligand (RANKL), thus causing inhibition of osteoclast formation, survival, and activity.

11.10.2 CALCIUM–PHOSPHATE METABOLISM IN CKD

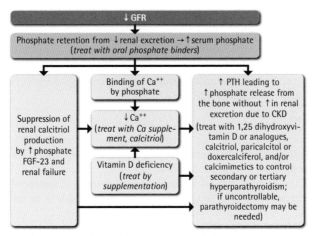

CKD, Chronic kidney disease; FGF-23, fibroblast growth factor-23
PTH, parathyroid hormone.

11.10.3 ROLE OF HYPERPHOSPHATEMIA IN CKD BONE DISEASE, PROGRESSION, AND COMORBIDITIES[39,40]

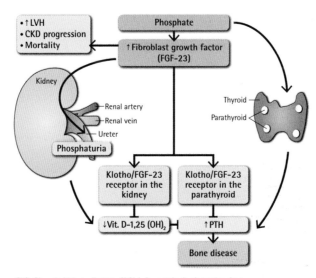

CKD, Chronic kidney disease; LVH, left ventricular hypertrophy;
PTH, parathyroid hormone.

11.10.4 ROLE OF FGF-23 AND KLOTHO

11.10.4.1 FGF-23

FGF-23 is a bone-derived hormone responsible for regulating phosphate balance through increased urinary phosphate excretion and inhibition of 1,25 dihydroxy-vitamin D synthesis. Concentrations of FGF-23 increase early in CKD and rise significantly throughout CKD progression. While helping to ameliorate hyperphosphatemia in early CKD, the contribution of FGF-23 to decreasing concentrations of 1,25 dihydroxy-vitamin D may implicate this hormone as a key pathogenetic factor in the development of secondary hyperparathyroidism.[41]

More recent studies have also shown that increased concentrations of FGF-23 are independently associated with cardiovascular disease (CVD) events, including left ventricular hypertrophy. This may be mediated by both abnormal calcium signaling in cardiac myocytes and upregulation of the renin-angiotensin-aldosterone system (RAAS).[42,43]

11.10.4.2 Klotho

Klotho is a transmembrane protein that functions as a coreceptor for FGF-23 and directly promotes the degradation of the sodium-phosphate cotransporters (NaPi2a) in the proximal tubule, leading to increased urinary phosphate excretion. The most common causes of Klotho deficiency are AKI and CKD. Potential clinical applications include early diagnosis of AKI/CKD and prognosis of AKI recovery or CKD progression, but reliable biomarkers are not yet available.[44]

11.10.5 CAUSES OF HIGH PTH LEVELS

- Hypocalcemia
- Decreased calcitriol activity
- Decreased sensitivity to Ca^{++} by parathyroid calcium-sensing receptor
- Hyperphosphatemia
- Skeletal resistance to the calcemic action of PTH
- Metabolic acidosis
- May develop autonomous tertiary hyperparathyroidism

11.10.6 FORMS OF HYPERPARATHYROIDISM

Type of Hyperparathyroidism	Mechanism
Primary: Adenoma (85%), hyperplasia (15%), or carcinoma (<1%) of the parathyroid glands	Primary elevated PTH production
Secondary: Hyperplasia or adenomatous hyperplasia	Elevated PTH secondary to other factors (low Ca^{++} levels, vitamin D deficiency, renal failure) causing ↑ PTH
Tertiary: Development of autonomous (hypercalcemic) hyperparathyroidism after a period of secondary (normocalcemic or hypocalcemic) hyperparathyroidism with an underlying cause such as malabsorption syndrome or chronic renal failure	After long-standing secondary hyperparathyroidism (because of prolonged overstimulation of parathyroid gland; may develop adenoma or adenomatous hyperplasia, now with persistent elevated Ca^{++})
Pseudohyperparathyroidism	Elevated PTH with resistance in end organs, causing hypocalcemia

PTH, Parathyroid hormone.

11.10.7 THERAPEUTIC OPTIONS FOR SECONDARY HYPERPARATHYROIDISM[45–47]

11.10.7.1 Phosphate Binders

- When eGFR is <25 mL/min, most patients require limitation of phosphate intake and oral phosphate binders to maintain serum phosphate below a normal level of 4.5 mg/dL or ≤5.5 mg/dL in severe CKD or ESKD patients.

- Calcium salts (less expensive, but risk of hypercalcemia, calciphylaxis, and vascular calcification; e.g., calcium carbonate [acetate, carbonate, citrate]): Start with one or two 500-mg pills with each meal; usually require 5–15 g/day). Hypercalcemia (serum Ca >10.2 mg/dL) is a side effect, which can be corrected by lowering dialysate Ca to 2.5 mEq/L or less.
- Calcium-free binders (sevelamer, lanthanum carbonate) reduce phosphate without increasing Ca level, but do not significantly reduce PTH.
- Aluminum-containing compounds: Cause accumulation in brain and bone, but may use for brief courses (e.g., <1 month) if calcium times phosphate (Ca × phos) solubility product >65.
- Mg containing antacids: May induce hypermagnesemia and cause diarrhea
- Iron-based binders[48]:
  - Ferric citrate: Provides additional iron for those with anemia of CKD, citrate may facilitate increased aluminum absorption
  - Sucroferric oxyhydroxide: Similar efficacy to sevelamer, but lower pill burden

11.10.7.2 Vitamin D and Vitamin D Analogues (Activate Vitamin D Receptor of Parathyroid)

- Calcitriol, paricalcitol, doxercalciferol, alfacalcidol, 22-oxacalcitriol
- Risk: Hypercalcemia, hyperphosphatemia, excessive suppression of PTH
- Should not be used in hypercalcemia or hyperphosphatemia (when total Ca × phos solubility product >70); will increase intestinal absorption of Ca and phos, exacerbating Ca × phos solubility product and possibly leading to extraskeletal calcification or calciphylaxis (calcific uremic arteriolopathy)
- For PTH suppression: Goal is to decrease PTH to 2 to 3 times normal (to about 150–300 pg/mL in stage 5 CKD) to decrease risk of osteitis fibrosa, yet not induce adynamic bone osteodystrophy
- Vitamin D analogues (e.g., paricalcitol), selective for PTH receptors, might affect intestinal receptors and Ca/phos absorption to a lesser extent than calcitriol, lessening rise of serum Ca and phos

11.10.7.3 Calcimimetics

- Activate/upregulate Ca-sensing receptor of parathyroid (e.g., cinacalcet orally or etelcalcetide by IV)
- May inhibit parathyroid hyperplasia
- Side effect: Hypocalcemia (managed with dose adjustment or vitamin D administration)

11.10.7.4 Bisphosphonates

- Limit the high rate of bone resorption as a bridge to more definitive treatment of secondary hyperparathyroidism or as a treatment for osteoporosis. Should be used selectively and with caution when eGFR <30 mL/min.

11.10.7.5 Parathyroidectomy

- Indicated for severe hyperparathyroidism, when medical treatment has failed.

11.11.7.6 Other Methods to Consider

- Percutaneous ethanol injected into the parathyroid to ↓PTH
- Correct metabolic acidosis to decrease bone resorption
- Estrogen supplements for osteoporosis (has risk of increased thrombosis)
- Denosumab was found to be effective to increase bone mineral density in dialysis and non-dialysis patients[49]

11.10.8 INDICATIONS FOR PARATHYROIDECTOMY

Uncontrolled levels of PTH + hypercalcemia + complications:

- Osteitis fibrosa
- Extraskeletal calcification
- Calciphylaxis (calcific uremic arteriolopathy)
- Persistent serum Ca >11.5 mg/dL
- Persistent uncontrollable hyperphosphatemia
- Skeletal pain or fractures
- Intractable pruritus

Effects of parathyroidectomy:

- Lower PTH
- Lower serum Ca
- Improved osteitis bone disease
- Resorption of extraskeletal calcifications
- Improved anemia
- Improved BP control
- May improve intractable pruritus

11.10.9 RENAL OSTEODYSTROPHY

High Turnover Bone Disease (↑ PTH)	Low Turnover Bone Disease (↓ PTH)
Osteitis fibrosa: ↑ osteoclast number, size, and activity; ↑ bone resorption, marrow fibrosis; ↑ osteoblastic activity; deposition of collagen is less ordered; ↑ rate of bone formation; and ↑ unmineralized bone matrix (osteoid)	• Osteomalacia: Reductions in bone turnover and number of bone-forming and bone-resorbing cells, and increase in osteoid formation and volume of unmineralized bone (rate of mineralization is slower than collagen synthesis). **Causes**: Vitamin D deficiency, aluminum intoxication, long-standing metabolic acidosis • Adynamic/aplastic bone lesions: Reduced bone turnover, no increase in osteoid formation (↓ mineralization, but normal amount of osteoid). **Causes**: Aluminum deposition (in a minority of cases), oversuppression of PTH, calcitriol (may directly suppress osteoblastic activity), use of oral Ca carbonate

11.10.10 OSTEOPOROSIS MANAGEMENT IN CKD

Diagnosis

Bone loss in osteoporosis compared with age-matched group (Z-score) and young group (T-score):
- 0 to 1 standard deviation about the mean: normal
- 1 to 2.5 standard deviation below the mean: osteopenia
- >2.5 standard deviation below the mean: osteoporosis

Treatment

Treatment nonspecific for osteoporosis in CKD

- Estrogen replacement
- Calcitonin
- Bisphosphonate (alendronate); use selectively and with caution in patients with CKD
- Denosumab (human monoclonal antibody to decrease osteoclast activity)

Treatment specific for osteoporosis in CKD

- Treat hyperparathyroidism and hyperphosphatemia
- Correct metabolic acidosis
- Encourage exercise, especially balance and weight-bearing

11.11 Uremic Coagulopathy[50,51]

As part of the uremic complications of severe renal failure, patients may develop bleeding. The coagulopathy is associated with diminished platelet adhesion and aggregation which may be manifested by a prolonged bleeding time. Multiple mechanisms related to circulating uremic toxins, anemia, vascular and platelet metabolic abnormalities of arachidonic acid metabolism, and defects in Factor VIII complex and von Willebrand factor activity may play a role in diminished platelet aggregation, fibrinogen, and vascular endothelial binding. Since dialysis only slowly reverses these defects, DDAVP or cryoprecipitate, which elevates Factor VIII and von Willebrand factor, is the mainstay of treatment when bleeding in uremic patients is active or anticipated.

11.11.1 TREATMENT OF UREMIC COAGULOPATHY

Treatment	Peak Action	Duration
DDAVP, 0.3 μg/kg IV in 50 mL over 15 min (or SC)	1 hour	4–8 hours
Cryoprecipitate, 7–10 units IV	2–4 hours	12–24 hours
Conjugated estrogens, 0.6 mg/kg IV or orally daily for 5 days	1–5 days	Up to 14 days
Dialysis	Days	Indefinite
EPO (+ iron as needed) to Hct >30%	Days	Indefinite

EPO, Erythropoietin; *Hct*, hematocrit; *SC*, subcutaneous.

11.12 Nutrition in CKD

11.12.1 ROLE OF LOW-PROTEIN DIET[52]

The role of protein restriction in progression of CKD remains controversial and evidence for use of protein restriction is inconclusive. However, if there is no safety concern regarding potential malnutrition, this maneuver can be implemented, often improving early uremic symptoms such as anorexia. Avoidance of high-protein intake seems beneficial.[53–56] While urea itself is not a toxic compound, it is a marker of other byproducts of protein metabolism that might lead to CKD progression (e.g., asymmetric dimethylargınıne [ADMA]).

11.12.2 NUTRITIONAL NEEDS

	Sufficient Protein Intake	Calorie Intake
Pre-ESKD patients	0.6–0.8 g/kg/day (increase to compensate for urinary protein losses)	35 kcal/kg/day
Adult HD patient	1.2 g/kg/day	35 kcal/kg/day
Adult PD patient	1.3 g/kg/day (needed for peritoneal protein loss)	35 kcal/kg/day

ESKD, End-stage kidney disease; *HD*, hemodialysis; *PD*, peritoneal dialysis.

As CKD progresses, restriction of sodium (<1.5–2 g/day) to prevent volume overload and edema,[25] potassium (<2 g/day) to prevent hyperkalemia (more fully discussed in Chapter 3 and Chapter 4), and phosphate (<800 g/day) is usually desirable to prevent edema/volume overload, hyperkalemia, hyperphosphatemia, hyperparathyroidism, and renal osteodystrophy (discussed above), respectively.

11.12.3 BICARBONATE THERAPY[57–61]

Correcting metabolic acidosis to serum HCO_3 >23 mEq/L with oral sodium bicarbonate 0.5 to 1.0 mEq/kg/day (usually 2.6–5.2 g/day) or sodium citrate 1 mEq/mL (30–60 mL/day, but citrate may enhance gastrointestinal [GI] absorption of aluminum, making it less desirable in severe CKD) helps to slow CKD progression, prevent bone buffering, improve nutritional status, and decrease mortality.

11.12.4 POTASSIUM RESTRICTION[62,63]

Hyperkalemia is common among individuals with CKD, given the decreased ability to excrete the filtered load of potassium in the diet. Additionally, medications that can lead to hyperkalemia are frequently prescribed in the CKD population, including renin-angiotensin-aldosterone inhibitors or aldosterone inhibitors. The treatment for hyperkalemia is discussed in Chapter 4.

Low-potassium diets are increasingly falling out of favor, given the positive health effects of a diet that includes potassium at least until kidney function has decreased to a level that risks hyperkalemia (eGFR approximately <30 mL/min/m²). Healthy, balanced diets, typically with higher amounts of potassium, have been associated with both improved BP and cardiovascular mortality overall in those with HTN.

References

1. Levin A, Stevens PE, Bilous RW, et al. Kidney Disease: Improving Global Outcomes (KDIGO) CKD work group. KDIGO 2012 clinical practice guideline for the evaluation and management of chronic kidney disease. *Kidney Int Suppl.* 2013;3(1):1–150. doi:10.1038/KISUP.2012.73.
2. National Kidney Foundation. K/DOQI clinical practice guidelines for chronic kidney disease: evaluation, classification, and stratification. *Am J Kidney Dis.* 2002;39(2 suppl 1):S1–S266.
3. Botev R, Mallié J-P, Wetzels JFM, Couchoud C, Schück O. The clinician and estimation of glomerular filtration rate by creatinine-based formulas: current limitations and quo vadis. *Clin J Am Soc Nephrol.* 2011;6(4):937–950. doi:10.2215/CJN.09241010.
4. Traynor J, Mactier R, Geddes CC, Fox JG. How to measure renal function in clinical practice. *BMJ.* 2006;333(7571):733–737. doi:10.1136/bmj.38975.390370.7C.
5. Cockcroft DW, Gault MH. Prediction of creatinine clearance from serum creatinine. *Nephron.* 1976;16(1):31–41. doi:10.1159/000180580.
6. Levey AS, Bosch JP, Lewis JB, Greene T, Rogers N, Roth D. A more accurate method to estimate glomerular filtration rate from serum creatinine: a new prediction equation. Modification of diet in renal disease study group. *Ann Intern Med.* 1999;130(6):461–470. doi:10.7326/0003-4819-130-6-199903160-00002.
7. Levey AS, Stevens LA, Schmid CH, et al. A new equation to estimate glomerular filtration rate. *Ann Intern Med.* 2009;150(9):604–612. doi:10.7326/0003-4819-150-9-200905050-00006.
8. Inker LA, Schmid CH, Tighiouart H, et al. Estimating glomerular filtration rate from serum creatinine and cystatin C. *N Engl J Med.* 2012;367(1):20–29. doi:10.1056/NEJMoa1114248.
9. Perrone RD, Steinman TI, Beck GJ, et al. Utility of radioisotopic filtration markers in chronic renal insufficiency: simultaneous comparison of 125I-iothalamate, 169Yb-DTPA, 99mTc-DTPA, and inulin. The modification of diet in renal disease study. *Am J Kidney Dis.* 1990;16(3):224–235. doi:10.1016/s0272-6386(12)81022-5.
10. Delgado C, Baweja M, Burrows NR, et al. Reassessing the inclusion of race in diagnosing kidney diseases: an interim report from the NKF-ASN Task Force. *J Am Soc Nephrol.* 2021;32(6):1305–1317. doi:10.1681/ASN.2021010039.

11. Delgado C, Baweja M, Crews D, et al. A unifying approach for GFR estimation: recommendations of the NKF-ASN Task Force on Reassessing the Inclusion of Race in Diagnosing Kidney Disease. *J Am Soc Nephrol.* 2021;32(12):2994–3015. doi:10.1681/asn.2021070988.

12. Inker LA, Eneanya ND, Coresh J, et al. New creatinine- and cystatin C–based equations to estimate GFR without race. *N Engl J Med.* 2021;385(19):1737–1749. doi:10.1056/nejmoa2102953.

13. Weinstein JR, Anderson S. The aging kidney: physiological changes. *Adv Chronic Kidney Dis.* 2010;17(4):302–307. doi:10.1053/j.ackd.2010.05.002.

14. Musso CG, Oreopoulos DG. Aging and physiological changes of the kidneys including changes in glomerular filtration rate. *Nephron Physiol.* 2011;119(suppl 1):p1–5. doi:10.1159/000328010.

15. Yang H, Fogo AB. Cell senescence in the aging kidney. *J Am Soc Nephrol.* 2010;21(9):1436–1439. doi:10.1681/ASN.2010020205.

16. O'Sullivan ED, Hughes J, Ferenbach DA. Renal aging: causes and consequences. *J Am Soc Nephrol.* 2017;28(2):407–420. doi:10.1681/ASN.2015121308.

17. Delanaye P, Jager KJ, Bökenkamp A, et al. CKD: a call for an age-adapted definition. *J Am Soc Nephrol.* 2019;30(10):1785–1805. doi:10.1681/ASN.2019030238.

18. Liu P, Quinn RR, Lam NN, et al. Accounting for age in the definition of chronic kidney disease. *JAMA Intern Med.* 2021;181(10):1359–1366. doi:10.1001/JAMAINTERNMED.2021.4813.

19. O'Hare AM, Rodriguez RA, Rule AD. Overdiagnosis of chronic kidney disease in older adults—an inconvenient truth. *JAMA Intern Med.* 2021;181(10):1366–1368. doi:10.1001/JAMAINTERNMED 2021.4823.

20. Kidney Disease: Improving Global Outcomes (KDIGO) Blood Pressure Work Group. KDIGO 2021 Clinical Practice Guideline for the Management of Blood Pressure in Chronic Kidney Disease. *Kidney Int.* 2021;99(3S):S1–S87. doi:10.1016/J.KINT.2020.11.003.

21. Zhuo M, Yang D, Goldfarb-Rumyantzev A, Brown RS. The association of SBP with mortality in patients with stage 1–4 chronic kidney disease. *J Hypertens.* 2021;39(11):2250–2257. doi:10.1097/hjh. 0000000000002927.

22. Wright EM. SGLT2 inhibitors: physiology and pharmacology. *Kidney360.* 2021;2(12):2027–2037. doi:10.34067/KID.0002772021.

23. Brown E, Heerspink HJL, Cuthbertson DJ, Wilding JPH. SGLT2 inhibitors and GLP-1 receptor agonists: established and emerging indications. *Lancet.* 2021;398(10296):262–276. doi:10.1016/S0140-6736(21) 00536-5.

24. Bakris GL, Agarwal R, Anker SD, et al. Effect of finerenone on chronic kidney disease outcomes in type 2 diabetes. *N Engl J Med.* 2020;383(23):2219–2229. doi:10.1056/NEJMOA2025845.

25. Mills KT, Chen J, Yang W, et al. Sodium excretion and the risk of cardiovascular disease in patients with chronic kidney disease. *JAMA.* 2016;315(20):2200–2210. doi:10.1001/jama.2016.4447.

26. McMurray JJV, Parfrey PS, Adamson JW, et al. Kidney disease: Improving global outcomes (KDIGO) anemia work group. KDIGO clinical practice guideline for anemia in chronic kidney disease. *Kidney International Supplements* 2012;2(4):279–335. doi:10.1038/kisup.2012.37.

27. Babitt JL, Eisenga MF, Haase VH, et al; Conference Participants. Controversies in optimal anemia management: conclusions from a Kidney Disease: Improving Global Outcomes (KDIGO) Conference. *Kidney Int.* 2021;99(6):1280–1295. doi: 10.1016/j.kint.2021.03.020.

28. Macdougall IC, Bircher AJ, Eckardt K-U, et al. Iron management in chronic kidney disease: conclusions from a "Kidney Disease: Improving Global Outcomes" (KDIGO) Controversies Conference. *Kidney Int.* 2016;89(1):28–39. doi:10.1016/J.KINT.2015.10.002.

29. Drüeke TB, Parfrey PS. Summary of the KDIGO guideline on anemia and comment: reading between the (guide)line(s). *Kidney Int.* 2012;82(9):952–960. doi:10.1038/ki.2012.270.

30. Portolés J, Martín L, Broseta JJ, Cases A. Anemia in chronic kidney disease: from pathophysiology and current treatments, to future agents. *Front Med (Lausanne).* 2021;8:642296. doi:10.3389/FMED.2021. 642296.

31. Babitt JL, Eisenga MF, Haase VH, et al. Controversies in optimal anemia management: conclusions from a Kidney Disease: Improving Global Outcomes (KDIGO) Conference. *Kidney Int.* 2021;99(6): 1280–1295. doi:10.1016/J.KINT.2021.03.020.

32. Drüeke TB, Locatelli F, Clyne N, et al. Normalization of hemoglobin level in patients with chronic kidney disease and anemia. *N Engl J Med.* 2006;355(20):2071–2084. doi:10.1056/NEJMoa062276.

33. Singh AK, Szczech L, Tang KL, et al. Correction of anemia with epoetin alfa in chronic kidney disease. *N Engl J Med*. 2006;355(20):2085–2098. doi:10.1056/NEJMoa065485.

34. Pfeffer MA, Burdmann EA, Chen C-Y, et al. A trial of darbepoetin alfa in type 2 diabetes and chronic kidney disease. *N Engl J Med*. 2009;361(21):2019–2032. doi:10.1056/NEJMoa0907845.

35. Chertow GM, Pergola PE, Farag YMK, et al. Vadadustat in patients with anemia and non–dialysis-dependent CKD. *N Engl J Med*. 2021;384(17):1589–1600. doi:10.1056/NEJMOA2035938.

36. Fishbane S, El-Shahawy MA, Pecoits-Filho R, et al. Roxadustat for treating anemia in patients with CKD not on dialysis: results from a randomized phase 3 study. *J Am Soc Nephrol*. 2021;32(3):737–755. doi:10.1681/ASN.2020081150.

37. Wish JB. Treatment of anemia in kidney disease: beyond erythropoietin. *Kidney Int Rep*. 2021;6(10):2540–2553. doi:10.1016/J.EKIR.2021.05.028.

37A. Singh AK, Carroll K, Perkovic V, et al. Daprodustat for the Treatment of Anemia in Patients Undergoing Dialysis. *N Engl J Med*. 2021;385(25):2325-2335. doi:10.1056/NEJMoa2113379.

37B. Singh AK, Carroll K, McMurray JJV, et al. Daprodustat for the Treatment of Anemia in Patients Not Undergoing Dialysis. *https://doi.org/101056/NEJMoa2113380*. November 2021. doi:10.1056/NEJMOA2113380

37C. Parfrey P. Hypoxia-Inducible Factor Prolyl Hydroxylase Inhibitors for Anemia in CKD. *N Engl J Med*. 2021;385(25):2390-2391. doi:10.1056/NEJMe2117100.

38. KDIGO 2017 Clinical Practice Guideline Update for the Diagnosis, Evaluation, Prevention, and Treatment of Chronic Kidney Disease-Mineral and Bone Disorder (CKD-MBD). 2017. www.kisupplements.org. Accessed September 6, 2021.

39. Kuro-O M. Phosphate and klotho. *Kidney Int Suppl*. 2011;79(121):S20–S23. doi:10.1038/ki.2011.26.

40. Jüppner H. Phosphate and FGF-23. *Kidney Int Suppl*. 2011;79(121):S24–S27. doi:10.1038/ki.2011.27.

41. Gutiérrez OM. Fibroblast growth factor 23 and the last mile. *Clin J Am Soc Nephrol*. 2020;15(9):1355–1357. doi:10.2215/CJN.13631119.

42. Marthi A, Donovan K, Haynes R, et al. Fibroblast growth factor-23 and risks of cardiovascular and noncardiovascular diseases: a meta-analysis. *J Am Soc Nephrol*. 2018;29(7):2015–2027. doi:10.1681/ASN.2017121334.

43. Faul C. Cardiac actions of fibroblast growth factor 23. *Bone*. 2017;100:69–79. doi:10.1016/J.BONE.2016.10.001.

44. Neyra JA, Hu MC, Moe OW. Klotho in clinical nephrology. *Clin J Am Soc Nephrol*. 2020;16(1):162–176. doi:10.2215/CJN.02840320.

45. Cunningham J, Locatelli F, Rodriguez M. Secondary hyperparathyroidism: pathogenesis, disease progression, and therapeutic options. *Clin J Am Soc Nephrol*. 2011;6(4):913–921. doi:10.2215/CJN.06040710.

46. Negri AL, Ureña Torres PA. Iron-based phosphate binders: do they offer advantages over currently available phosphate binders? *Clin Kidney J*. 2015;8(2):161–167. doi:10.1093/ckj/sfu139.

47. Scialla JJ, Kendrick J, Uribarri J, et al. State-of-the-art management of hyperphosphatemia in patients with CKD: an NKF-KDOQI controversies perspective. *Am J Kidney Dis*. 2021;77(1):132–141. doi:10.1053/j.ajkd.2020.05.025.

48. Negri AL, Spivacow FR, Del Valle EE, Forrester M, Rosende G, Pinduli I. Role of overweight and obesity on the urinary excretion of promoters and inhibitors of stone formation in stone formers. *Urol Res*. 2008;36(6):303–307. doi:10.1007/s00240-008-0161-5.

49. Kunizawa K, Hiramatsu R, Hoshino J, et al. Denosumab for dialysis patients with osteoporosis: A cohort study. *Sci Rep*. 2020;10:2496. doi:10.1038/s41598-020-59143-8.

50. Jubelirer SJ. Hemostatic abnormalities in renal disease. *Am J Kidney Dis*. 1985;5(5):219–225. doi:10.1016/s0272-6386(85)80112-8.

51. Molino D, De Lucia D, Gaspare De Santo N. Coagulation disorders in uremia. *Semin Nephrol*. 2006;26(1):46–51. doi:10.1016/j.semnephrol.2005.06.011.

52. Kalantar-Zadeh K, Jafar TH, Nitsch D, Neuen BL, Perkovic V. Chronic kidney disease. *Lancet*. 2021;398(10302):786–802. doi:10.1016/S0140-6736(21)00519-5.

53. Molina P, Gavela E, Vizcaíno B, Huarte E, Carrero JJ. Optimizing diet to slow CKD progression. *Front Med (Lausanne)*. 2021;8:654250. doi:10.3389/FMED.2021.654250.

54. Hahn D, Hodson EM, Fouque D. Low protein diets for non-diabetic adults with chronic kidney disease. *Cochrane Database Syst Rev*. 2020;10(10):CD001892. doi:10.1002/14651858.CD001892.pub5.

55. Rhee CM, Ahmadi SF, Kovesdy CP, Kalantar-Zadeh K. Low-protein diet for conservative management of chronic kidney disease: a systematic review and meta-analysis of controlled trials. *J Cachexia Sarcopenia Muscle.* 2018;9(2):235–245. doi:10.1002/JCSM.12264.

56. Yan B, Su X, Xu B, Qiao X, Wang L. Effect of diet protein restriction on progression of chronic kidney disease: a systematic review and meta-analysis. *PLoS One.* 2018;13(11). doi:10.1371/JOURNAL.PONE.0206134.

57. Goraya N, Simoni J, Jo C-H, Wesson DE. Treatment of metabolic acidosis in patients with stage 3 chronic kidney disease with fruits and vegetables or oral bicarbonate reduces urine angiotensinogen and preserves glomerular filtration rate. *Kidney Int.* 2014;86(5):1031–1038. doi:10.1038/ki.2014.83.

58. de Brito-Ashurst I, Varagunam M, Raftery MJ, Yaqoob MM. Bicarbonate supplementation slows progression of CKD and improves nutritional status. *J Am Soc Nephrol.* 2009;20(9):2075–2084. doi:10.1681/ASN.2008111205.

59. Kittiskulnam P, Srijaruneruang S, Chulakadabba A, et al. Impact of serum bicarbonate levels on muscle mass and kidney function in pre-dialysis chronic kidney disease patients. *Am J Nephrol.* 2020;51(1):24–34. doi:10.1159/000504557.

60. Raphael KL. Metabolic acidosis in CKD: core curriculum 2019. *Am J Kidney Dis.* 2019;74(2):263–275. doi:10.1053/J.AJKD.2019.01.036.

61. Madias NE. Metabolic acidosis and CKD progression. *Clin J Am Soc Nephrol.* 2021;16(2):310–312. doi:10.2215/CJN.07990520.

62. Aburto NJ, Hanson S, Gutierrez H, Hooper L, Elliott P, Cappuccio FP. Effect of increased potassium intake on cardiovascular risk factors and disease: systematic review and meta-analyses. *BMJ.* 2013;346:f1378. doi:10.1136/bmj.f1378.

63. Lemann JJ, Pleuss JA, Gray RW, Hoffmann RG. Potassium administration reduces and potassium deprivation increases urinary calcium excretion in healthy adults [corrected]. *Kidney Int.* 1991;39(5):973–983. doi:10.1038/ki.1991.123.

CHAPTER 12

Kidney Replacement Therapy: Dialysis

Mark E. Williams ▨ Alexander Goldfarb-Rumyantzev ▨ Robert Stephen Brown

12.1 Indications for Acute/Chronic Dialysis

Treatment options for both end-stage kidney disease (ESKD) and acute kidney injury (AKI) include extracorporeal hemodialysis-based options, and peritoneal dialysis (PD).[1] Important elements in the decision to initiate dialysis include interpreting the signs and symptoms of uremic syndrome (Table 12.1).

Assessment should include the specific indication(s) for initiating dialysis, the appropriateness of initiating dialysis as opposed to conservative management, the best method of dialysis, and the appropriate timing of initiation of dialysis.[2–4]

In some cases, the initiation should be done on a trial basis, leaving open the possibility of later withdrawing the patient from dialysis support. An increasingly popular strategy in the chronic setting is active conservative chronic kidney disease (CKD) management, to forestall the need for dialysis. In addition, withholding of dialysis is increasingly a part of the nephrologist's evaluation in the AKI or ESKD setting.[5,6] Examples include patients with profound, irreversible neurological impairment, terminal illness, inability to cooperate with the procedure, and those with markedly impaired functional status.[2] Such a decision requires appropriate input from the patient/healthcare proxy/family members, including the option for them to pursue a second opinion.

TABLE 12.1 ■ **Symptoms and Signs of the Uremic Syndrome**

Symptoms
- Poor appetite, weight loss
- Diminished taste
- Pruritus
- Muscle cramps
- Fatigue
- Nausea/vomiting
- Cold intolerance
- Sleep disturbance
- Impaired cognition

Signs
- Hypervolemia, edema, congestive heart failure
- Neuropathy
- Pericarditis
- Encephalopathy, confusion, seizures
- Coagulopathy, bleeding

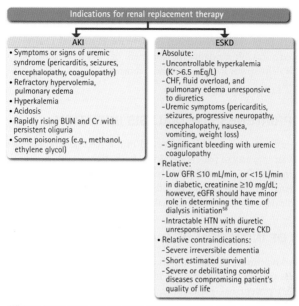

AKI, Acute kidney injury; BUN, blood urea nitrogen; CHF, congestive heart failure; CKD, chronic kidney disease; Cr, creatinine; eGFR, estimated glomerular filtration rate; ESKD, end-stage kidney disease; HTN, hypertension.

Figure 12.1   Indications for renal replacement therapy.

12.1.1 INDICATIONS FOR DIALYSIS INITIATION

Several indications for initiating dialysis are common, and they are similar in acute or chronic renal failure: to alleviate symptoms or signs of uremia, correct abnormalities of electrolyte or acid-base balance, or reverse uncontrolled hypervolemia (Figure 12.1).

Dialysis may be started in severe acute renal failure when no quick recovery is expected, to avoid "impending uremia." Typical indications for initiating renal replacement therapy (RRT) are related to hyperkalemia, acidemia, volume overload, and symptomatic azotemia.

12.2 Dialysis Modalities for Acute Kidney Injury

Guidelines state that intermittent hemodialysis (IHD) and continuous renal replacement therapy (CRRT) are complementary therapies, with no clear superiority of one over the other (PD is currently rarely used for AKI). In a recent meta-analysis of 21 studies comparing clinical outcomes among critically ill adults with AKI treated with CRRT, IHD, or sustained low efficiency dialysis (SLED), for example, no modality had a distinct advantage.[7] For clinically stable AKI patients, IHD is the standard modality. For more compromised patients in the intensive care unit (ICU) in whom either hemodialysis (HD) or CRRT is a consideration, continuous therapies do not appear to result in superior key outcomes such as patient survival, ICU length of stay, or ventilator days.[8]

Meta-analyses have compared outcomes without an overall survival benefit to either modality. Several, but not all, analyses of observational data have shown a higher rate of nonrecovery from AKI among survivors treated with IHD.[9] Conventional HD may be assumed to be contraindicated in severely compromised ICU patients (e.g., those with hypotensive circulatory failure, for whom CRRT is the standard modality). In patients with acute brain injury or fulminant hepatic failure, better preservation of cerebral perfusion may be achieved with CRRT.

Recent guidelines from the International Society for Peritoneal Dialysis suggested that PD should be considered a suitable modality for treatment of AKI in all settings,[10] citing studies that demonstrated equivalent survival and possibly a shorter need for RRT with PD compared to other modalities.[11,12]

12.2.1 APPROPRIATENESS OF DIALYSIS INITIATION

Whether or not to offer dialysis must be addressed in the AKI patient, just as it is in the ESKD patient. While the vast majority of patients could undergo dialysis with current technology, feasibility must first be addressed. The potential for dialysis recovery should be evaluated. Advance directives must be accommodated. The patient must be informed about the procedure and potential outcomes, including the possible dependence on chronic dialysis.[13] Professional guidelines should be reviewed.[14]

12.2.2 TIMING OF INITIATION OF DIALYSIS IN AKI

The evidence regarding timing of dialysis initiation in sick patients with AKI remains relatively weak, and guidelines remain nonspecific.[15] It is generally accepted that dialysis is urgently indicated when the AKI patient has pericarditis, altered mental status, seizures, severe metabolic derangements, uncontrollable symptomatic hypervolemia, or treatable intoxications.

When the case to initiate dialysis is less compelling, considerations may include the likelihood of recovery and the risks of doing dialysis. Elective initiation of dialysis for AKI may be required when symptoms or laboratory derangements are less severe. Multiple clinical trials have compared an early initiation approach when there is no specific indication, with a delayed approach (i.e., initiating when relevant but nonsevere signs or symptoms) have developed.

In recent years, a few randomized controlled trials have attempted to resolve the issue of initiation of dialysis for AKI with mixed results (Table 12.2).[16]

Two randomized controlled trials have recently reported data on the timing of RRT in critically ill patients with AKI, while demonstrating the difficulties of such trials. In the Artificial Kidney Initiation in Kidney Injury (AKIKI)[17] multicenter trial from France, 620 patients were initiated either "early" (KDIGO stage 3) or "late" (KDIGO stage 3 and clinical indications), to determine whether late dialysis initiation improved mortality risk. There was no difference in the primary outcome of 60-day all-cause mortality. Importantly, however, half of patients randomized to late initiation did not receive RRT, either recovering kidney function or dying. Nonetheless, a post-hoc analysis indicated that, for patients in the late-start group actually treated with RRT, mortality was higher in comparison with the early group.

In the Standard Versus Accelerated Initiation of Renal-Replacement Therapy in Acute Kidney Injury (STARRT-AKI) trial,[18] the most definitive study to date, over 3000 AKI patients without a specific indication for dialysis were randomized. Dialysis was initiated in most of the early-initiation patients, but only about two-thirds of the late-initiation patients. Adverse events, continued dialysis dependence, and rehospitalization, but not mortality, were higher in the early-initiation group. In the AKIKI-2 trial, critically ill AKI patients were allowed to be more azotemic before randomization to early or late strategies, with mixed results.[19]

The single-site Early Versus Late Initiation of KRT in Critically Ill Patients With AKI (ELAIN) trial in Germany[20] compared early (KDIGO AKI stage 2) with late (KDIGO AKI stage 3). To diminish the likelihood that enrollees would actually recover kidney function and not need dialysis, clinical AKI criteria were combined with levels of the biomarker NGAL. In the late group, only 5% recovered from AKI without needing dialysis. The early group had a lower 90-day all-cause mortality; the ELAIN trial is the only recent randomized trial to demonstrate mortality benefit.

TABLE 12.2 ■ Comparison of Recent Randomized Clinical Trials of Timing of KRT in AKI

Variable[a]	ELAIN (N = 231)	AKIKI (N = 620)	IDEAL-ICU (N = 488)	STARRT-AKI (N = 3019)
Study design	Single-center RCT	Multicenter RCT	Multicenter RCT	Multicenter multinational RCT
Early group	Within 8 hr of stage 2 AKI and NGAL > 150 ng/mL; median: 6 hr	Within 6 hr of stage 3 AKI; median: 2 hr	Within 12 hr of stage 3 AKI; median: 7.6 hr	Within 12 hr of stage 2 or 3 AKI; median: 6.1 hr
Delayed/standard group (time from eligibility)	Within 12 hr of stage 3 AKI or clinical indication; median: 25.5 hr	After 72 hr in stage 3 AKI or clinical indication; median: 57 hr	After 48 hr in stage 3 AKI or clinical indication; median: 51.5 hr	After 72 hr in AKI or clinical indication; median: 31.1 hr
Key exclusions	eGFR < 30	Severe lab abnormalities	Emergent need for dialysis	eGFR < 20
KRT protocol	Prescribed protocol using CVVHDF	Discretion of site providers, guideline based	Discretion of site providers, guideline based	Recommendations provided based on guidelines
Primary outcome	90-day mortality: 39.3% vs. 54.7% (P = 0.03)	60-day mortality: 48.5% vs. 49.7% (P = 0.79)	90-day mortality: 57.7% vs. 53.8% (P = 0.38)	90-day mortality: 43.9% vs. 43.7%; RR, 1.00 (95% CI, 0.93–1.09)
Proportion not requiring KRT	0% vs. 9.2%	1.9% vs. 49.0%	2.8% vs. 38.4%	3.2% vs. 38.2%
Dialysis dependence (among survivors)	At 90 days: 13.4% vs. 15.1% (P = 0.80)	At 60 days: 1.9% vs. 5.2% (P = 0.12)	At 90 days: 2.0% vs. 2.7% (P = 1.00)	At 90 days: 10.4% vs. 6.0%; RR, 1.74 (95% CI, 1.24–2.43)
Adverse events	No significant differences	CRBSIs: 10.0% vs. 5.2%; P = 0.03	Hyperkalemia: 0% vs. 4.1%; P = 0.03	Any: 23.0% vs. 16.5% (P < 0.001); no difference in serious adverse events

[a]All comparisons are early versus delayed/standard groups.

AKI, Acute kidney injury; CI, confidence interval; CRBSIs, catheter-related bloodstream infections; CVVHDF, continuous veno-venous hemodiafiltration; eGFR, estimated glomerular filtration (in mL/min/1.73 m²); KRT, kidney replacement therapy; NGAL, neutrophil gelatinase-associated lipocalin; RCT, randomized controlled trial; RR, relative risk. (Table 1.[16])

Few studies have examined initiation of dialysis for AKI in specific settings. For elective initiation of dialysis in cases of AKI after major abdominal surgery, there is a suggestion that early initiation of dialysis might be beneficial to patient mortality.[21]

Finally, a recent meta-analysis showed that mortality did not differ significantly according to whether dialysis was initiated early or delayed in AKI, and suggested initiation only when a specific clinical indication emerges as an acceptable approach.[22]

Taken together, these studies have diminished enthusiasm for aggressive initiation of dialysis for AKI in the absence of a compelling indication.

12.2.3 WITHDRAWAL FROM DIALYSIS

The principal justification for dialysis is to improve quality of life and to prolong life. However, dialysis in vulnerable patients may be associated with deteriorating physical function, increasing dependence, and deteriorating quality of life. Withdrawal from dialysis may then be appropriately discussed with the patient and family, with emphasis placed on symptom control and addressing end-of-life goals.[13]

12.2.4 RECOVERY FROM AKI

The dialysis- or CRRT-dependent AKI patient should be monitored for recovery of kidney function, but the optimal strategy and timing for actually weaning from dialysis remain uncertain.[23]

The obvious clinical clues include increase in urine output (UO) before dialysis (usually detected in the interdialytic interval), slowed postdialytic rise in creatinine (Cr), or a functional test such as responsiveness to diuretics. In the future, renal biomarkers may be shown to be independent predictors of recovery.

12.2.5 ADEQUACY OF CONVENTIONAL HEMODIALYSIS IN AKI

Assessment of adequacy of IHD is conventionally based on urea kinetic modeling. In the chronic setting, a calculated single-pool Kt/V urea of 1.2 is accepted as the minimal goal for adequate dialysis. Kt/V (urea) (the fractional urea clearance) is regarded as the most clinically valid small-solute measure of dialysis dose at the current time. It is a biochemical outcome measure. Kt/V (urea) refers to clearance of urea in a given time period (Kt = clearance × time), individualized to patient size, with this calculation based on the patient's total body water volume (V) as estimated from the patient's weight, leading to the expression Kt/V. In the setting of AKI, however, the volume of distribution of urea may be highly variable. Kidney Disease: Improving Global Outcomes (KDIGO) guidelines recommend delivering a Kt/V of 3.9 per week for IHD.[24] The Veterans Adminstration/National Institutes of Health (VA/NIH) ATN study[25] randomized patients to receive either intensive or less intensive dialysis; for those on intermittent dialysis, the less intensive group were treated 3 times per week, and the more intensive group 6 times per week. Intensive renal support did not improve outcomes. The best evidence, such as from the Acute Renal Failure Trial Network (ATN) Study (VA/NIH), suggests that patients with dialysis-dependent AKI should receive at least 3 HD treatments per week, each with a delivered Kt/V value of 1.2. A simpler approach may be to target a urea reduction ratio (URR = [predialysis BUN—postdialysis BUN] / predialysis BUN) of >0.67.[26]

12.2.6 CONTINUOUS RENAL REPLACEMENT THERAPY

The choice of renal replacement modality is commonly determined by the patient's hemodynamic status. However, CRRT for AKI in gradually undergoing a paradigm shift beyond just those patients too unstable to tolerate conventional HD, to becoming the treatment of choice for all with multiorgan failure.[27] CRRT is an ICU-based therapy intended to be applied on a continuous but short-term basis.

CRRT is the preferred dialysis modality in patients with AKI and hemodynamic instability.[28] A typical indication for CRRT is the need for RRT (fluid overload, uremia, uncorrectable acidosis, hyperkalemia, some intoxications) in a hemodynamically unstable patient. It may also have advantages for the AKI patient with increased intracranial pressure,[29] severe hypo/hypernatremia,[30] or drug intoxications. Typical indications for CRRT are shown in Table 12.3.

There are multiple CRRT options, as shown below in Table 12.4.

Most CRRT is done by continuous veno-venous hemofiltration (CVVH), rather than continuous arterio-venous hemofiltration (CAVH), as CVVH without dialysis or with concomitant dialysis, through a process called continuous veno-venous hemodialysis or hemodiafiltration (CVVHD). Balanced hemofiltration and dialysis with larger volumes of hemofiltration and large volumes of replacement fluid, together with dialysis, can be achieved with CVVHDF (also known as continuous hemodiafiltration) when the hemofiltration rate is set at 20% and the effluent target ranges from 20 to 35 mL/kg/hr. They should be viewed as complementary therapies for the AKI/ESKD population.

CRRT offers several advantages over intermittent HD in critically ill patients: greater hemodynamic stability, increased fluid removal, and continuous solute (uremic toxins, electrolytes) control.[31] CRRT clearance is based on a combination of diffusion (dialysis), convection (ultrafiltration), and to a lesser degree, adsorption by the membrane. It is similar to clearance by intermittent dialysis, although less efficient per unit time.

Compared to HD, blood flow is slower, the throughput of fluid (i.e., administered and removed) is much larger than for HD, and the dialysate rate is slower. Because filter clearance for small solutes is equal to the product of the total effluent (i.e., postfilter fluid) amount and

---

TABLE 12.3 ■ Typical Indications for CRRT

- Oliguria with hypotension
- AKI/ESKD with fluid overload
- Cardiogenic shock with pulmonary edema
- AKI/ESKD with acute brain injury
- ARDS
- Severe sepsis
- Refractory congestive heart failure

AKI, Acute kidney injury; *ARDS*, acute respiratory distress syndrome; *CRRT*, continuous renal replacement therapy; *ESKD*, end-stage kidney disease.

TABLE 12.4 ■ CRRT Options

Option	Clearance	Dialysis	Replacement	UF Goals	Clearance
SCUF	Convection	No	No	Modest	Low
CVVH	Convection	No	Yes	Large	Medium
CVVHD	Convection and diffusion	Yes	No	Modest	Higher
CVVHDF	Convection and diffusion	Yes	Yes	Large	Highest

CRRT, Continuous renal replacement therapy; *CVVH*, continuous veno-venous hemofiltration; *CVVHD*, continuous veno-venous hemodialysis; *CVVHDF*, continuous veno-venous hemodiafiltration; *SCUF*, slow continuous ultrafiltration; *UF*, ultrafiltration.

TABLE 12.5 ■ Examples of Available Substitution Fluid and Dialysate Solutions in the United States for CRRT by Manufacturer

	GAMBRO (BAXTER)		NXSTAGE	B. BRAUN
	[a]PrismaSol BGK/B22K/BK	[b]PrismaSATE3 BGK/B22K/BK	[b]RFP 400–456	[b]Duosol 4551– 4556
Na+, mEq/L	140	140	130–140	140–136
K+, mEq/L	0–4	0–2–4	0–4	0–4
Cl−, mEq/L	108–113	108–120.5	108.5–120.5	109–117
Lactate, mEq/L	3	3	0	0
Bicarbonate, mEq/L	22–32	22–32	25–35	35–25
Ca++, mEq/L	0–2.5–3.5	0–2.5–3.5	0–3	3–0
Mg+, mEq/L	1.0–1.2–1.5	1.0–1.2–1.5	1–1.5	1–1.5
Dextrose, g/dL	0–1	0–1.1	1	1–0

[a]Substitution fluid.
[b]Dialysate solutions.
CRRT, Continuous renal replacement therapy.
From Macedo E, Mehta RL. Continuous dialysis therapies: core curriculum 2016. Am J Kidney Dis. 2016 Oct;68(4):645–657. doi:10.1053/j.ajkd.2016.03.427.

the concentration of solute in that effluent is relative to plasma (i.e., the sieving coefficient)—which reaches 1 for small solutes—clearance adequacy can be measured as actual solute removal. Adequacy is therefore determined by the total effluent fluid rate (replacement fluid, dialysate, net fluid removal), which is recommended to be 25 mL/kg body weight per hour.

The fluids utilized for replacement and dialysate are premixed, sterile, and free of bacterial endotoxins. Depending on the product, they generally contain calcium, magnesium, sodium, potassium, bicarbonate, lactate, and dextrose. An additional fluid replacement option contains phosphate. A few of the options do not contain dextrose; loss of endogenous glucose in the ultrafiltrate may place some critically ill, catabolic patients at risk for euglycemic ketosis during CRRT.[32] Typical replacement and dialysate solutions are shown in Table 12.5.[27]

A typical order set for CVVHDF would include blood flow rate 100 to 250 mL/min; dialysate flow rate 1000 to 2000 mL/hr; replacement flow rate 1000 to 2000 mL/hr; and ultrafiltration rate 33 to 66 mL/min.[27]

Replacement fluids may be administered pre- or postfilter. Prefilter administration is associated with decreased filter clotting and increased filter lifespan. (The blood pump will usually have its rate increased to compensate for the added fluid and to achieve sufficient clearances.) Postfilter administration is associated with improved solute clearances.

As a motor-driven system involving flow of fluid, key pressure measurements are determined at four points in the CRRT extracorporeal circuit. Abnormal pressure alarms require clinical correlation. Pressures are used to calculate the transmembrane pressure (TMP) and pressure drop from one end of the filter to the other. Pressure measurements that may require troubleshooting are shown in Figure 12.2.

12.2.7 CHARACTERISTIC PRESSURE MEASUREMENTS AND COMMON ABNORMALITIES

■ Access line: Preblood pump; pressure always negative (−50 to −150); high due to catheter clotting, line kinked.

Pressure monitoring

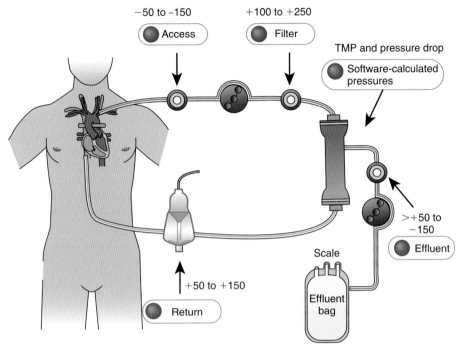

TMP, Transmembrane pressure.

Figure 12.2 The CRRT extracorporeal circuit and typical pressure readings obtained at the points in the circuit shown to determine the status of the dialysis access outflow, the CRRT filter, the effluent collection system, and the dialysis access venous return.

- Filter (prefilter): At postblood pump; always positive (+50 to +150); detects resistance to flow to patient, or clotting.
- Effluent line: Before effluent pump; usually negative but may be positive; −150 to +50; used to calculate TMP.
- Return line: Pressure of return circuit before catheter; high pressure due to catheter clotted/line kinked.

The filtration fraction is the fractional volume of plasma removed from the dialyzed blood in the process of ultrafiltration (i.e., the ratio of the ultrafiltration rate to the plasma flow rate). Filtration fraction is calculated as follows:

12.2.8 FILTRATION FRACTION

- FF(%) = (UFR × 100)/Qp
- where Qp = BFR × (1—hct) = filter plasma flow rate in mL/min (FF, filtration fractio; UFR, ultrafiltration rate; Hct, hematocrit)
- Example: BFR = 100 mL/min
  - Hct = 30%
  - UFR of .21 (21%) = FF 30%

Experts recommend keeping the filtration fraction below 20% to 30% in order to reduce the risk of premature filter clotting.[33] However, there are limitations of using the filtration fraction as an index of risk of hemofilter clotting, including the rate of administration of prefilter replacement fluids. So the use of end-of-hemofilter hematocrit is an alternative, but needs to be validated.

Removal of medications by CRRT, since it is a form of continuous dialysis, may be significant, and may even exceed that of normal kidney function. Multiple citations are available as guides to drug dosing in CRRT.[34]

Some antimicrobial agents do not require dose modification during CRRT (Table 12.6)[34].

CRRT allows for increased volumes of nutritional support but may result in loss of some nutrients.

The CRRT system typically requires anticoagulation, in the form of regional citrate anticoagulation with calcium replacement (Figure 12.3)[27], or, less commonly, systemic or regional heparin anticoagulation (Figure 12.4).

Citrate infused into the arterial port of the circuit chelates calcium, resulting in anticoagulation of the filter. Replacement parenteral calcium is administered separately. Guidelines now advocate citrate anticoagulation as first-line therapy for CRRT.[24] Trisodium citrate is typically administered prefilter at a fixed ratio between blood and citrate infusions. Replacement calcium

---

TABLE 12.6 ■ **Antimicrobials With No Dosage Adjustment in CRRT**

- Amphotericin
- Azithromycin
- Ceftriaxone
- Clindamycin
- Doxycycline
- Linezolid
- Metronidazole
- Micafungin
- Oxacillin
- Rifampin
- Tigecycline
- Voriconazole

CRRT, Continuous renal replacement therapy.
From Thompson AJ. Drug dosing during continuous renal replacement therapies. *J Pediatr Pharmacol Ther.* 2008 Apr;13(2):99–113. doi:10.5863/1551-6776-13.2.99.

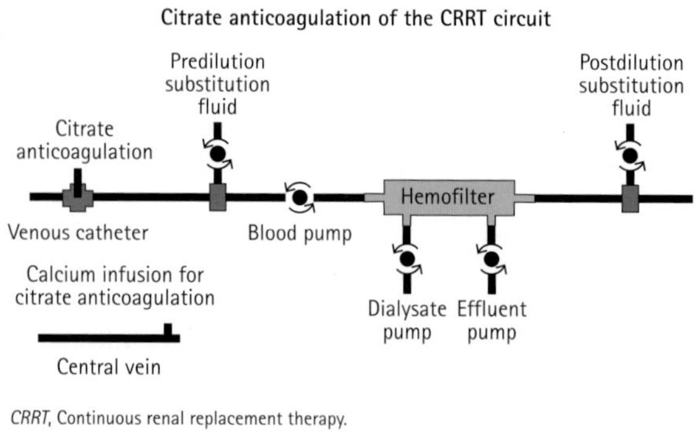

CRRT, Continuous renal replacement therapy.

Figure 12.3 Citrate anticoagulation of the CRRT circuit. (Modified from Macedo E, Mehta RL. Continuous dialysis therapies: core curriculum 2016. *Am J Kidney Dis.* 2016 Oct;68[4]:645–657. doi:10.1053/j.ajkd. 2016.03.427.)

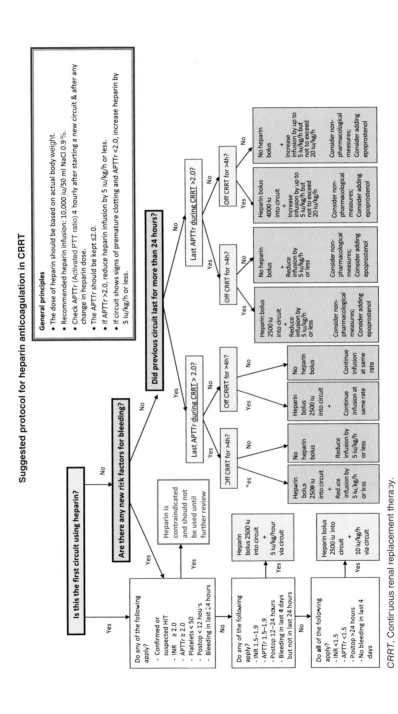

Figure 12.4 Suggested protocol for heparin anticoagulation in CRRT. *HIT*, heparin-induced thrombocytopenia. (From Dickie H, Tovey L, Berry W, Ostermann M. Revised algorithm for heparin anticoagulation during continuous renal replacement therapy. *Crit Care.* 2015 Oct 27;19:376. doi:10.1186/s13054-015-1099-y.)

CRRT, Continuous renal replacement therapy.

TABLE 12.7 ■ Common Complications of CRRT

- Hypotension
- Arrhythmias
- Bleeding
- Citrate intoxication
- Hypothermia
- Underdosing of drugs
- Hypocalcemia
- Hypophosphatemia
- Hypokalemia
- Nutrient losses

CRRT, Continuous renal replacement therapy.

is administered systemically. Dosing protocols for using unfractionated heparin vary widely; a typical approach would be a systemic loading dose of 500 to 1000 IU followed by 500 units hourly, and adjusted according to the activated partial thromboplastin time (Figure 12.4).

The results of a recent large randomized trial comparing anticoagulation strategies for CRRT favored citrate compared to heparin anticoagulation, with greater efficacy (filter lifespan) and safety (lower risk of bleeding complications).[35] Several regional citrate anticoagulation protocols are available.[36] CRRT in COVID-19 patients may be complicated by thromboembolic events and disseminated intravascular coagulation. Frequent clotting of CRRT filters and dialysis catheters in many cases has required both systemic heparin and prefilter citrate anticoagulation as well.[37,38]

From the above description of the CRRT procedure, several complications would be predicted. Common complications are shown in Table 12.7.

CRRT is intensive and complex therapy. Key quality metrics in CRRT commonly used include delivery of adequate dose of dialysis, adequate fluid removal, actual compared to prescribed dialysis dose, filter life, and preventable significant errors. Strategies have been described to bring process-based metrics to quality improvement of CRRT delivery.[39]

Few studies have evaluated strategies for weaning the AKI patient off of CRRT.[40] Clinical considerations should include evidence of impending renal recovery (UO monitoring, improvement in kidney function tests), as well as goals of care. Increased UO before CRRT cessation is a common predictor.

Between CVVH and CVVHDF, there is little evidence to support one modality over the other in the overall CRRT population. Several studies have addressed both renal recovery and mortality outcomes of CRRT relative to HD in AKI, with no consensus.

While no improvement with CVVH in mortality was shown in a meta-analysis, hemofiltration did increase the clearance of medium to larger molecules.[41]

Data on mortality and other outcomes related to the amount of CRRT delivered are limited.[42] The RENAL study assessed CRRT at two levels of intensity in critically ill patients with AKI (replacement): lower (effluent flow of 25 mL/kg/hr) or higher (40 mL/kg/hr).[43] High intensity (35–48 mL/kg/hr) was not associated with benefit in terms of mortality or renal recovery in a meta-analysis.[44]

A summary of basic reminders for the dialysis prescription is shown in Table 12.8.

12.2.9 SUSTAINED LOW-EFFICIENCY DIALYSIS

SLED has been increasingly used recently, related to patient surges exceeding the availability of CRRT machines in the ICU setting. The 2012 KDIGO guidelines for AKI noted that SLED

TABLE 12.8 ■ What the Clinician Needs to Know to Write Orders for CRRT

Pumps:
- Blood flow rate 120–250 (average 180) mL/min.
- UF rate 1–2 L/hr total, but net UF depends on patient volume status and overall goals of treatment.

Replacement fluids:
- If standard commercial replacement fluid is not available, peritoneal dialysis fluid, Ringer's lactate, normal saline, or pharmacy made solutions can be used.

Dialysis fluid:
- The composition of dialysis fluid is selected based on the same principles as for intermittent hemodialysis; peritoneal dialysate solutions are often used, though calcium-free dialysate may be preferable for citrate anticoagulation.

Anticoagulation:
- Systemic heparin or regional citrate anticoagulation.
- Citrate anticoagulation:
  - ACD-A solution of 3% trisodium citrate infused at a rate of 150% in mL/hr of the blood flow rate (Q_B) in mL/min (e.g., 225 mL/hr for a Q_B of 150 mL/min)
  - Ca^{++} infusion rate is calculated based on the principle of giving about 1 mmol of Ca for each mmol of citrate, then adjust infusion rate based on ionized calcium (iCa^{++}) level (e.g., calcium gluconate 20 g in 500 mL D5W at 30 mL/hr with an increase for $iCa^{++} < 1.0$ mmol/L or a decrease for $iCa^{++} > 1.1$ mmol/L).

Parameters to monitor:
- Serum electrolytes, iCa^{++}, Mg^{++} every 12–24 hr.
- For citrate anticoagulation, iCa^{++} every 4 hr initially until stable, then every 6 hr and total calcium every 12 hr to assess for citrate toxicity (by an increasing gap between total and ionized calcium levels).
- Activated clotting time measured at the post-filter maintained between 180 and 200 sec with either heparin or citrate is usually adequate.

CRRT, Continuous renal replacement therapy; *UF*, ultrafiltration.

TABLE 12.9 ■ Suggested SLED Prescription

Blood Flow	Dialysate Flow	Duration	UF Rate	Frequency
150–300 mL/min	100–300 mL/min	6–12 hr	Up to 500 mL/hr	3–6 times per week

SLED, Sustained low efficiency dialysis; *UF*, ultrafiltration.

was suitable for hemodynamically unstable patients, but noted the lack of scientific evidence necessary to support it as a modality alternative to CRRT.[24] At some centers, it is employed as a prolonged therapy instead of CRRT.

The same dialysis machines for intermittent HD are used for SLED; alternatively, CRRT machines may be used for this hybrid therapy. A typical SLED prescription would include blood flow 250 to 300 mL/min, dialysate flow 100 to 300 mL/min, a duration of 6 to 12 hours, fluid removal less than 500 mL/hr, and treatment frequency 3 to 6 times per week. Metabolic clearance goals are achieved in less time than with CRRT. There is less need for anticoagulation than with CRRT (i.e., prefilter heparin 1000 u bolus, then 500 u/hr would be typical). Potential advantages of SLED include faster correction of acidemia, less anticoagulation, and uninterrupted therapy (i.e., CRRT patients have the treatments paused not infrequently for radiology, etc.) so that clearance goals are more likely to be met than with CRRT.

Typical parameters for a SLED prescription are shown in Table 12.9.

SLED and CRRT have demonstrated equivalence in outcomes such as hemodynamic tolerance, fluid removal, ICU stays, renal recovery, pressor requirement, and mortality rates.[45,46]

Practical disadvantages include cost of supplies, limited flow rates, and dependence on dialysis nursing because conventional HD machines are used.

12.2.10 PERITONEAL DIALYSIS FOR AKI

PD should be considered a suitable modality for treatment of AKI. In fact, potential advantages include simplicity, lower cost, gradual solute removal, no need for anticoagulation, better hemodynamic tolerance, and possibly shorter time to renal recovery. Disadvantages may include catheter-related mechanical problems, risk of peritonitis, lack of adequacy in hypercatabolic or hypoperfused patients, undesirable effects on mechanical ventilation, glucose absorption, and protein loss. The main concern of physicians may be inadequate clearances with PD.[47]

Because of insufficient good-quality clinical data, selection of PD for AKI patients needs to be individualized.

Commercially available PD solutions typically contain significant lactate, which may accumulate in critically ill patients or those with liver failure. Emergent placement of PD catheters should be used where resources and expertise exist.[48]

The appropriate dose of PD in the AKI patient remains uncertain. The application of standard urea kinetic modeling has not been validated for use of PD in AKI. Recent guidelines indicate that targeting a weekly Kt/V urea of 3.5 provides outcomes comparable to those of daily HD in critically ill patients.[48]

Recent meta-analyses have shown that PD is not inferior to other extracorporeal therapies in the management of patients with AKI,[47] and additional experience has been gained during the COVID-19 pandemic,[49,50] though the need for prone positioning to improve oxygenation posed a challenge for some COVID-19 patients.

12.3 Dialysis for ESKD

Characteristics of currently available dialysis modalities are shown in Table 12.10. (adapted from Table 1[51]).

TABLE 12.10 ■ Characteristics of Dialysis Modalities

Characteristic	Conventional Hemodialysis	Short Daily Hemodialysis	Nocturnal Hemodialysis	Continuous Ambulatory Peritoneal Dialysis	Automated Peritoneal Dialysis
Location	In-center	In-center or home	In-center or home	At home	At home
Sessions per week	3	5–6	5–6	Daily	Daily
Time per session	4 hr	2–3 hr	6–9 hr	3–5 hr per exchange	8–9 hr at night
Contraindications	No vascular access; CV instability	No vascular access; CV instability; inadequate home support	No vascular access; CV instability; inadequate home support	Abdominal surgeries; nonfunctional membrane; inadequate home support	Abdominal surgeries; nonfunctional membrane; inadequate home support

CV, Cardiovascular.

Conventional HD is by far the most common modality. Compared to the standard 3 weekly in-center treatments, frequent (6 weekly) treatments appear to reduce long-term mortality and benefit select patients.[52] Longer session times appear to improve hospitalization and mortality rates.[53] HD intensification with extended-duration nocturnal treatments modestly improves overall metabolic profiles of uremic toxins[54] but is more effective in clearing small toxins, and studies suggest improved quality of life and patient survival.[55] Results from recent studies have revealed concerns inherent in the 3-times weekly intermittent HD schedule, which obligates one longer, 3-day interdialytic interval each week. These include increased arrhythmias, hospitalizations, and mortality on the day of the dialysis treatment that follows the longer interdialytic interval.[56]

12.3.1 TIMING OF DIALYSIS INITIATION IN ESKD

Older studies established a trend for early initiation of dialysis in ESKD.[57] The definition of early and late was based on the degree of renal dysfunction, measured by creatinine clearance (CrCl) or Cr-based estimated glomerular filtration rate (eGFR). More recently there has been much uncertainty about the timing of chronic dialysis initiation (early vs. late start).

Several studies have found that there is no benefit of early initiation of dialysis, and that it may lead to dialysis of patients who might not require it. Furthermore, there is a suggested benefit of a late start based on symptoms or signs of uremia. The results of the Initiating Dialysis Early and Late (IDEAL) study, the only randomized trial to have tested the impact of dialysis initiation at two different levels of kidney function on outcomes, demonstrated no significant difference in survival or other patient-centered outcomes between treatment groups.[58] Another large retrospective analysis concluded that late initiation of dialysis (classified by eGFR at the time of initiation) was associated with a reduced risk of mortality.[59]

These data have challenged the established paradigm of using estimates of glomerular filtration as the primary guide for initiation of maintenance dialysis and illustrate the compelling need for research to optimize the high-risk transition period from CKD to ESKD. That is, the solute and volume control achievable by dialysis may be offset by the potential risks of dialysis. Risk equations for predicting the time frame to needing maintenance kidney replacement therapy have been developed.[60]

12.3.2 APPROPRIATENESS OF DIALYSIS INITIATION

The appropriateness of starting dialysis in a particular patient applies especially to the chronic setting, and should be based upon two considerations: expected patient survival with or without dialysis, and quality of life.[61,62]

Elderly patients (>80 years) with significant comorbidities might need to be informed that chronic HD may extend life only 2 to 3 months more than conservative medical management without improving quality of life, although that should be decided individually on a case-by-case basis.[63,64]

12.3.3 CONSERVATIVE MANAGEMENT OF THE ESKD PATIENT

Conservative (nondialytic) care of the patient with advanced kidney failure is increasingly recognized as an alternative and appropriate approach for certain patients.[65,66] Key features while attempting to delay late progression of kidney disease include minimizing ESKD complications and improving symptom burden and life satisfaction. Advanced care planning and shared decision-making should be incorporated.

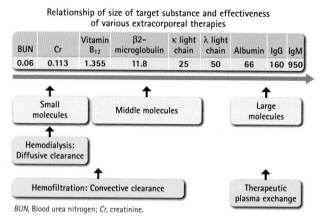

Figure 12.5   Relationship of size of target substance and effectiveness of various extracorporeal therapies.[69]

12.3.4 DIALYSIS MEMBRANES

HD membranes are manufactured with cellulose, modified cellulose, or synthetic polymers.[67] A variety of membrane compositions continue to be tested in order to bring solute removal closer to that of native kidneys.

Dialyzer clearance specifications are determined by the surface area (A) and mass transfer coefficient of a given solute, which is a function of the membrane composition. Ideal features of an HD membrane include nonthrombogenic, selective permeability, biologically compatible, adequate surface area, tight pore size distribution, minimal thickness, and affordability.[68] Noncellulosic membranes are characterized as high flux (i.e., they are better able to remove fluid and moderate-sized molecules).

Solute removal in conventional HD occurs primarily by diffusion. The effectiveness of extracorporeal therapies in general is related to the size of the target substances being removed.[69] While smaller molecules are effectively removed by HD, clearance of "middle molecules" (0.5–60 kD), typically represented by beta2-microglobulin, is less effective (Figure 12.5)[69].

Middle molecules have been associated with inflammation, cardiovascular events (CVEs), and other ESKD comorbidities.[70] Compared to the previous generation of low-flux dialysis membranes, currently used high-flux membranes provide greater clearance of larger solutes. The clinical benefit of even newer "medium cutoff" dialysis membranes, which help remove larger middle molecules with minimal albumin leak, is under investigation.[71] This device has recently received FDA approval in the United States.

Dialysis membrane biocompatibility refers to specific interactions between the dialysis membrane and the patient's blood. The material of the dialysis membrane is the major determinant of the biological response to it.[72] Improved, biocompatible membranes elicit less of an inflammatory response. Synthetic membranes have higher biocompatibility than older cellulosic membranes.

Membrane characteristics are shown in Figure 12.6.

12.3.5 VASCULAR ACCESS FOR HEMODIALYSIS

While the intent of chronic dialysis is to clear uremic toxins from the entire body, quality HD starts with the existence of a reliable access to the patient's vascular system.[73] There are three main

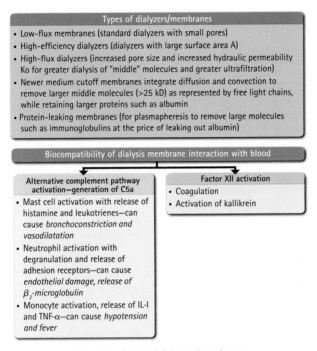

Figure 12.6 Types of dialyzers/membranes.

types of vascular access for HD: arteriovenous fistula (AVF), arteriovenous graft (AVG), and central venous catheter (CVC; tunneled or not). (Note that a "hybrid" access called the Hemodialysis Reliable Outflow [HeRO] involves a graft at one end, typically sutured to the brachial artery, and a tunneled central venous segment at the other end; it is designed to allow bypass of a central venous occlusion). The standard types of dialysis access are described below (Figure 12.7).

The "Fistula First" initiative emphasized the AVF as the optimal vascular access type,[74] while reevaluation of this strategy for all patients has increased awareness that this may not always be the best strategy, such as in elderly patients.[75] HD access should be able to provide a blood flow of at least 300 mL/min. Recent recommendations call for a more patient-focused approach to access planning and management.[76]

12.4 Dialysis Access Planning

Access care decisions involve protocols and an interdisciplinary team but must be individualized in order to determine the best access use for each patient[73,77] since there are advantages and disadvantages of all vascular access types.[78] In recent years, there have been shifts from AVGs to fistulas and from distal to upper arm fistula locations. Patients referred to the nephrologist prior to the need for dialysis are more likely to start dialysis with an AV fistula as their permanent access. Unfortunately, the CVC remains the first access used in as many as 75% of patients initiating dialysis in the United States.

Dialysis access planning begins with educating the patient about the basic types of kidney replacement therapy (HD, PD, transplantation). In patients not certain to choose PD or those unlikely to receive a timely kidney transplant, evaluation for an AVF should be initiated, while at the same time CKD management should continue, and the patient should understand that this does not mean dialysis is imminent.

Patient in need of access for hemodialysis

Types of dialysis access

AVF

An AVF is created by a surgical connection between a native artery and vein, usually in the arm or forearm; the subsequent growth of the venous segment constitutes the AVF. The AVF is the optimal dialysis access as it is associated with the best clinical outcomes ("fistula first"). The likelihood of AVF maturation should be an important consideration for vascular access planning. Failure of successful AVF use by 6 months after creation may be associated with a 50% increase in mortality (although some of the outcome advantage with the AVF may relate to comorbidities that led to lower odds of having an AVF in the first place). The AVF has lower rates of infection, and better long-term survival of the patient and of the access itself. However, it requires sufficient vasculature to create an adequate AVF that will mature and be usable to obtain satisfactory blood flow rates. It takes at least 3–4 weeks for an AVF to mature before being used, and more commonly, longer with many fistulae never maturing adequately. Failure of the AVF to mature results in long-term CVC exposure.

AVG

An AVG requires surgical interposition of graft material between a large artery and vein. An AVG is useful in patients for whom an AVF is not feasible due to poor veins. It provides good blood flow, and because it is internalized, it is less prone to infections than a CVC (but more so than the AVF). The AVG is considered to be inferior to the AVF in terms of patient survival (except in elderly patients with comorbidities). The AVG does not require much time to mature, and early cannulation grafts can often be used immediately or within days of placement.

CVC

A CVC is a double- or triple-lumen large catheter designed for dialysis. Temporary CVCs are not tunneled or cuffed, and are used for short-term acute dialysis. For ESKD, the CVC is a tunneled, cuffed, double-lumen catheter placed into a central vein, usually the internal jugular vein, and terminating near the heart. The CVC remains the first access used in the majority of ESKD patients in the United States. The CVC is considered to be the poorest choice for chronic dialysis access, to be used only after AVF and AVG options are not feasible, if there is no time for AVF/AVG maturation, for patients likely to recover from AKI, or if patient survival is likely to be short. Catheters are associated with poorer patient survival, are often complicated by infection, generally have lower blood flow rates, and are more prone to clotting than AVF/AVG. The benefit of a CVC is that it can be used immediately after placement.

AKI, Acute kidney injury; *AVF*, arteriovenous fistula; *AVG*, arteriovenous graft; *CVC*, central venous catheter; *ESKD*, end-stage kidney disease.

Figure 12.7   Types of dialysis access.

Since fistula maturation (i.e., maturation means the AVF can be cannulated and provide prescribed dialysis) may take at least 1 month, commonly, 3 to 12 months, and may require interventional procedures before use, each patient with progressive and/or an eGFR of 15 to 20 mL/min/1.73 m^2 should therefore begin access planning, including patient education and referral to the access surgery team.[79] (It is important that the patient understand that veins for potential AVF placement should not be used for venipuncture, placement of intravenous catheters, or overlying blood pressure [BP] cuff placement.) Imaging studies to determine the suitability of vessels for AV access creation, such as Doppler ultrasound, may be required.

12.4.1 ACCESS DYSFUNCTION/MONITORING/SURVEILLANCE

Access dysfunction occurs in several ways, most importantly resulting in reduction in access flow (Table 12.11).

TABLE 12.11 ■ **Dysfunction of the Dialysis Fistula/Graft**

- Inadequate dialysis achieved
- Excessive bleeding from needle sites
- Loss of thrill/bruit
- Pseudoaneurysms
- Localized arm swelling
- Inadequate blood flow delivered
- Recirculation (e.g., visible recirculation of saline)
- Arterial "steal" syndrome (i.e., vascular compromise below the access)

TABLE 12.12 ■ **Dialysis Access Surveillance (Clinical Assessment) and Monitoring (Special Testing)**

- Goal is to identify access with high likelihood of stenosis
- Patient education for signs and symptoms of access dysfunction
- Physical exam of pulse and bruit of AVF/AVG for abnormality
- Failure of AVF to collapse when the upper extremity is elevated
- Static venous pressure measurements at dialysis (at blood flow rate (Q^b) 200 mL/min, VP should be <130 mmHg with 15-g needle, <150 mmHg with 16-g needle)
- Recirculation study indicated when blood flow achieved during dialysis or dialysis adequacy (decreased Kt/V) is poor
- Direct Doppler volume blood flow measurements of AVF/AVG
- Angiography if surveillance/monitoring suggest abnormality

AVF, Arteriovenous fistula; *AVG*, arteriovenous graft; *VP*, venous pressure.

Recent guidelines emphasize the primary importance of clinical monitoring strategies such as inspection, palpation, and auscultation in early detection of access dysfunction.

Access recommendations now conclude that evidence supporting technical measures such as access blood flow, pressure monitoring, or imaging for stenosis as surveillance tools is inadequate.[73,80] Likewise, guidelines are not to recommend preemptive angioplasty of fistulas or grafts which have stenosis that is not associated with clinical indicators.

Key features of dialysis access surveillance and monitoring are shown in Table 12.12.

12.5 Hemodialysis Catheters

For both ESKD and (more commonly) AKI requiring urgent HD, the most efficient and achievable access remains the HD catheter. Tunneled dialysis catheters are in fact the most common vascular access used to initiate maintenance dialysis in many patients with ESKD, and may be appropriate in cases of AKI with some likelihood of recovery from longer-term dialysis dependence. The ideal dialysis catheter would deliver adequate blood flow, be resistant to infection and thrombosis, and not cause vascular injury,[81] but currently available catheters are imperfect.

Duration of optimal catheter use to minimize infection risk is shown in Table 12.13.

TABLE 12.13 ■ **Standard Duration of Use for Hemodialysis Catheters**

- Temporary (not tunneled) femoral vein catheters, inserted with sterile technique and meticulously cleaned daily in bedbound patients, can usually be left in place safely for 3–7 days, occasionally longer, but are not suitable for ambulatory patients and may be undesirable in morbidly obese patients.
- Subclavian and internal jugular temporary catheters (not tunneled) may be left in place for 2–4 weeks.
- Silastic/silicone cuffed catheters (tunneled) are suitable for long-term use.

Early complications of catheter insertion are mainly related to insertion, as shown in Table 12.14. Subsequent complications of the HD catheter use are shown in Table 12.15.

An additional management challenge is a poorly functioning catheter. The differential diagnosis may include not only thrombotic occlusion, but also growth of a fibrin sheath, malpositioning of the catheter tip, or kinking of the catheter. Mechanical problems are more common shortly after insertion whereas thrombotic occlusion or fibrin sheath formation is more likely 2 weeks or more after catheter insertion.[82] The approach to malfunction is indicated in Figure 12.8.

Note that evidence does not support the routine use of prophylactic systemic anticoagulation in order to prevent catheter thrombosis episodes.

TABLE 12.14 ■ Complications of Hemodialysis Catheter Insertion

- Arterial, rather than venous, puncture
- Exogenous or subcutaneous hemorrhage
- Hemothorax
- Pneumothorax
- Air embolism
- Atrial and ventricular arrhythmias
- Perforation of central vein or cardiac chamber
- Pericardial tamponade
- Venous thrombosis

TABLE 12.15 ■ Later Complications of Hemodialysis Catheters

- Infection (see more detailed discussion below).
- Clotting of catheter or formation of a fibrin sheath. Minimize by instillation of heparin or tPA following hemodialysis. Unclear role of systemic warfarin or low molecular weight heparin. Treatment: tPA - 2 mg of rtPA into each port. Some cases may require catheter stripping to remove clot and fibrin sheaths that adhere to the catheter, or exchanging the catheter over a guidewire.
- Central vein thrombosis or stricture (30%–40% in subclavian, 2%–10% IJ), which may cause loss of ipsilateral arm use for AVF. KDOQI recommends avoidance of subclavian vein unless no other options exist, or the ipsilateral extremity can no longer be used for permanent dialysis access (AVF or AVG) if occlusion occurs.
- IVC thrombosis with lumbar catheter.
- Arteriovenous fistula formation as rare complication.

AVF, Arteriovenous fistula; *AVG*, arteriovenous graft; *IJ*, internal jugular vein; *IVC*, inferior vena cava; *KDOQI*, Kidney Disease Outcomes Quality Initiative; *rtPA*, recombinant tissue plasminogen activator; *tPA*, tissue plasminogen activator.

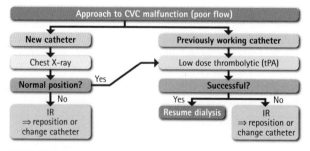

CVC, Central venous catheter; *IR*, interventional radiology; *tPA*, tissue plasminogen activator.

Figure 12.8 Approach to CVC malfunction.

12.6 Hemodialysis Catheter Infections

Prophylaxis: Catheter infection may occur via contamination of external or internal tunneled catheter surfaces. In addition to routine surveillance and monitoring, methods to prevent catheter-related bloodstream infections (CRBSIs) include extraluminal strategies and the use of intraluminal antibiotic lock solutions.[73] The approach to prophylaxis is shown in Table 12.16.

CRBSIs contribute significantly to morbidity and mortality in HD patients.[83] Common risk factors include impaired immune system, skin colonization with *Staphylococcus*, prolonged catheter duration, and a history of prior catheter-related bacteremia episodes.

Blood cultures should be drawn as an initial step to confirm the presence of bloodstream infection. Determination that bacteremia is secondary to the HD catheter is likely when there is obvious infection of the external portion of the catheter by the same organism.

Confirmation that the catheter is the culprit in a bacteremic patient, according to recent guidelines, may also be determined by criteria involving cultures obtained from blood samples through the catheter or directly from the catheter tip (at removal), compared to results from a peripheral venous culture.[73]

There are four main options for CVC management (in addition to systemic antibiotic treatment) in the setting of CRBSI, as shown in Table 12.17.

Immediate empiric catheter removal may be indicated in the presence of high-grade bacteremia, severe sepsis, metastatic infection, or concurrent exit-site/tunnel infection.

Empiric therapy should include both Gram-positive (vancomycin) and Gram-negative (ceftazidime/aminoglycoside) coverage.

Subsequent antibiotic coverage should be based on identification and antibiotic sensitivity of the offending pathogen.[84]

The KDOQI algorithm for CVC-related infection is shown in Figure 12.9.[73]

TABLE 12.16 ■ **Hemodialysis CVC Infection Prophylaxis**

- Using tunneled rather than nontunneled dialysis catheters
- Strict aseptic technique during connection and disconnection procedures
- Exit site and hub care with a chlorhexidine-based solution or alcohol swabs
- Topical triple antibiotic ointment or mupirocin ointment to exit site with each dressing change
- Antimicrobial barrier catheter caps
- Protection of exit site from wet and dirty environments
- Filling the lumen with antibiotic-anticoagulant after dialysis ("antibiotic lock") in high-risk patients (a large number of antibiotic CVC lock solutions are available)

CVC, Central venous catheter.

TABLE 12.17 ■ **Management Options for Catheter-Related Infection**

1. CVC removal with exchange over a guidewire at the same site
2. CVC removal with a new CVC placed at a new site
3. CVC removal with delayed placement of a new CVC
4. Retention of CVC, without or with use of antibiotic lock solution

CVC, Central venous catheter.

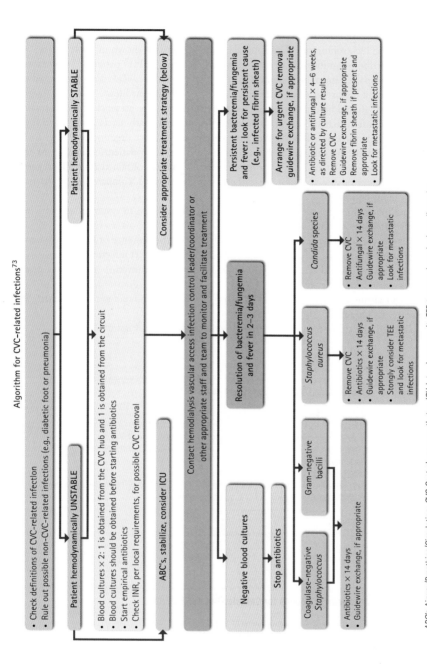

Figure 12.9 Algorithm for CVC-related infections.

ABC's, Airway/Breathing/Circulation; *CVC,* Central venous catheter; *ICU,* intensive care unit; *TEE,* transesophageal echocardiography.

12.7 Anticoagulation in Hemodialysis

Anticoagulation is an important part of the dialysis procedure itself.[85] Most common options for anticoagulation are unfractionated heparin and, less commonly, low molecular weight heparin. While there is no need to adjust dosing of unfractionated heparin in ESKD, dosage reduction is necessary for low molecular weight heparin. Other agents are available when heparin is not an option (e.g., in heparin-induced thrombocytopenia). The pharmacokinetic properties of anticoagulants in the setting of ESKD are shown in Table 12.18.

The need for systemic anticoagulation is also common in ESKD apart from the dialysis procedure. A common example is atrial fibrillation. The proper use of anticoagulation unrelated to the dialysis procedure in ESKD begins with assessment of bleeding risk (Table 12.19).

The site of action of oral anticoagulants in the coagulation cascade is noted in Figure 12.10.[86]

The use of vitamin K antagonists has long been the standard of care in CKD patients at risk for thromboembolic complications, but the risk of bleeding is disproportionately increased.[87] For ESKD patients requiring systemic anticoagulation such as atrial fibrillation, initiation and maintenance of anticoagulation is complex. For example, doses of warfarin required may be 20% lower,

---

TABLE 12.18 ■ **Pharmacokinetic Properties of Anticoagulants in Renal Failure**

Anticoagulant	Chemical Composition	Mechanism	Follow-Up Indicator
Unfractionated heparin	Mixture of glycosaminoglycan chains 5000–30,000 Da; renal excretion 10%	Binds to antithrombin III, inhibits clotting factors IIa and Xa	PTT; anti-Xa heparin assay (therapeutic range 0.3–0.7 U/mL); 1%–5% heparin-induced thrombocytopenia
Low molecular weight heparin	Fragments of larger heparins, 4000–8000 Da; renal excretion 40%	Binds to antithrombin III, inhibits clotting factor Xa	Anti-Xa (therapeutic range 0.5–1.2 U/mL, prophylactic 0.2–0.5 U/mL); 0%–3% heparin-induced thrombocytopenia
Citrate	Citrate 2.4 mEq/L in dialysate acid concentrate or trisodium citrate solution, 3% (ACD-A solution)	Citrate chelates calcium to disrupt the coagulation cascade	Visual inspection for clots in dialysis circuit; ionized calcium (therapeutic <0.4 mmol/L in the dialyzer) or an activated clotting time of 1.5–2.0 times baseline (180–250 sec)

PTT, Partial thromboplastin time.

TABLE 12.19 ■ **Assessing Bleeding Risk During Hemodialysis Anticoagulation**

Serious risk	Moderate risk
Major surgery <72 hr	Already anticoagulated
Active bleeding	Recent tunneled hemodialysis catheter placed
Bleeding diathesis	Pericarditis
Recent intracranial hemorrhage	Minor surgery <72 hr
	Major surgery <7 days

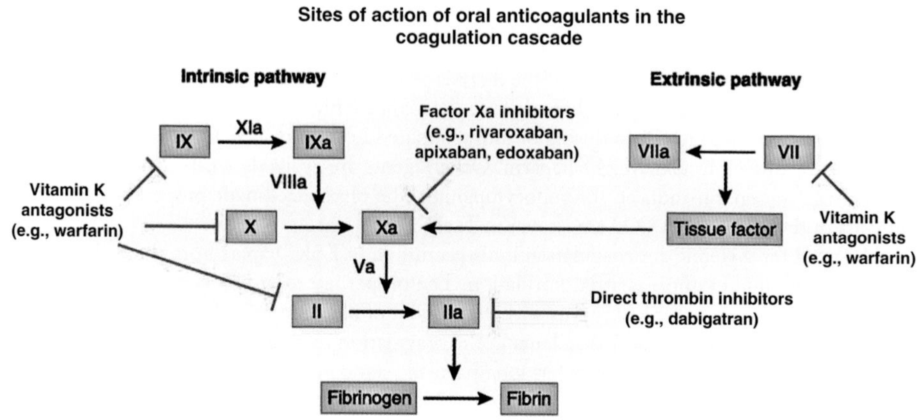

Sites of action of oral anticoagulants in the coagulation cascade

Figure 12.10 Sites of action of oral anticoagulants in the coagulation cascade. (From Jain N, Reilly RF. Clinical pharmacology of oral anticoagulants in patients with kidney disease. *Clin J Am Soc Nephrol*. 2019 Feb 7;14[2]:278–287. doi:10.2215/CJN.02170218.)

and ESKD patients spend less time in the therapeutic INR range. Note that warfarin is considered a risk factor for calcific uremic arteriolopathy (calciphylaxis). Non–vitamin K-dependent oral anticoagulants are increasingly used, primarily for atrial fibrillation, and would be expected to have an improved risk–benefit profile.[88] Apixaban 2.5–5 mg twice daily may be administered in ESKD, but the dosage should be reduced to 2.5 mg twice daily if the patient is over 80 years old or weighs less than 60 kg. Apixaban appears to be associated with reduced mortality and embolic events and is safer than warfarin treatment in dialysis patients. In a recent randomized trial, rivaroxaban reduced fatal/nonfatal CVEs and major bleeding complications compared to a vitamin K antagonist in HD patients with atrial fibrillation.[89]

The pharmacokinetic properties of oral anticoagulants are shown in Table 12.20.[86]

12.8 Hemodialysis Emergencies

Maintenance HD safety has improved significantly over time and is now considered a routine procedure.[90] Nonetheless, serious complications can occur and require emergency evaluation and management. Some are reviewed below (Table 12.21).

12.8.1 DIALYZER REACTIONS

Allergic or even anaphylactic reactions may occur in the dialysis patient, usually within the first 5 to 10 minutes (Type A, commonly related to ethylene oxide used as a sterilant, or less commonly to the dialyzer membrane), but in some cases up to 30 minutes after initiation. Dialyzer reactions occurring after 30 minutes and up to 60 minutes after initiation (Type B) are usually less severe and most commonly related to reactions to the dialyzer membrane that are often complement mediated. Less commonly, reactions are related not to the sterilant or membrane, but to heparin or other medications administered, such as iron, rarely erythropoiesis stimulating agents (ESAs), or blood products.

Presentation may include acute bronchial constriction with respiratory distress or chest tightness, vasodilation with hypotension, anxiety, abdominal cramping/diarrhea, or in the worst cases, cardiac arrest.[91]

TABLE 12.20 ■ **Summary of Pharmacokinetic and Pharmacodynamic Properties of Commonly Used Oral Anticoagulants (adapted from Table 1[86])**

| OAC | Type | Prodrug | PHARMACOKINETICS | | | Pharmaco-dynamics: Binding to Effector |
			Metabolism	Renal Dose Adjustment	Dialyzable	
Warfarin	Vitamin K–dependent factor inhibitor	No	Extensive metabolism by CYP2C9	Minor	No	Irreversible
Dabigatran	Direct thrombin inhibitor	Yes	Metabolized by esterases, 80% excreted by kidney	Yes	Yes	Reversible
Apixaban	Free and clot-bound Xa inhibitor	No	Metabolized in liver by CYP3A4, then excreted in feces and kidney (25%), no active metabolite	Yes for some	Small	Reversible
Rivaroxaban	Free and clot-bound Xa inhibitor	No	66% excreted by kidney, 36% unchanged, minimal in feces	Yes	No	Reversible
Edoxaban	Free Xa inhibitor	No	50% excreted unchanged by the kidney, 10% hydrolyzed by carboxyesterase 1	Yes	No	Reversible

CYP2C9, Cytochrome P450 type 2C9; *CYP3A4*, cytochrome P450 type 3A4; *OAC*, oral anticoagulant; *Xa*, factor Xa.

TABLE 12.21 ■ **Major Hemodialysis Emergencies**

- Dialyzer reaction
- Dialysis disequilibrium syndrome
- Venous air embolism
- Pyrogenic reactions
- Arrhythmias

Dialysis in such severe cases should be terminated without returning blood to the patient; provide aggressive fluids for hypotension, call for emergency assistance, and administer antihistamines, corticosteroids, or epinephrine.

For subsequent episodes, switch to a dialyzer with a non-ethylene oxide sterilizer, such as a gamma ray–sterilized dialyzer; use an alternative dialysis membrane; prime the dialyzer well, and pretreat with antihistamines/steroids as needed.

12.8.2 DIALYSIS DISEQUILIBRIUM SYNDROME

Neurological signs and symptoms of dialysis disequilibrium syndrome can include nausea, vomiting, confusion, or seizures during or shortly after the initial dialysis session(s).

Risk factors are very high BUN/Cr, rapid reduction of BUN/Cr by the dialysis treatment, older age, liver disease, abnormal serum sodium, and metabolic acidosis.[92]

Prevention measures for the initial 3 HD treatments include lower blood flow, shortened dialysis sessions, and higher dialysate sodium, or consideration of CRRT.[90]

12.8.3 VENOUS AIR EMBOLISM

A venous air embolism occurs when air enters the patient's bloodstream from the extracorporeal circuit due to a loose connection or defect in the components of the blood circuit.

A venous air embolism may cause hypoxia, hypotension, pulmonary hypertension (HTN), or cardiac arrest; if it coexists with a patent foramen ovale, it may enter the arterial circulation and result in ischemic injury, usually cerebral.

In cases of venous air embolisms, stop dialysis, place the patient in the left lateral recumbent position, and treat for hypoxia and hypotension.

12.8.4 PYROGENIC REACTIONS

Symptoms of pyrogenic reactions include fever, chills, hypotension, headache, and myalgias during HD. Such reactions are usually caused by Gram-negative bacteria that produce endotoxins in the dialysate. A pyrogenic reaction may lead to systemic infection and death. The dialysis machine, extracorporeal circuit including dialysis membrane, and water treatment system should be evaluated.

12.8.5 ARRHYTHMIAS

Arrhythmias and cardiac arrest account for almost one-third of deaths in ESKD patients, the most common single cause. Furthermore, the risk of sudden cardiac death is highest following the longer interdialytic period. Unlike in the general population, bradyarrhythmias appear to be more common than ventricular arrhythmias.[90] Potential triggering factors include rapid electrolyte changes (potassium, calcium).[93]

12.9 ESKD Comorbidities/Coexisting Conditions

ESKD is a state of multiple comorbidities. Conditions variously included as comorbidities in the incident/prevalent ESKD patient population include HTN, diabetes, ischemic heart disease, congestive heart failure, hyperlipidemia, cerebrovascular disease, anemia, gout, and others.

12.9.1 ISCHEMIC HEART DISEASE

Atherosclerosis is accelerated in patients with ESKD, due to both traditional and nontraditional (uremia-related) factors, such as vascular calcification, endothelial dysfunction, inflammation, anemia, and insulin resistance.[94] Changes in ventricular function chronically or temporally related to the dialysis procedure (see Intradialytic Hypotension section below) may be a result of myocardial hypoperfusion. ESKD patients with severe coronary artery disease may require coronary bypass surgery.

12.9.2 HYPERTENSION

HTN affects a majority of ESKD patients. Multiple mechanisms are involved, although the predominant one is sodium and volume excess. HTN contributes to cardiovascular morbidity and mortality in ESKD. Control of extracellular volume is the primary therapeutic strategy. The linear relationship between systolic BP and mortality in the general population is not seen in ESKD. In fact, data suggest a U-shaped relationship, with increased mortality risk at low systolic ($<$~110 mmHg) and at high systolic ($>$165 mmHg).[95]

Control of HTN in ESKD patients, especially if documented in home or ambulatory readings, is associated with improvement in cardiovascular outcomes. Dialysis patients also suffer greater adverse consequences of hypotension than the general population. Trials done in ESKD patients suggest that treatment may be important, but have not led to firmly established BP treatment targets. Guidelines suggest that predialysis BP should be 140/90 and postdialysis BP 130/80, but goals must be individualized.

Medications commonly used are listed in Table 12.22.[96]

TABLE 12.22 ■ Antihypertensive Medications Used in Hemodialysis[96]

Medication	Usual Dose Range	Removal With Hemodialysis (%)
Alpha-blockers		
Doxazosin	1–16 mg daily	None
Prazosin	1–10 mg twice daily	None
Terazosin	1–20 mg daily	None
ACEi		
Benazepril	5–40 mg daily	20–50
Enalapril	2.5–10 mg daily	35–50
Fosinopril	10–80 mg daily	None
Lisinopril	2.5–40 mg every 24–48 hr	50
Perindopril	2–8 mg daily	50
Quinapril	10–20 mg daily	25
Ramipril	2.5–10 mg daily	20–30
Trandolapril	0.5–4 mg daily	30
ARBs		
Candesartan	4–32 mg daily	None
Irbesartan	75–300 mg daily	None
Losartan	50–100 mg daily	None
Olmesartan	10–40 mg daily	None
Telmisartan	40–80 mg daily	None
Valsartan	80–320 mg daily	None
Beta-blockers		
Atenolol	25–100 mg every 24–48 hr	50–75
Carvedilol	6.25–25 mg twice daily	None

Continued on following page

TABLE 12.22 ■ **Antihypertensive Medications Used in Hemodialysis** (Continued)

Medication	Usual Dose Range	Removal With Hemodialysis (%)
Labetalol	100–1200 mg twice daily	None
Metoprolol	50–200 mg twice daily	High
Nadolol	40–240 mg daily	50
Propranolol	40–160 mg twice daily	None
CCBs		
Amlodipine	2.5–10 mg daily	None
Diltiazem CD	180–360 mg daily	None
Felodipine	2.5–10 mg daily	None
Nifedipine XL	30–120 mg daily	None
Verapamil	180–360 mg daily	None
Diuretics		
Bumetanide	0.5–2 mg twice daily	None
Ethacrynic acid	50–200 mg twice daily*	None
Furosemide	40–160 mg twice daily	None
Metolazone	5–10 mg daily	None
MRAs		
Eplerenone	50–100 mg daily	None
Spironolactone	25–100 mg daily	None
Others		
Clonidine (oral)	0.1–0.4 mg three times daily	5
Hydralazine	10–100 mg three times daily	None
Minoxidil	2.5–30 mg daily	Yes

*Ethacrynic acid is not generally used due to concern for hearing loss.
ACEi, Angiotensin-converting-enzyme inhibitors; *ARBs*, angiotensin II receptor blockers; *CCBs*, calcium channel blockers; *MRAs*, mineralocorticoid receptor antagonists.

Drug selection should take into consideration patient comorbidities for which specific agents are also indicated. The approach to drug selection should include factors such as comorbid conditions, adverse effects, pharmacokinetics in ESKD, and effects of the dialysis treatment on BP.

Note that most angiotensin-converting-enzyme inhibitors (ACEi), metoprolol, atenolol, and nadolol are removed by HD.

12.9.3 CHRONIC FLUID OVERLOAD

Controlling fluid overload in ESKD patients should be viewed as another component of dialysis adequacy. Pulmonary congestion is a predictor of cardiac events and mortality in ESKD.[97] Clinical assessment of fluid overload may be difficult. While fluid overload carries risk, so does the need for excessive ultrafiltration during the dialysis procedure in an ongoing attempt to achieve euvolemia. Fluid removal rates higher than 13 mL/hr/kg body weight are associated with poor outcomes.[98] The use of diuretics between HD treatments to control hypervolemia was initially considered controversial, but they are now being used successfully by many nephrologists.

Dialysis can potentially relieve heart failure. There is no consensus for treatment of systolic heart failure. The benefit of beta-blocker therapy was indicated in a recent observational study showing lower mortality in HD patients with heart failure.[99] Atenolol, metoprolol, nadolol, and bisoprolol are dialyzed off. Some studies have shown increased risk for diabetes, stroke, or hyperkalemia with beta blockade.

12.9.4 PULMONARY HYPERTENSION

Pulmonary HTN is a progressive pulmonary circulatory disease that accompanies either left or right ventricular failure and volume overload.[100] It is underrecognized in ESKD patients, though causes and mechanisms of right heart failure have now been well described.[101] However, awareness of right-sided heart failure and pulmonary HTN in the ESKD population is increasing.[102]

Treatment consists of control of HTN, use of beta-blockers, ACEi/angiotensin II receptor blockers (ARBs), mineralocorticoid receptor antagonists (MRAs), correction of anemia, reassessment of target weight, treatment of arrhythmias, and evaluation and treatment of coronary ischemia.

12.9.5 PERIPHERAL ARTERY DISEASE

The prevalence of peripheral artery disease (PAD) is 25% to 35% in incident patients. The risk in prevalent patients is higher in association with intradialytic hypotension (IDH).[103] Predictors include advanced age, male sex, diabetes, current smoking, coronary artery disease, and malnutrition.[104] Presentation includes gangrene, ischemic ulceration, and pain at rest; classic symptoms of claudication are uncommon. Guidelines recommend evaluation for PAD at initiation of chronic dialysis. Calcification of vessels may reduce the success of endovascular therapy. Increased postoperative mortality after surgical revascularization is a risk.

12.9.6 INTRADIALYTIC HYPOTENSION

Intradialytic hypotension (IDH) is one of the most frequent complications of HD, affecting 10% to 30% or more of treatments, depending on its definition. During an HD treatment, the majority of patients experience some overall decline in BP. Commonly used definitions of IDH include a decrease in systolic BP of 20 mmHg, a nadir systolic BP below 90 mmHg, or any hypotensive event that requires an immediate corrective measure. The ultrafiltration goals for an HD treatment in the United States are commonly up to 3 L (roughly 1 total plasma volume).[105]

The evaluation should begin with a full assessment of the patient's condition and comorbidities that may contribute to hypotension with HD fluid removal (Figure 12.11).[106]

The mechanism of IDH in the absence of the underlying conditions described above usually involves failed compensations of cardiac output and arteriolar tone for fluid removal. Compensation may be hindered by impaired sympathetic activation. Major risk factors are diabetes, large interdialytic weight gains, and lower body weight.[107]

The most common symptoms of IDH include muscle cramps, nausea, vomiting, and dizziness. Severe episodes may be complicated by loss of residual renal function, hypotensive seizures, stroke events, coronary and cerebral ischemia, vascular access occlusion, and increased mortality risk.[108] Repeated episodes are now known to result in damage to the heart with myocardial fibrosis, central nervous system (CNS) cerebral ischemia, kidneys, and gastrointestinal (GI) tract related to end-organ hypoperfusion.[109,110]

Multiple interventions may be utilized to prevent IDH, but because of inadequate longitudinal trials, treatment is individualized and frequently empiric. Refractory patients should be evaluated for undiagnosed cardiac disease and undergo autonomic testing. Note that the full

Differential diagnosis of intradialytic hypotension

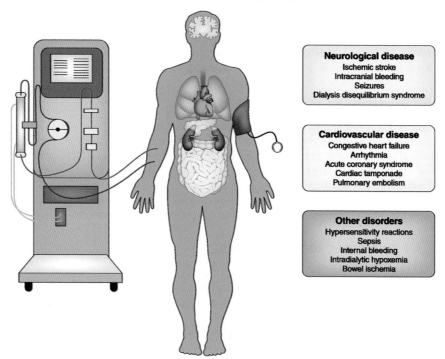

Neurological disease
Ischemic stroke
Intracranial bleeding
Seizures
Dialysis disequilibrium syndrome

Cardiovascular disease
Congestive heart failure
Arrhythmia
Acute coronary syndrome
Cardiac tamponade
Pulmonary embolism

Other disorders
Hypersensitivity reactions
Sepsis
Internal bleeding
Intradialytic hypoxemia
Bowel ischemia

Figure 12.11   Underlying factors to be considered in the patient with HD treatments complicated by IDH.

TABLE 12.23 ■ **Prevention and Treatment of Intradialytic Hypotension**

Dialysis-Related Modalities	Extra–Dialysis-Related Modalities
Confirm accuracy of blood pressure reading	Adjust antihypertensive dosing and timing
Establish an accurate target weight	Limit intradialytic weight gain
Reduce ultrafiltration rate	Improve anemia
Reduce intradialytic blood flow	Predialysis midodrine
IV fluid administration	Predialysis pseudoephedrine
Ultrafiltration modeling	Predialysis caffeine consumption
Prohibit food consumption during dialysis	Fludrocortisone (extrarenal effect)
Oxygen administration	Oral carnitine (if deficient)
Increase dialysate calcium	
Cool dialysate to 36°C	

Trendelenburg position is no longer recommended. Both hyperoncotic (25%) and isooncotic (5%) intravenous albumin have been used in place of isotonic saline for hypotension, but resultant volume expansion appears to be ineffective despite its oncotic properties.[111]

Prevention and treatment of IDH is outlined in Table 12.23.

12.10 Anemia Management

Comorbid anemia occurs in over half of ESKD patients, and a substantial portion of ESKD patients initiate dialysis with very low hemoglobin (Hgb) levels.[112] Anemia at initiation of dialysis is associated with increased fatigue, weakness, and an increased risk of cardiovascular mortality. The multifactorial etiology includes decreased endogenous erythropoietin (EPO) production, functional or absolute iron deficiency, resistance to EPO in uremia related to suppression of hypoxia-inducible factors, and shortened red cell lifespan.

Initial anemia evaluation should be similar to that in the non-ESKD patient, and should consider factors such as the patient's history, complete blood count (CBC), iron studies, and reticulocyte count (Table 12.24).

Determination of iron deficiency is of relevance not only as a primary diagnosis, but as a factor in the response to ESAs.

Anemia is treated with ESAs (e.g., epoetin), intravenous iron, and, infrequently, blood transfusions. Note that management in the dialysis facility is usually facilitated by the use of approved protocols. KDOQI Guideline Recommendations for HD Patients[113] are shown in Table 12.25.

Concerns regarding toxicity of ESAs began to emerge with their initial regulatory trials. Several adverse effects of ESAs were reported early, when Hgb targets were near normal or normal, including CVEs, malignancy, seizures, exacerbation of HTN, dialysis access thrombosis, and mortality.

Harmful effects were related to the use of large ESA doses and maintaining higher Hgb levels.[114] As a result, clinically acceptable target for Hgb with ESAs are in the range of 10 to 12 g/dL. Several treatments are now available to treat patients with ESKD. Doses are titrated based on the patient's response to ESA treatment.

ESA hyporesponsiveness is found in up to 20% of HD patients, and is associated with higher ESA requirements, increased major CVEs, and mortality. Causes include iron deficiency, inflammation, hyperparathyroidism, and systemic infection. Rarely, neutralizing antibodies to ESAs will result in severe anemia.[113]

Parenteral iron is also known to raise or help sustain Hgb levels in ESKD.

Current treatment options for anemia management in the ESKD patient are shown in Table 12.26.[115-121]

TABLE 12.24 ■ **Evaluation of Anemia in the ESKD Patient**

Initial anemia evaluation (Hgb <12 g/dL)
Iron deficiency—iron indices (transferrin saturation <20%; serum ferritin <200 ng/mL)
Reticulocyte count
RBC indices
Serum folate level
Vitamin B$_{12}$ level
Stool for occult blood

ESKD, End-stage kidney disease; *Hgb*, hemoglobin; *RBC*, red blood cell.

TABLE 12.25 ■ **Considerations in Initiating ESA in ESKD Patients**

- Determine hemoglobin goal.
- Monitor hemoglobin level.
- Adjust ESA dose every 2–4 weeks.
- Consider contraindications to ESA administration.

ESA, Erythropoiesis stimulating agent; *ESKD*, end-stage kidney disease.

TABLE 12.26 ◼ ESA Options for Treating Anemia in ESKD

EPO alfa (epoetin): genetically engineered recombinant human EPO. Initial dose 50 units/kg three times weekly.
EPO alfa-epbx: biosimilar of EPO alfa, identical in amino acid sequence and comparable in carbohydrate
   composition. Shown to be equivalent to EPO alfa in efficacy and similar to EPO alfa in safety when
   given intravenously to HD patients, and more recently when each was administered subcutaneously.[a,b]
Darbepoetin: extended dosing intervals. Can be given less often than EPO alfa; has a half-life three
   times longer than EPO alfa. Studies show noninferiority to EPO alfa, with potential cost savings.[c]
HIF PHIs: a new class of oral agents able to increase Hgb levels in patients naïve to ESAs or converted
   from ESA treatment.[d–f] Roxadustat is approved in a number of countries for use in adult CKD and
   ESKD patients. In the United States, an FDA advisory committee has recommended not approving
   roxadustat because of safety concerns, primarily CVEs.
CERA: longer-acting ESA, lower frequency of administration; recent meta-analysis suggested CERA is
   similar to EPO alfa and darbepoetin in outcomes such as mortality, major adverse CVEs, or need for
   transfusions/iron therapy.[g]

[a]Fishbane S, Spinowitz BS, Wisemandle WA, Martin NE. Randomized controlled trial of subcutaneous epoetin
   alfa-epbx versus epoetin alfa in end-stage renal disease. *Kidney Int Rep*. 2019 May 22;4(9):1235–1247.
   doi:10.1016/j.ekir.2019.05.010.
[b]Fishbane S, Singh B, Kumbhat S, Wisemandle WA, Martin NE. Intravenous epoetin alfa-epbx versus epoetin
   alfa for treatment of anemia in end-stage kidney disease. *Clin J Am Soc Nephrol*. 2018 Aug 7;13(8):
   1204–1214. doi:10.2215/CJN.11631017.
[c]Sinha SD, Bandi VK, Bheemareddy BR, et al. Efficacy, tolerability and safety of darbepoetin alfa injection for
   the treatment of anemia associated with chronic kidney disease (CKD) undergoing dialysis: a randomized,
   phase III trial. *BMC Nephrol*. 2019 Mar 13;20(1):90. doi:10.1186/s12882-019-1209-1.
[d]Chen N, Hao C, Liu B-C, et al. Roxadustat treatment for anemia in patients undergoing long-term dialysis.
   N Engl J Med. 2019 Sep 12;381(11):1011–1022. doi:10.1056/NEJMoa1901713.
[e]Akizawa T, Iwasaki M, Yamaguchi Y, Majikawa Y, Reusch M. Phase 3, randomized, double-blind, active-
   comparator (darbepoetin alfa) study of oral roxadustat in CKD patients with anemia on hemodialysis in
   Japan. *J Am Soc Nephrol*. 2020 Jul;31(7):1628–1639. doi:10.1681/ASN.2019060623.
[f]Singh AK, Carroll K, Perkovic V, et al. Daprodustat for the treatment of anemia in patients undergoing dialysis.
   N Engl J Med. 2021;385(25):2325–2335. doi:10.1056/NEJMoa2113379.
[g]Saglimbene VM, Palmer SC, Ruospo M, Natale P, Craig JC, Strippoli GFM. Continuous erythropoiesis
   receptor activator (CERA) for the anaemia of chronic kidney disease. *Cochrane Database Syst Rev*. 2017
   Aug 7;8(8):CD009904. doi:10.1002/14651858.CD009904.pub2.
CERA, Continuous erythropoiesis receptor activator; *CKD*, chronic kidney disease; *CVEs*, cardiovascular
events; *EPO*, erythropoietin; *ESA*, erythropoiesis stimulating agent; *ESKD*, end-stage kidney disease; *HIF*,
hypoxia-inducible factor; *PHIs*, prolyl hydroxylase inhibitors.

12.11 Management of Hyperkalemia

Hyperkalemia, defined as serum potassium greater than 5.0 to 5.5 mEq/L, is the most frequent electrolyte disturbance requiring urgent treatment in kidney failure and dialysis patients. Dietary noncompliance and insufficient dialytic removal are the main contributing factors. Other factors may include internal shifts of potassium due to acidosis or medications; tissue breakdown; decreased colonic potassium loss due to constipation; and loss of residual renal function.

Pseudohyperkalemia is when an elevated serum potassium does not reflect the *in vivo* plasma potassium levels. It may result from an improper collection process, hemolysis (within the extra-corporeal dialysis circuit or after collection), or thrombocytosis. This can be confirmed with a normal plasma (whole blood) potassium level.[122]

Reverse pseudohyperkalemia, a rare occurrence in which the serum potassium is normal but the heparinized plasma potassium is falsely elevated, occurs with hematological malignancies and extreme leukocytosis from heparin-induced potassium loss from white blood cells (WBCs) elevating the plasma potassium after whole blood collection.[122]

An elevated risk of adverse events has been demonstrated in dialysis patients with serum potassium levels >5.5 or 6.0 mEq/L, although an even lower threshold for risk of hospitalization and

TABLE 12.27 ■ **Medical Management of Hyperkalemia**

Purpose of Treatment	Agent	Dose	Comments/Side Effects
Stabilization of cardiac membrane	Calcium gluconate	1–2 g IV over minutes, can be given peripherally	Rapid cardiac effect in <5 min
	Calcium chloride	10 mL of 10% solution; preferably given centrally	
Shift K into cells	Regular insulin	10 U IV	K⁺ decreases in 15–30 min, Given with 25–50 g IV dextrose to avoid hypoglycemia
	Beta-2 adrenergics	Nebulized; 5–20 mg in 4 mL over 10 min	K⁺ decreases in 30 min,
	Sodium bicarbonate	50–150mEq IV	K⁺ decreases in 1–4 hr especially if severe acidemia; sodium load
Removal from body	Loop diuretic	Furosemide 80 mg IV	Effective if diuretic-responsive
	Cation exchange resin	SPS 15 g orally 1–4 times daily	Associated with colonic necrosis; avoid if history of GI problems; less effective per rectum
		Patiromer 8.4 g 1–2 times daily with food; separate from other meds by 3 hr	Hypomagnesemia, constipation, impaired absorption of some drugs, slow onset of action
		SZC 10 g three times daily, then reduce to daily	Edema, fluid overload; onset in 1 hr; separate from other meds by 2 hr; 400-mg sodium/5-g dose
	Mineralocorticoid agonist	Fludrocortisone	Limited kaliuretic effect in ESKD

ESKD, End-stage kidney disease; *GI*, gastrointestinal; *IV*, intravenously; *SPS*, sodium polystyrene sulfonate; *SZC*, sodium zirconium cyclosilicate.

mortality may exist for some patients.[123] Hyperkalemia may lead to symptomatic muscle weakness, cardiac conduction delay, and cardiac arrhythmias. The main consequence of severe hyperkalemia is decreased myocardial conduction velocity, acceleration of repolarization, and possible cardiac arrest.

Mineralocorticoid receptor antagonists, of proven benefit in heart failure patients, have attracted growing attention in the ESKD population. A meta-analysis noted improvements in CV and all-cause mortality.[124] Their application of HD patients has been limited by concern about hyperkalemia. One U.S. data analysis indicated a higher risk of death with MRA use in ESKD.[125] A recent trial of spironolactone showed that 50 mg but not lower doses increased the risk of hyperkalemia.[126]

Medical management of hyperkalemia, added to dietary potassium restriction and dialysis (the gold standard), may be urgently or emergently required (Table 12.27).

Polystyrene resins such as sodium polystyrene sulfonate (SPS, Kayexalate), which act by exchanging a cation for potassium within the intestinal lumen and are administered orally or rectally, have long been used to treat hyperkalemia. However, there have been concerns about weak evidence regarding efficacy, and well-known concerns about severe but rare adverse events such as bowel necrosis. A black box FDA warning from 2009 has warned against its use, particularly against coadministration with sorbitol to offset its constipating effects, as sorbitol appears to increase the risk of bowel toxicity. A recent systematic review reported a relative risk of 2.1 and a hazard ratio of 1.25 to 1.94, with a low absolute risk because of event rates of about 20/1000 person-years.[127] SPS crystals may be visible in rectal ulcer pathology.

Patiromer and sodium zirconium cyclosilicate (SZC) are now important alternatives to SPS.[128] In patients in need of acute management of hyperkalemia, SZC is preferred because of a more rapid effect, although the onset of action may be several hours and the effect modest.[129] Edema may result from its sodium content. Patiromer may be the drug of choice for chronic management, but may cause hypomagnesemia and constipation.

12.12 Bone and Mineral Disorders

ESKD-mineral bone disorder is a systemic disorder involving laboratory and skeletal abnormalities, vascular calcifications, or calcific uremic arteriolopathy (calciphylaxis). The clinical consequences are increased risk of bone fractures, CVEs, and mortality. The therapeutic approach must primarily address hyperparathyroidism and hyperphosphatemia.[130]

12.12.1 MANAGEMENT OF SECONDARY HYPERPARATHYROIDISM

The related bone and mineral abnormalities of ESKD commonly manifest as progressive secondary hyperparathyroidism. Because of uremic resistance to the skeletal actions of parathyroid hormone (PTH), target PTH levels are 2 to 9 times the normal range. Secondary hyperparathyroidism may lead to progressive bone pain and fractures, refractory pruritus, accelerated vascular and cardiac valvular calcification, and myopathy. In tertiary hyperparathyroidism, progressive autonomous parathyroid production of PTH results in hypercalcemia.

Treatment options involve use of synthetic vitamin D analogues and calcimimetics. With the publication of the 2017 KDIGO guidelines,[130] the approach to controlling secondary hyperparathyroidism has evolved toward the first-line use of calcimimetic agents in addition to, or even instead of, starting vitamin D analogues. However, in most ESKD patients, a vitamin D analogue will also be required to correct vitamin D deficiency. Calcimimetics reduce parathyroid levels by increasing the sensitivity of the parathyroid calcium-sensing receptor to calcium. While effective at lowering PTH (especially if PTH is not very elevated), activated vitamin D administration may increase intestinal absorption and thereby serum concentrations of calcium and phosphorus; both are associated with increased cardiovascular risk. In contrast, calcimimetics are known to reduce both serum calcium and phosphorus levels, while lowering PTH.

Available calcimimetics include oral cinacalcet and IV etelcalcetide. Benefits of calcimimetics include lowering of serum PTH levels, but long-term effectiveness on cardiovascular and bone complications are uncertain. Both oral and IV forms are associated with nausea, vomiting, and hypocalcemia. Pooled data from initial regulatory trials indicated that oral cinacalcet in HD patients could reduce CVEs, fractures, and the need for surgical parathyroidectomy, compared to standard care with vitamin D analogues.[131] Subsequently, in the Evaluation of Cinacalcet Hydrochloride Therapy to Lower Cardiovascular Events (EVOLVE) study, patient outcomes such as death or major CVEs were not demonstrated in an unadjusted analysis,[132] although a beneficial effect in older patients appeared to occur. In a secondary analysis which included changes in the statistical analysis, the rate of clinical fractures was shown to be reduced.[133] Significant lowering of serum calcium with either calcimimetic may cause significant QT prolongation and ventricular arrhythmias.

Etelcalcetide IV is an effective alternative to oral cinacalcet.[134] It has been associated with hypersensitivity reactions, hypotension, congestive heart failure, prolonged QT interval, and decreased myocardial function. It may produce GI side effects similar to oral cinacalcet.

While fewer patients now appear to require parathyroidectomy, those with refractory hyperparathyroidism may nonetheless be best managed with surgical subtotal parathyroidectomy.

Activated vitamin D analogues are known to decrease parathyroid levels in dialysis patients, and may have other "pleotropic" effects.[135] Vitamin D analogues may increase both calcium and phosphorus levels, promoting soft tissue and vascular calcification. Commonly available analogues include calcitriol, paricalcitol, and doxercalciferol. No data indicate superiority of any single agent. Some,[136] but not all, observational studies have indicated a reduction of mortality in ESKD patients on active vitamin D treatment.

12.12.2 MANAGEMENT OF HYPERPHOSPHATEMIA

Hyperphosphatemia is almost ubiquitous in patients on maintenance dialysis. Reduced adherence to phosphate-binder therapy, reported in over half of treated patients, contributes to poor control. The serum phosphorus goals are based on the guidelines of KDOQI ($\leq$5.5 mg/dL)[137] and KDIGO ($\leq$4.5 mg/dL).[130] The three key elements in the management of phosphate balance in ESKD are dietary restriction, oral phosphate binders, and adequate dialysis. Dietary phosphate absorption in the intestine is now known to involve not only active transcellular transport, but also passive paracellular absorption through tight junctions between enterocytes.

Basic research data on hyperphosphatemia suggest calcification toxicity to vasculature, and observational studies have indicated a positive association between elevated serum phosphate levels and mortality. Hyperphosphatemia has been associated with severity of coronary artery calcification, which is itself a predictor of mortality in dialysis patients. The recent EPISODE trial indicated that strict phosphate control toward the normal range may mitigate this effect.[138]

The standard dietary phosphate restriction for ESKD patients is 900 to 1000 mg/day. However, there are very limited data on the benefit of restricted dietary phosphate intake on ESKD clinical outcomes.[139] A large observational study indicated treatment with phosphate binders was associated with improved survival among incident HD patients.[140]

Conventional HD does not remove sufficient phosphate to achieve goal levels, so patients are managed with dietary phosphate restriction and, in most cases, with phosphate binders.[141]

Contemporary guidelines, although opinion based, strongly support the use of phosphate binders for serum phosphate lowering, to less than 5.5 mg/dL. For all prescribed binders, the lowest effective dose should be used.

In addition, the 2017 update of the KDIGO clinical practice guideline suggested restricting use of calcium-based phosphate binders in patients with ESKD, regardless of baseline serum calcium levels.[130] However, a subsequent trial did not suggest increased cardiovascular safety of the costlier sevelamer compared with calcium acetate.[142]

It may be underappreciated that phosphate binders differ significantly in features, such as their phosphate-binding capacity and the range of pHs in which they are effective. For example, the binder sucroferric oxyhydroxide binds about 260 mg of phosphorus in the gut, compared to binding of 21 mg by an equivalent amount of sevelamer.[143] A reduced pill burden may result. Characteristics of oral phosphate binders are shown in Table 12.28.

Current clinical approaches involve use of non–calcium-containing phosphate binders as the preferred choice, when possible, with an optimal clinical target goal of normalization of serum phosphate levels (3.5–4.5 mg/dL or at least <5.5 mg/dL). A recent study was the first randomized trial to demonstrate that normalization of serum phosphate levels was associated with improvement in cardiovascular health.[138] Analysis of Dialysis Outcomes and Practice Patterns Study (DOPPS) data indicates that worse phosphorus control may be strongly associated with cardiovascular mortality.[144]

The fundamental clinical benefit of phosphate control in HD patients, however, remains unanswered, with a large clinical trial underway to look at the beneficial effects of higher or lower serum phosphate goals in the U.S. dialysis population.[145]

12.12.3 CALCIFIC UREMIC ARTERIOLOPATHY (CALCIPHYLAXIS)

Calcific uremic arteriolopathy is more commonly referred to as calciphylaxis. The incidence in ESKD patients is in the range of 1% to 4%; it is far less commonly described in predialysis patients. While not fully understood, the fundamental pathology is progressive arterial calcification

TABLE 12.28 ■ **Management of Hyperphosphatemia**[141]

Phosphate Binder	Mechanism of Action	Dosage Strength	Initial/Maximum Recommended Dose (With Meals)	Advantages	Disadvantages
Aluminum hydroxide	Forms insoluble phosphate complexes	600-mg tablets	1–3 tablets three times/day	Inexpensive; calcium-free; effective at wide range of pH	Constipation; osteomalacia; CNS toxicity; anemia. For short-term use or with monitoring of aluminum levels.
Sevelamer carbonate	Cationic polymer/anion exchange resin	800-mg tablet, 800- or 2400-mg powder packet	800–2400 mg three times/day	No calcium loading; may lower lipid levels	GI intolerance
Calcium acetate	Binds with PO_4 to form insoluble calcium phosphate in stool	667-mg tablet, 667-mg/5-mL solution; 25% elemental calcium	1–4 tablets three times/day (considered advisable to keep total elemental calcium dose to 1500 mg/day = 3-tablet dose)	Inexpensive; generally well tolerated	GI intolerance; positive calcium balance; possible risk of calcification
Lanthanum carbonate	Binds PO_4 to form lanthanum phosphate in stool	500-, 750-, 1000-mg chewable tablet; 750- and 1000-mg oral powder	500–1000 mg three times/day	Potent; smaller pill burden; binds at lower pH	More costly; must be chewed; GI intolerance; tasteless
Ferric citrate	Iron-based phosphate binder	210-mg tablet	2–4 tablets three times/day	Provides bioavailable iron	More costly; avoid in iron overload; GI intolerance; dark stool
Sucroferric oxyhydroxide	Iron-based ligand exchange	500-mg chewable tablet	2–4 tablets three times/day	Potent; works in wide range of pH; smaller pill burden	More costly; flavored; may stain teeth; dark stool

CNS, Central nervous system; *GI*, gastrointestinal.

involving arterioles and capillaries in the dermis and subcutaneous adipose tissue, and affecting not only skin but at times other organs such as muscle, lungs, and brain.[146] In cutaneous calciphylaxis, painful and nonhealing violaceous skin ulcers may be preceded by nonulcerative subcutaneous plaques/nodules, and typically progress to tissue necrosis and gangrene.

Risk factors include female sex, obesity, elevated calcium/phosphorus levels, hyperparathyroidism, and hypercoagulable states.[147] Warfarin-associated calciphylaxis is a variant that is well described in the absence of CKD/ESKD. The drug promotes vascular calcification by inhibiting vitamin K–dependent matrix Gla protein, which normally prevents calcium deposition in arterioles.[148]

The differential diagnosis of calciphylaxis may include ulcers related to peripheral vascular disease, cellulitis, atheroembolic disease, vasculitis, cryoglobulinemia, bacterial endocarditis, disseminated intravascular coagulation, and hypercoagulable states. The diagnosis is best established by skin biopsy of the peripheral area of the lesion, revealing the characteristic finding of diffuse calcification of small capillaries in adipose tissue, often with fibrin thrombi and dermal/epidermal necrosis, and inflammatory cell infiltration. However, the biopsy procedure itself may create a painful new lesion with bleeding and necrosis. Noninvasive support indicating the likelihood of the diagnosis may be found when a bone scan reveals increased technetium uptake in areas of involvement. Management considerations for calcific uremic arteriolopathy are shown in Table 12.29.

Calciphylaxis is associated with a mortality rate of 40% or more, but there have been encouraging reports of intravenous sodium thiosulfate producing improvement or even symptomatic resolution of lesions.[149] There are reports of intradermal injections and even intraperitoneal administration of sodium thiosulfate as well. Multiple clinical trials of other agents are currently underway.[146] Treatment options utilized for the management of calcific uremic arteriolopathy are shown in Table 12.29.

TABLE 12.29 ■ **Management of Calcific Uremic Arteriolopathy (Calciphylaxis)**

- Sodium thiosulfate
- Stop vitamin D analogues
- Stop calcium supplements
- Lower dialysate calcium concentration
- Change warfarin to an NOAC (also called DOAC), if possible
- Increase dialysis intensity
- Treat hyperparathyroidism (PTH >800 pg/mL despite medical therapy)
- Consider vitamin K 10 mg orally (if not on warfarin)

DOAC, Direct oral anticoagulant; *NOAC*, new oral anticoagulant; *PTH*, parathyroid hormone.

12.13 Management of the ESKD Patient With Diabetes Mellitus

ESKD problems special to the patient with diabetes are shown in Table 12.30.

12.13.1 GLYCEMIC MANAGEMENT

In fundamental ways, glycemic management in the ESKD patient is different and more complex.[150] Insufficient glycemic monitoring has been identified as one of the gaps in care for HD patients with diabetes mellitus. However, the role of tight glycemic control in ESKD patients remains controversial. The 2020 KDIGO guidelines on diabetes indicate that glycemic control must be individualized, based on comorbidities, risk of hypoglycemia, and other factors.[151,152] The optimal target hemoglobin A1c (HbA1c) range for patients with diabetes on dialysis differs from that of the general population.[153] Suggested factors to consider in the spectrum of tighter (HbA1c <6.5%) or looser (HbA1c <8%) control in ESKD patients are shown in Table 12.31.[152]

TABLE 12.30 ■ **ESKD Problems in Patients With Diabetes**

Problem	Evaluation
Glycemic control	Hemoglobin A1c, continuous glucose monitoring, home fingerstick monitoring
Vascular access	Preservation of arterial and venous vasculature and early assessment for native fistula options
Coronary ischemia	Exercise tolerance test, P-thallium nuclear imaging, echocardiogram, heart catheterization, if indicated
Visual impairment	Ophthalmology evaluation and follow-up
Foot ulcers	Podiatry evaluation and follow-up
Peripheral vascular disease	Regular foot exams, podiatry care, Doppler flow studies of lower extremities
Gastroparesis/dysmotility	Gastric emptying study for symptoms
Neuropathy	Neurology evaluation, electromyography, if indicated
Malnutrition	Serum albumin, dietary counseling

ESKD, End-stage kidney disease.

TABLE 12.31 ■ **Factors to Consider in Determining Hemoglobin A1c Goal in ESKD Patients With Diabetes and CKD**

Factors	GOAL HEMOGLOBIN A1c FOR BETTER OUTCOMES	
	<6.5%	<8.0%
CKD severity	Lower (e.g., eGFR stage 1)	Higher (e.g., eGFR stage 5)
Macrovascular complications	None or mild	Severe
Comorbidities	None or few	Many
Life expectancy	Long	Short
Hypoglycemia awareness	Good	Diminished
Resources for hypoglycemia management	Available	Limited
Likelihood of treatments causing hypoglycemia	Low	High

CKD, Chronic kidney disease; *eGFR*, estimated glomerular filtration rate; *ESKD*, end-stage kidney disease.
Based on information in Chen TK, Sperati CJ, Thavarajah S, Grams ME. Reducing kidney function decline in patients with CKD: core curriculum 2021. *Am J Kidney Dis*. 2021 Jun;77(6):969–983. doi:10.1053/j.ajkd.2020.12.022.

12.13.2 METHODS OF MEASURING GLYCEMIA

Continuous glucose monitoring, the most effective method to determine ongoing glucose exposure in patients with diabetes, appears to be accurate in CKD,[154] but chronic data in the ESKD population are not available. Levels of HbA1c, generally the gold standard, are affected by factors unrelated to glycemic control in ESKD, leading to a potential overestimation of glycemic control. Reduction in glycosylation of erythrocyte Hgb in anemic ESKD patients treated with ESAs accounts for the lowering of HbA1c. Diabetic HD patients with HbA1c measured below 6.5% and over 8.0% appear to have higher mortality risk.[155–157] Guidelines recommend a target HbA1c of 7.0% to 8.0%.[151] Glycated albumin has been suggested as the preferred alternative glycemic marker in HD patients. The normal reference range for glycated albumin is 11.9% to 15.8%. There is limited evidence that the target range for glycated albumin should also exceed the reference range.[158]

12.13.3 MANAGEMENT OF HYPERGLYCEMIA

The high prevalence of diabetes mellitus in the ESKD population means that the nephrologist should have some expertise in glycemic management.[159] A summary of drug selection would be as follows (Table 12.32). Note that sodium-glucose cotransporter-2 (SGLT2) inhibitors would not be effective in ESKD patients and should not be used.

A detailed accounting of diabetes treatments is shown in Tables 12.33 and 12.34.[160]

Of note, a recent small study evaluating the benefit of a fully automated closed-loop insulin delivery system simulating the artificial pancreas (continuous glucose monitoring, insulin pump, diabetes control algorithm) demonstrated safe and effective glucose control over 24 hours.[161]

12.13.4 RISK OF HYPOGLYCEMIA

Hypoglycemia is a cause of morbidity and mortality in patients with diabetes, and affects the approach to treatment of diabetes in ESKD. Several factors, including diminished clearance of insulin, failure of renal gluconeogenesis, and inadequate nutrition, increase the risk of hypoglycemia in ESKD.[162] Periods of hypoglycemia may be severe and prolonged.

The consequences of hypoglycemia are shown in Table 12.35.

Hypoglycemia may also be associated with stress-induced myocardial ischemia, thrombosis, proinflammatory events, and prolonged QT interval. With ESKD, more intense glucose monitoring is indicated in order to avoid hypoglycemic episodes.[163]

12.14 Seizures

Acute seizures may occur as a complication of ESKD, or occur in patients with epilepsy that is exacerbated by uremia. The association with kidney failure may relate to many factors, such as hyponatremia, hypernatremia, hypocalcemia, acid-base disorders, azotemia, dialysis disequilibrium, uncontrolled HTN, and, rarely, ESAs.

For acute seizures, IV benzodiazepines can be used to halt seizure activity. Laboratory evaluation should include glucose, calcium, potassium, sodium, magnesium, blood urea nitrogen (BUN), and Cr. Options for antiepileptic drug treatment of seizures in ESKD patients are shown in Table 12.36.[164]

Table 12.36 lists the properties of antiepileptic drugs used as therapy for chronic seizure control in the ESKD patient. Commonly used medications in ESKD are levetiracetam and lacosamide.[164]

TABLE 12.32 ■ **Oral Hypoglycemic Agents and ESKD**

- Avoid metformin
- Glipizide is the preferred oral sulfonylurea
- No dose adjustment for repaglinide
- No dose adjustment for Pioglitazone or Roziglitazone
- No dose adjustment for exenatide
- Need decreased dose of sitagliptin

ESKD, End-stage kidney disease.

TABLE 12.33 ■ Detailed Characteristics of Oral Hypoglycemic Agents

Class	Compound	Drug Name	Formulations	Mechanism of Action	Primary Physiological Action	Advantages	Disadvantages	Renal Metabolism/ Elimination	Eskd Dose Range
Sulfonylureas	Glipizide	Glucotrol	5, 10 mg	Close K$_{ATP}$ channels on β-cell membrane	• ↑Insulin secretion	• Common use	• Hypoglycemia • Weight gain • Low durability • ?Cardiovascular risk	10% excreted unchanged in urine	2.5–10 mg daily
		Glucotrol XL	2.5, 5, 10 mg						
	Glimepiride	Amaryl	1, 2, 4 mg				• Drug interactions	Weekly active and inactive metabolites excreted in urine	1–4 mg daily
Meglitinides	Repaglinide	Prandin	0.5, 1, 2 mg	Close K$_{ATP}$ channels on β-cell membrane	• ↑Insulin secretion	• ↓Postprandial glucose excursions • Dosing flexibility • Relative safety	• Hypoglycemia • Weight gain • Frequent dosing • High cost	Limited excretion of inactive metabolites	0.5–1.0 mg three times daily w/meals
Thiazolidinediones	Pioglitazone	Actos	15, 30, 45 mg	Activate the nuclear transcription factor PPAR-γ	• ↑Insulin sensitivity	• No hypoglycemia • Durability of effect • Favorable effect on lipid profile	• Weight gain • Possible fluid retention • ?Bladder cancer • Fractures • High cost	Limited excretion of active metabolites	15–30 mg daily

Class	Drug	Brand	Dose forms	Mechanism	Benefits	Concerns	Excretion	Dose
DPP-4 inhibitors	Sitagliptin	Januvia	25, 50, 100 mg	Inhibit the inaction of endogenous incretins by DPP-4	• ↑Insulin secretion • ↓Glucagon secretion	• Well tolerated • No weight gain • Less hypoglycemia	• Effect is modest • ?Pancreatitis • Urticaria/angioedema	Excreted mostly unchanged in urine	25 mg daily
	Saxagliptin	Onglyza	2.5, 5 mg					Renal excretion of drug and metabolites	2.5 mg daily
	Linagliptin	Tradjenta	5 mg					Very limited urinary excretion	5 mg daily
	Vildagliptin	Galvus	50 mg					Some excretion of drug by kidneys	50 mg daily
Incretin mimetics	Liraglutide	Victoza	18 mg/3 mL	Activates GLP-1 receptor	• ↑Insulin secretion • ↓Glucagon Secretion • ↓ Gastric emptying • ↑Satiety	• Weight loss • No hypoglycemia	• GI side effects • No experience in renal failure • Injection required • ?Medullary thyroid cancer • ?Pancreatitis • High cost • Weight loss	Endogenous enzymes throughout the body	0.6–1.8 mg SQ daily

GI, Gastrointestinal; *SQ*, subcutaneously.
Adapted from Garg R, Williams M. Diabetes management in the kidney patient. *Med Clin North Am.* 2013 Jan;97(1):135–156. doi:10.1016/j.mcna.2012.11.001.

TABLE 12.34 ■ **Characteristics of Insulin Analogues**

Insulin Type	Name	Example	Onset of Actions	Peak Effect	Duration
Basal	NPH	Humulin N Novolin N	1–2 hr	4–8 hr	12–18 hr
	Glargine	Lantus	2 hr	No peak	20–24 hr
	Detemir	Levemir	2 hr	3–9 hr	16–24 hr
Prandial	Regular	Humulin R Novolin R	30 min	2–4 hr	6–8 hr
	Lispro	Humalog	5–15 min	1–2 hr	4–6 hr
	Aspart	NovoLog	5–15 min	1–2 hr	4–6 hr
	Glulisine	Apidra	5–15 min	1–2 hr	4–6 hr

Adapted from Garg R, Williams M. Diabetes management in the kidney patient. *Med Clin North Am*. 2013 Jan;97(1):135–156. doi:10.1016/j.mcna.2012.11.001.

TABLE 12.35 ■ **Consequences of Hypoglycemia**

Neurogenic	Neuroglycopenic
Tremulousness	Confusion/odd behavior
Palpitations	Drowsiness
Anxiety	Weakness
Sweating	Warmth
Tingling	Clumsiness
Hunger	Seizure
	Coma

TABLE 12.36 ■ **Antiepileptic Drug Use in ESKD**

Drug	Daily Dose in ESKD
Levetiracetam	500–1000 mg; 50% of daily dose as a post-HD supplement
Valproic acid	30–60 mg/kg/day as BID or TID
Lamotrigine	100–500 mg as QD or BID
Topiramate	100–200 mg BID; 50% supplement of BID dose as a post-HD
Zonisamide	100–600 mg/day as QD or BID; give post-HD
Phenytoin	150–200 mg BID or TID; follow free phenytoin levels
Phenobarbital	60–100 mg BID or TID
Carbamazepine	200 mg BID, maximum 800 mg BID
Oxcarbazepine	300 mg BID, maximum 1200 mg BID
Gabapentin	300 mg TID, maximum 1800 mg; give 200–300 mg post-HD dose
Pregabalin	150–600 mg/day as BID or TID, give 25–150 mg post-HD dose
Lacosamide	50 mg BID, maximum 200 mg BID; give 50% of BID dose as post-HD supplement

BID, Twice daily; *ESKD*, end-stage kidney disease; *HD*, hemodialysis; *QD*, daily; *TID*, three times daily.

12.15 Gout

Although the incidence of gout may be low in the ESKD patient, it is associated with a 1.5-fold increased risk of mortality.[165] Its incidence is increased with advancing age, obesity, alcohol use, female sex, and in the Black population. Hyperuricemia is almost universal in the patient with gout. Uric acid accumulates in kidney failure, but has a low molecular weight and is water soluble and not protein bound, so clearance with HD is excellent (and superior when HD is compared with PD). Nonetheless, hyperuricemia occurs in a large percentage of patients on dialysis. The mechanisms for the association with mortality risk are not well understood.

Gout should be considered in the differential diagnosis of acute joint complaints, although it may be mimicked by conditions such as pseudogout, septic monoarthritis, or localized cellulitis. Gout may resolve on its own, but it usually requires treatment, the sooner, the better.

The management of gout flares in the ESKD patient is challenging due to nephrotoxicity or contraindications of available agents.[166] The usual duration of therapy is 5 to 7 days. As described by Vargas-Santos et al.,[166] the treatment for gout can be separated into management of acute flares and prophylactic lowering of serum urate levels.

12.15.1 FOR ACUTE GOUT FLARES

Glucocorticoids: Treatment of choice in most ESKD cases; usually oral prednisone. Avoid if septic arthritis needs to first be ruled out. Initial dose is 30 to 40 mg. Avoid excessive dosing if gout occurs frequently. Will affect glycemic control in patients with diabetes. Intraarticular glucocorticoids may be preferred if oral agents are contraindicated.

Colchicine: Narrow therapeutic margin; should generally be avoided in ESKD. Poorly tolerated, dose must be adjusted; not removed by dialysis; increased risk of myo/neurotoxicity. Note that medications that inhibit the cytochrome P450 system component CYP3A4 (HIV protease inhibitors, clarithromycin, others) or the membrane P-glycoprotein drug efflux pump (cyclosporine, tacrolimus, amiodarone, verapamil, others) may dangerously raise colchicine levels and cause toxicity. FDA label limits dosing (in both HD and PD) to 0.3 mg twice weekly or a single 0.6-mg dose, not to be repeated in 2 weeks. Commonly causes diarrhea and abdominal cramping. ESKD patients should be monitored closely for colchicine toxicity if the drug is used.

NSAIDs: Relatively contraindicated in ESKD; available without a prescription; risk of acute gastritis and GI bleeding; systemic bleeding tendency due to impaired thromboxane-dependent platelet aggregation; may result in loss of any residual renal function. Aspirin, especially at low doses (<2–3 g/day), is contraindicated in treating gout flares because of elevation of serum uric acid levels that may result from the medication.

12.15.2 FOR URATE-LOWERING THERAPY

Allopurinol: Dose adjusted so that serum levels of oxypurinol do not rise; do not give during active flare; significant toxicity such as allopurinol hypersensitivity syndrome (related to the initial dose and whether the patient is a carrier of the HLA-B*5801 allele); risk is greatest in first 6 months of use; initial dose 50 mg/day to reduce risk of gout flare and allergic reaction with up-titration to maximum of 100 mg daily or 300 mg twice weekly. Should be discontinued at first appearance of skin rash or other signs of allergy. Dose limitation may reduce efficacy. Continue during flare without interruption. Do not initiate or reintroduce during flare as might predispose to another flare. If patient is on azathioprine, reduce its dose to one-fourth of pre-azathioprine allopurinol dose.

Febuxostat: Xanthine oxidase inhibitor; prohibitive cost; few case reports in ESKD showing reduction in uric acid levels; risk of severe adverse cutaneous reactions such as drug rash with eosinophilia and systemic symptoms (DRESS) syndrome, Stevens-Johnson syndrome, and toxic epidermal necrolysis may be increased in CKD.

Pegloticase: Recombinant PEGylated uricase, converts uric acid to the more soluble allantoin; dosing IV every 2 weeks; no dose adjustment; G6PD deficiency is contraindication; anaphylaxis and infusion reactions have been reported.[167]

Rasburicase: Recombinant urate oxidase that can be used for acute hyperuricemia in patients with hematological and solid tumor malignancies who are receiving anticancer therapy to prevent or treat tumor lysis syndrome[168]; [on line] can cause anaphylaxis, hemolysis (G6PD deficiency is a contraindication), or methemoglobinemia.

Dialysis: Increasing dialysis frequency in order to reduce uric acid levels.

12.16 Cancer Screening in ESKD

The overall cancer risk in ESKD patients is increased (standardized incidence ratio = 1.42), particularly kidney/bladder, breast, lymphoma, lung, and colon cancer.[169] Cancer screening guidelines developed for the general population may not apply to ESKD patients, related to the performance characteristics of the screening tests and the potential benefits related to reduced life expectancy. A screening algorithm for cancer in ESKD is shown in Figure 12.12.[169]

A specific challenge is related to the increased incidence of acquired renal cystic disease with time on dialysis (over 50% by 10 years), and the association of the acquired cysts with renal cell carcinoma. Periodic screening by initial ultrasound (US), followed by CT scan when indicated, is recommended for ESKD patients who are transplant candidates or who have longer expected survival.[169,170]

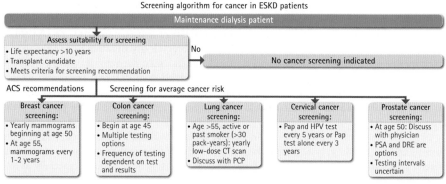

ACS, American Cancer Society; DRE, digital rectal exam; ESKD, end-stage kidney disease; HPV, human papillomavirus; PCP, primary care physician; PSA, prostate-specific antigen.

Figure 12.12 Screening algorithm for cancer in ESKD patients. (From Rosner MH. Cancer screening in patients undergoing maintenance dialysis: who, what, and when. *Am J Kidney Dis*. 2020 Oct;76[4]:558–566. doi:10.1053/j.ajkd.2019.12.018.)

12.17 COVID-19 and ESKD

Patients with CKD/ESKD have been severely affected by the COVID-19 pandemic.[171,172] Chronic dialysis patients have specific risk factors for COVID-19, including older age, obesity, diabetes, HTN, and Black/Hispanic demographics, as well as risk of person-to-person exposure during transportation and in the crowded dialysis venue. Outbreaks in dialysis units and clustering of cases on specific dialysis shifts have been reported.

ESKD patients are particularly susceptible to COVID-19,[173] only in part related to overrepresentation of the elderly and Blacks relative to the general population. Universal screening indicates a high prevalence of positive RT-PCR results from nasopharyngeal swabs in both patients and staff. The overall dialysis seropositivity rates in patients have been 2 to 3 times those of the general population. Despite implementation of stringent policies and procedures to reduce risk in the HD setting, overall seropositivity rates averaged around 6% during the pandemic,[174] with geographic variation ranging between 2% and 24%. Black and Hispanic patients had rates over twice as high as White patients. The seropositivity rate was surprisingly lower in older patients, possibly due to their higher mortality risk. The overall rate of patients clinically diagnosed with COVID-19 was 3.3%, making the seropositivity rate about 1.7 times the clinical diagnosis rate.

Patients on dialysis appeared to have fewer unknown COVID-19 infections than the general population, although many cases are subclinical or asymptomatic.[175] Reports from around the world have indicated a fatality rate of 20% to 30% among patients with ESKD.[176] All-cause mortality among dialysis patients during the 2020 COVID-19 surge was about 50% higher than the same time in preceding years. Maintenance dialysis patients needing ICU care for COVID-19 have a hospital mortality rate of 50%. In addition, 20% to 40% of COVID-19 patients in the general population have developed AKI, many of them intensive care patients requiring dialysis. Patients who recover from symptomatic episodes have prolonged viral shedding, although they do develop an IgG antibody response to the virus.

During the 2020 crisis phase of the pandemic, one result of shortages of supplies and trained staff was a reduction for some acute patients in the number of HD treatments to twice weekly. Also, data indicate that a reduction in CKD care during the peak months of the pandemic occurred that may lead to a downstream impact of reduced RRT preparedness.

By comparison, the incidence of symptomatic disease is reduced by at least half in home hemodialysis (HHD) patients and is only slightly above that of the general population in PD patients.[172] A transition toward greater utilization of home dialysis modalities may also be a legacy of the COVID-19 pandemic.

Importantly, prevention of transmission in the HD unit setting has been shown to be achievable using universal COVID-19 testing along with universal droplet and contact precautions.[177] Strategies to reduce COVID-19 risk in chronic dialysis patients[178] are shown in Table 12.37.

A variety of treatment options for COVID-19 have been tested (chloroquine, IL-6 blockade, interferon, corticosteroids, convalescent plasma, remdesivir, favipiravir, therapeutic plasma exchange, monoclonal antibodies, and new oral antiviral drugs), but data in the ESKD population are sparse in part due to exclusion of patients from clinical trials.[179] Remdesivir pharmacokinetics predict an accumulation of the parent compound, an active metabolite, and the vehicle compound with sustained use in the setting of kidney failure.[180] Nirmatrelvir-ritonavir (Paxlovid) is significantly renally excreted, but can be utilized at reduced dosage for patients with CKD. It is generally not recommended for those with advanced kidney failure, but has been increasingly used in symptomatic dialysis patients at reduced dosages. For dialysis, heightened anticoagulation necessary to

---

TABLE 12.37 ■ **Strategies to Reduce Risk of COVID-19 Infection in ESKD Patients[178]**

Risk reduction through patient and family education
Expanded testing in high-risk community settings
Universal mask use among dialysis patients and staff
Reduced waiting-room exposure
Routine primary screening before entry to the facility, for signs and symptoms or known exposure to COVID-19
Cohorting of patients with symptomatic or asymptomatic COVID-19 status
Mandatory screening of nursing home residents and new hospital admissions

ESKD, End-stage kidney disease.

prevent filter clotting has been well demonstrated in those on CRRT.[181] Acute PD has emerged as an alternative emergency therapy due in part to HD machine/staff shortages in surges. For chronic dialysis therapy, PD has been promoted when possible, to avoid hospitalization time and reduce the risk of hospital-acquired infections.[182]

The ability of current vaccines to provide protective capacity in ESKD patients, who are known to have a suboptimal acquired immunity from other vaccines, remains to be determined.[183] Dialysis patients appear to develop lower titers of protective antibody than control groups.[184] However, evidence suggests that over 80% will respond to 2 doses of an mRNA vaccine. Nonetheless, elderly ESKD patients are especially advised to receive a third vaccine dose. Effects on the severity of the disease and long-term safety remain to be determined. Seroconversion, which occurs after infection, approaches 100% in the dialysis population, but titers may decline after a few months; natural immunity to COVID-19 among chronic HD patients occurs, but is incomplete and is of reduced magnitude compared to healthy individuals.[185] However, acquired immunity significantly reduces risk of subsequent COVID-19 infection among ESKD patients.

12.18 Symptom Management in ESKD Patients

Even less objectively assessable than dialysis adequacy, but increasingly considered a relevant measure of it, are patient-reported outcomes such as symptom control (Table 12.38[186]). Patients with ESKD experience many physical and psychological symptoms, and their physical state typically deteriorates over time. This may be underrecognized by the physician. Regular symptom management should be assessed through available survey tools.[186]

Fatigue: Fatigue is a common complaint, diminishes quality of life, and may not improve with the dialysis procedure.[187] Little is actually understood about the pathogenesis and treatment of fatigue.[188] Almost three-quarters of patients report some degree of fatigue, and it is severe in one-third of them. Postdialysis fatigue may be the most intolerable part of dialysis dependence. A new fatigue measure (tiredness, energy level, limits on usual activities) may be useful.[189] Empiric treatment includes increasing physical activity, maximizing the target Hgb level, correcting acidemia, and evaluating/treating depression. More frequent dialysis sessions may actually diminish fatigue.

TABLE 12.38 ■ Symptoms Reported in ESKD Patients

Fatigue/weakness: 68%
Dry skin: 72%
Pruritus: 54%
Pain: 50%
Dry mouth: 45%
Insomnia: 44%
Muscle cramps: 43%
Diarrhea: 17%
Anxiety: 28%
Shortness of breath: 19%
Poor appetite: 29%
Depression: 24%
Restless legs: 29%
Nausea: 26%
Constipation: 21%
Vomiting: 11%

ESKD, End-stage kidney disease.
Adapted from Gelfand SL, Scherer JS, Koncicki HM. Kidney supportive care: core curriculum 2020. *Am J Kidney Dis*. 2020 May;75(5):793–806. doi:10.1053/j.ajkd.2019.10.016.

Pain: Dialysis patients experience a high pain symptom burden.[190] Avoidance of NSAIDs in ESKD has led to increased administration of opioids and other adjuvant therapies to manage pain. Dialysis patients with residual renal function may face the same NSAID risks as other stage 5 CKD patients, including AKI, loss of residual kidney function, hypervolemia, and hyperkalemia. If NSAIDs are to be used in ESKD, low doses of short half-life agents restricted to 5 or fewer days are appropriate.[191] Opioid prescribing in ESKD patients has increased,[192] but has been associated with increased hospitalizations, death risk, and other adverse outcomes. Dosing for preferred opioids in advanced CKD is shown in Table 12.39.[192]

Pharmacokinetics and clearance vary among parent opioid compounds. Hydromorphone (0.5 mg every 6 hr), fentanyl (12.5-mcg patch every 72 hr), methadone, and buprenorphine (5-mcg patch every 7 days) are preferred; not recommended are morphine, hydrocodone, codeine, and extended-release tramadol.

Pruritus: Uremic pruritus is common, and is associated with poorer quality of life as well as higher mortality.[193] Its prevalence is underestimated by physicians, and many patients remain untreated. It frequently exists with dry skin, and often is precipitated by the dialysis procedure. Other dermatological conditions, such as contact dermatitis or scabies infestation, and systemic conditions such as cholestasis and postherpetic neuralgia, should be ruled out.

Treatment generally targets high phosphate levels, hyperparathyroidism, or inadequate dialysis, based on weak evidence. In addition, all sufferers should receive a topical emollient (such as 1% pramoxine hydrochloride lotion) and reapply after bathing; in addition, sufferers should avoid hot-water bathing, use moisturizers regularly, and take low-dose gabapentin or pregabalin. Use of

TABLE 12.39 ■ Suggested Starting Doses of Preferred Opioids for Use in Advanced CKD[192]

Opioid	Normal Kidney Function (eGFR > 100)	CKD Stage 4 (eGFR 15–30)	CKD Stage 5 (eGFR <15)
Hydromorphone (short-acting)	2- to 4-mg oral tab every 4–6 hr	1-mg oral tab every 6 hr	0.5-mg oral tab every 6 hr
Fentanyl (long-acting)	Not recommended in opioid-naïve patients; dose may be variable based on oral opioid equivalent dose	12.5- or 25-mcg patch transdermally every 72 hr (decrease to 50%-75% of normal dose)	12.5-mcg patch transdermally every 72 hr (decrease to 50% of normal dose)
Methadone	Recommend referral to specialist; requires pretreatment and follow-up ECG monitoring for QT interval prolongation		
Buprenorphine	5-mcg patch transdermally every 7 days; may precipitate withdrawal in patients already receiving opioids; should discontinue other long-acting opioids; may need to continue short-acting analgesics until adequate analgesia from buprenorphine is achieved	5-mcg patch transdermally every 7 days (no clear evidence for dosage adjustments; use with caution)	5-mcg patch transdermally every 7 days (no clear evidence for dosage adjustments; use with caution)
Oxycodone	10–30 mg every 4–6 hr; use with caution	5 mg every 6–8 hr; use with caution	2.5–5 mg every 8–12 hr; use with caution

CKD, Chronic kidney disease; ECG, electrocardiogram; eGFR, estimated glomerular filtration rate (in mL/min/1.73 m^2).

TABLE 12.40 ■ **Treatment of Uremic Pruritus**

1. Optimization of dialysis: maximize Kt/V; use of high-flux dialyzer
2. Treatment of hyperphosphatemia
3. Parathyroidectomy for hyperparathyroidism if calcimimetic treatment fails
4. Topical emollients, capsaicin, and pramoxine
5. Antihistamines and gabapentin
6. Opioid receptor modulators (naltrexone or naloxone; difelikefalin or nalfurafine)
7. Ultraviolet B phototherapy for resistant cases

antihistamines such as hydroxyzine is based on weak evidence and may result in sedation. With the exception of gabapentin, the evidence for benefit is weak.[194]

Stimulators of the υ-opioid receptor (morphine) in the brain lead to pruritus, and κ-opioid receptor stimulation leads to inhibition of υ-receptors, making modulation an attractive therapeutic target. Opioid receptor antagonists include naltrexone, nalfurafine, and difelikefalin. A recent regulatory trial using the Worse Itching Intensity Numerical Rating Scale indicated superiority over placebo of the intravenous agent difelikefalin, a selective κ-opioid receptor agonist.[195] In select patients, narrow-band ultraviolet B phototherapy, parathyroidectomy, or acupuncture may be appropriate. Treatment for uremic pruritus is indicated in Table 12.40.

12.18.1 DEPRESSION

Depression affects at least one-quarter of ESKD patients and affects their outcomes.[196] The Institute for Health and Care Excellence (NICE) guidance for depression in adults with chronic health problems recommends a stepped care approach to treatment, including medications for mild to moderate depression.

Management of dialysis patients is mandated to include annual screening and follow-up by the dialysis team for depression. Screening tools have been validated in ESKD. Treatment is similar to the general population, with evidence suggesting the benefit of psychosocial interventions in addition to medications. However, in many instances, renal providers are unwilling to prescribe antidepressants, or patients do not accept treatment.

Selective serotonin reuptake inhibitors (SSRIs) are first-line therapy in ESKD patients. Paroxetine clearance is significantly reduced in renal failure. No antidepressants are cleared by dialysis. Therefore, no dose adjustment is required with sertraline and fluoxetine in dialysis patients, while the dose of paroxetine is reduced by at least half. Evidence indicates that cognitive behavioral treatment as well as exercise therapy are beneficial.

12.18.2 SLEEP DISORDERS

Up to 80% of ESKD patients experience sleep disturbances, including insomnia, restless leg syndrome, sleep-disordered breathing, and periodic limb movement disorder. Furthermore, there are associations between sleep disorders and cognitive impairment.[197] Parasomnias refer to sleep states of partial arousal with abnormal movements and dreams. Obesity and neck circumference (>40 cm) are risk factors. Mechanisms in uremia include fluid accumulation, systemic inflammation, and disturbed respiratory drive. The normal evening surge of melatonin is inadequate in ESKD patients. Sleep apnea improves in patients with intensive dialysis such as nocturnal HD. In addition to optimization of the dialysis regimen, treatment of insomnia in ESKD is the same as in the general population. Benzodiazepines should be avoided in older patients or those with a history of substance use disorder. Contributing factors such as dementia, obstructive sleep apnea, and heart failure should be ruled out.

12.19 Home Dialysis Options

Much effort has been put into correcting a perceived underutilization of home dialysis therapy, including both HHD and PD, in recent years.[198] Incentivized by health policy changes and regulatory efforts, the home dialysis option has recently increased to its highest point in 2 decades.[199] Close to 90% of patients undergoing dialysis use in-center HD, and the probability of switching to home dialysis decreases from 7% in the first month to <1% by the fourth month of dialysis. If home dialysis is likely to expand further in the future to meet current goals, predialysis planning will need to fundamentally change.

There are no randomized clinical trials comparing home and in-center dialysis. Home modalities do appear to offer the potential for improved clinical outcomes, increased patient satisfaction and autonomy, and increased employment. Regarding health-related quality of life (HRQoL), a recent analysis showed better physical HRQoL with home dialysis than in-center dialysis, while mental HRQoL was comparable.[200] Barriers include reduced patient referrals, workforce shortages, lack of professional expertise, patient costs, and patient/caregiver burdens. A recent NKF-KDOQI conference concluded that policy and reimbursement changes to better empower patients to make informed choices about home dialysis are necessary.[201] Potential advantages of a home dialysis regimen are shown in Table 12.41.[201]

12.20 Home Hemodialysis

Growth in home dialysis is particularly evident in HHD, which is being given high priority by dialysis organizations. While for many nephrologists, a barrier to HHD is their lack of familiarity with the modality, intensive efforts are being made to educate both physicians and patients regarding the full scope of this treatment option and whether the patient can manage it. Patient-perceived barriers include need for self-cannulation of AVFs or AVGs and fear of a catastrophic event. More user-friendly machine technology has contributed to the growth in HHD.

Recent practice guidelines suggest an individualized prescription for HHD, taking into account lifestyle goals, with the same dose and time target considerations each week as for in-center–based patients.[202] Current clinical practice guidelines for weekly HD adequacy suggest a target standard ($stdKt/V_{urea}$) of 2.3, with a minimum delivered dose of 2.1. This stdKt/V formula is used for higher home dialysis frequencies than the single-pool ($spKt/V$) formula used for thrice-weekly in-center HD.[203]

Potential benefits of HHD include regression in left ventricular (LV) mass, reduced depressive symptoms, improved volume control with liberalized diet, superior bone/mineral parameters, decreased postdialysis recovery time, improved quality of life, and reduced mortality risk. One

---

TABLE 12.41 ■ Potential Advantages of Home Dialysis

Improved patient satisfaction
Flexibility in scheduling
Employment more likely
Superior physical health-related quality of life
Intensified dialysis regimen
Shorter interdialytic period
Fewer hospital visits
Regression of left ventricular hypertrophy
Longer life expectancy

Adapted from Chan CT, Collins K, Ditschman EP, et al. Overcoming barriers for uptake and continued use of home dialysis: an NKF-KDOQI conference report. *Am J Kidney Dis*. 2020 Jun;75(6):926–934. doi:10.1053/j.ajkd.2019.11.007.

landmark study comparing three conventional weekly HD sessions to somewhat shorter, 6-weekly sessions reported a 40% mortality reduction in the frequent HD group.[204] In a randomized controlled trial, patients who switched from conventional HD to HHD performed overnight 5 to 6 times weekly showed improvements in LV mass, BP, and mineral metabolism.[205]

12.21 Hemodialysis Adequacy

According to the most recent KDOQI clinical practice guideline,[206] Kt/V monitoring is done on a monthly basis for the majority of chronic HD patients. The current convention is a minimum delivered single-pool Kt/V of 1.2, three times per week for chronic HD patients, with a target Kt/V of 1.4[202,206]; the contribution from residual kidney function is no longer generally measured or included. Targeting a Kt/V over 1.4 does not appear to improve outcomes.[207] In a simpler but less tested alternative fashion, the dialysis dose may also be expressed as a percent reduction in plasma urea concentration (urea reduction ratio or URR). Recommendations for dialysis adequacy with schedules other than conventional 3 times weekly HD (such as HHD or nocturnal dialysis) are less certain. KDOQI guidelines[199] suggest a minimum delivered Kt/V dose of 2.1 with a method that includes residual kidney function and ultrafiltration volume.[208]

Virtually all randomized controlled trials on HD outcomes have used Kt/V or URR to reflect dialysis adequacy. Several observational studies[209,210] have indicated a correlation between Kt/V and mortality outcomes. A major shortcoming of KtV (urea) is its reliance on the clinical importance of urea despite the presence of numerous other uremic toxins. In addition, data to indicate that "patient-relevant" outcomes relate to better Kt/V results are largely lacking.[211] As a result, determining the adequate dose of dialysis for an individual patient remains somewhat uncertain, and there is growing consensus that the totality of adequacy in dialysis involves more than just small solute removal.[212] The assessment of dialysis adequacy for ESKD is seen in Figure 12.13.

12.22 Peritoneal Dialysis

INTRODUCTION

PD is the major alternative modality to HD, and is the most common form of home dialysis. Modality choice is typically determined by patient preference. Although associated with similar mortality, higher quality of life, lower rates of complications, and lower costs compared to HD, PD has been underutilized.[213] Use has increased in the United States since Medicare payment reform in 2011.[214]

A disadvantage of PD is a number of infectious and mechanical complications specific to the modality, such as peritonitis, catheter malfunction, ultrafiltration failure, hydrothorax, and others.

Factors to be overcome in expanding the use of PD have included an incorrect perception that clinical outcomes are inferior, that peritonitis rates are high, that small-solute clearances are inadequate, and that ultrafiltration failure rates are high. Note that PD has emerged as an attractive alternative to HD for some ESKD patients with COVID-19 infection, by minimizing healthcare facility visits, reducing exposure in congregate settings, and improving social distancing. PD can be delivered at lower costs than the costs for HD.[215] "Assisted" PD utilizes a paid caregiver model and is being developed to allow this home modality for those with physical or cognitive barriers to self-care PD at home.

Recent publications have suggested a role for PD in non-ESKD patients with cardiorenal syndrome, although the benefit of hemofiltration itself when compared to diuretic therapy in that setting was inconsistent in three trials (UNLOAD, RAPID-CHF, and CARRESS-HF).[216] PD should be considered in patients with volume overload related to chronic cardiorenal syndrome.[217]

Recent guidelines emphasize incorporating quality of life into the assessment of care; preserving residual renal function; utilizing incremental PD; and prescribing PD for older people with frailty.[218]

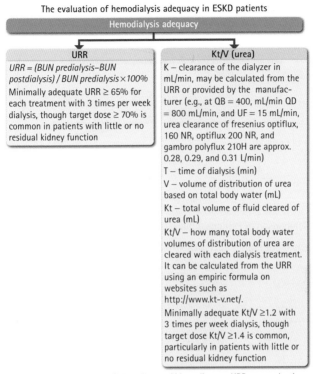

The evaluation of hemodialysis adequacy in ESKD patients

Hemodialysis adequacy	
URR	**Kt/V (urea)**
URR = (BUN predialysis–BUN postdialysis) / BUN predialysis × 100% Minimally adequate URR ≥ 65% for each treatment with 3 times per week dialysis, though target dose ≥ 70% is common in patients with little or no residual kidney function	K – clearance of the dialyzer in mL/min, may be calculated from the URR or provided by the manufacturer (e.g., at QB = 400, mL/min QD = 800 mL/min, and UF = 15 mL/min, urea clearance of fresenius optiflux, 160 NR, optiflux 200 NR, and gambro polyflux 210H are approx. 0.28, 0.29, and 0.31 L/min) T – time of dialysis (min) V – volume of distribution of urea based on total body water (mL) Kt – total volume of fluid cleared of urea (mL) Kt/V – how many total body water volumes of distribution of urea are cleared with each dialysis treatment. It can be calculated from the URR using an empiric formula on websites such as http://www.kt-v.net/. Minimally adequate Kt/V ≥1.2 with 3 times per week dialysis, though target dose Kt/V ≥1.4 is common, particularly in patients with little or no residual kidney function

BUN, Blood urea nitrogen; ESKD, end-stage kidney disease; URR, urea reduction ratio.

Figure 12.13 The evaluation of hemodialysis adequacy in ESKD patients. (From Windpessl M, Prischl FC, Prenner A, Vychytil A. Managing hospitalized peritoneal dialysis patients: ten practical points for the nonnephrologist. *Am J Med*. 2021 Jul;134[7]:833–839. doi:10.1016/j.amjmed.2021.02.007.)

12.22.1 PERITONEAL DIALYSIS INITIATION

PD takes advantage of the peritoneum to act as a dialysis "membrane" for solute and fluid removal. Location of the peritoneal catheter is depicted in Figure 12.14.[213]

The catheter consists of a visible external portion, the mid-portion of which is tunneled through the abdominal wall and ultimately penetrates the peritoneal cavity, and the intraabdominal portion. Optimal catheter tip location is in the pelvis. Connected to the external end of the catheter is a transfer set (not shown), to which the dialysis bag's tubing is connected.

It is ideal to have the PD catheter placed at least 2 weeks before the anticipated need for initiation of PD, mainly to prevent fluid leakage from the peritoneal cavity.[219] Alternatively, PD may need to be initiated on an "urgent" basis (see below).

12.22.2 PERITONEAL DIALYSIS SOLUTIONS

Commercially available peritoneal dialysate solutions are composed of an osmotic agent, electrolytes, and a buffer (Table 12.42).

The glucose-based solutions are hypertonic-containing dextrose, a monosaccharide, as the primary osmotic agent in a concentration of 1.5%, 2.5%, and 4.25%. The solutions contain the electrolytes sodium, chloride, calcium, and magnesium, but no potassium. As a buffer, they

The peritoneal dialysis catheter[213]

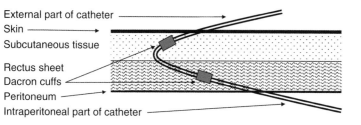
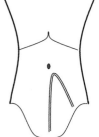

External part of catheter
Skin
Subcutaneous tissue
Rectus sheet
Dacron cuffs
Peritoneum
Intraperitoneal part of catheter

Figure 12.14   The peritoneal dialysis catheter.

TABLE 12.42 ■ **Comparison of Peritoneal Dialysis Solutions**

Solution	1.5% Dextrose	2.5% Dextrose	4.25% Dextrose	7.5% Icodextrin
Dextrose	15 g/L	25 g/L	42.5 g/L	0 (75 g/L icodextrin)
Sodium	132 mEq/L	132 mEq/L	132 mEq/L	132 mEq/L
Chloride	95 mEq/L	95 mEq/L	95 mEq/L	96 mEq/L
Calcium	2.5 mEq/L	2.5 mEq/L	2.5 mEq/L	3.5 mEq/L
Magnesium	0.5 mEq/L	0.5 mEq/L	0.5 mEq/L	0.5 mEq/L
Lactate	40 mEq/L	40 mEq/L	40 mEq/L	40 mEq/L
Osmolarity	344 mOsm/L	395 mOsm/L	485 mOsm/L	285 mOsm/L
pH	4.0–6.5	4.0–6.5	4.0–6.5	5.0–6.0

contain significant concentrations of lactate. The glucose exposure has been linked to adverse metabolic consequences related to significant systemic glucose absorption.

Icodextrin is an isosmotic glucose-sparing solution derived from maltodextrin and is used in the long dwell to improve fluid removal, particularly in patients with fast peritoneal solute transfer rates ("rapid transporters").[220] Icodextrin-containing solutions enable the long dwell and promote more sustained ultrafiltration capacity, for up to 8 to 12 hours. Compared to crystalloid solutions which induce ultrafiltration through aquaporin and large/small pores (the former producing water-only ultrafiltration), icodextrin induces more sodium removal through colloid osmosis, acting predominantly through large/small pores, with minimal absorption. It also prevents nonfluid (presumed fat) weight gain and improves insulin resistance. In PD therapy for diabetic kidney disease patients, the use of icodextrin-containing solutions has a beneficial effect on technique survival.[221] Note that only glucose-specific monitors and test strips to monitor blood glucose should be used in patients on icodextrin; other devices may show falsely elevated glucose levels. Icodextrin is contraindicated in patients with lactic acidosis or in patients with a known allergy to cornstarch or icodextrin itself. Serious reactions such as toxic epidermal necrolysis, angioedema, or erythema multiforme may result. Rarely, encapsulating peritoneal sclerosis, which may be fatal, has been reported with icodextrin.

Icodextrin may improve metabolic control in patients with diabetes, and may also lower serum insulin levels in patients without diabetes, although patients should be monitored for volume overload.[222]

12.22.3 PERITONEAL DIALYSIS TECHNIQUES

PD exchanges may be done manually or with an automated cycler, or in combination usually performed 6 to 7 days per week:

Manual technique
- CAPD: Continuous ambulatory peritoneal dialysis (CAPD); continuous technique with about 4 sequential 2- to 3-liter exchanges per day, 4- to 6-hour dwell cycles

Techniques requiring a cycler machine or automated PD (APD)
- CCPD: Continuous cycling peritoneal dialysis using a cycler machine, usually during the night; with shorter dwell times than CAPD but more exchanges and commonly with an additional long dwell, or even a manual exchange, during the day
- CCPD with abdomen dry during the day may be called intermittent PD (IPD) or nocturnal intermittent PD (NIPD) performed as frequent, short cycles during the night with no daytime dwell
- TPD: Tidal peritoneal dialysis (series of quick fills with incomplete drains so that some residual volume (15%–25% of usual dwell volume) remains in the peritoneal space; used infrequently as a peritoneal "conditioning" regimen or for patients with abdominal/rectal/pelvic pain when completely drained

12.22.4 PERITONEAL DIALYSIS PRESCRIPTION

The fill volume and dwell time of PD should be tailored to the individual patient's needs.[223] The initial PD prescription is based on clinical assessment of the patient. An adequate "prescription" of PD should be designed to provide adequate clearance and volume removal, while fitting the patient's lifestyle/schedule. The components of the PD prescription include PD modality, number of exchanges, volume of exchanges, and dialysate solution osmolarity ("strength" of PD dialysate to ultrafilter off fluid is usually determined by dextrose concentration, though icodextrin is available). In "incremental" PD, the initial prescription takes advantage of residual kidney function to limit the solute transfer required to meet treatment goals.

A key tool for assessing peritoneal membrane function, and therefore the dialysis prescription, is the peritoneal equilibration test (PET).[224] The PET is typically performed several weeks after initiation of chronic PD. The dialysis prescription is then modified, based on the transport characteristics of the peritoneal membrane determined by the PET results.

Note that, in addition to forming the basis for the initial PD prescription, the PET may be used later in the course of PD when poor fluid removal or inadequate dialysis suggests membrane dysfunction.

Importantly, when membrane dysfunction subsequently occurs, additional PET evaluation may be an important tool in providing an explanation for the dysfunction.

12.22.5 PET INTERPRETATION AND DIALYSIS MODALITY SELECTION

The purpose of the PET is to characterize the rate of transfer of solute and water across the peritoneal membrane.[225] The test yields data on Cr and glucose levels and ultrafiltration volume. The results of the PET are used to maximize solute clearances and fluid removal for individual patients. Limited data are available to validate the impact of the PET on outcomes such as hospitalization and mortality.

Details of PET administration are standardized.[226] After morning drain, 2L of dialysate containing 2.5% dextrose (2500 mg/dL) are infused and dwelled for 4 hours, and samples of dialysate and serum are taken at time 0, 2, and 4 hours. Dialysate (D) and plasma (P) Cr and dialysate glucose are measured to calculate the Cr D/P ratio and glucose Dt/D0 ratio. The results can be

TABLE 12.43 ■ Peritoneal Equilibration Test Results Used to Determine PD Transport Type

Transport Type	D/P Creatinine 4 hr	D_{4hr}/D_0 Glucose	PD Modality
High	0.82–1.03	<0.26	CAPD or CCPD with rapid short exchanges is needed
High average	0.66–0.81	0.26–0.38	Standard CAPD or CCPD will be effective
Low average	0.5–0.64	0.38–0.49	If residual renal CrCl >2 mL/min: standard CAPD or CCPD will be effective
			If residual renal CrCl <2 mL/min: high-dose CAPD or CCPD with day dwell is needed
Low	0.34–0.49	>0.49	High-dose CAPD, consider HD

CAPD, Continuous ambulatory peritoneal dialysis; *CCPD*, continuous cycling peritoneal dialysis; *CrCl*, creatinine clearance; *D/P*, dialysate/plasma; *HD*, hemodialysis; *PD*, peritoneal dialysis.
Adapted from Mehrotra R, Ravel V, Streja E, et al. Peritoneal equilibration test and patient outcomes. *Clin J Am Soc Nephrol.* 2015 Nov 6;10(11):1990–2001. doi:10.2215/CJN.03470315.

plotted on a graph to assess the peritoneal transport characteristics of the patient as a high or rapid transporter, average transporter, or low or slow transporter. Recent guidelines have also suggested incorporating a "sodium dip" or sodium sieving ratio to evaluate ultrafiltration adequacy.[224,227]

The 4-hour values and suggested PD modality based membrane transport characteristics are shown in Table 12.43.[225]

12.23 Peritoneal Dialysis Adequacy

As with forms of HD, the minimum effective dose of PD is determined by measurements of urea clearance. Both the KDOQI guidelines[228] and the International Society for Peritoneal Dialysis (ISPD) guideline[229] recommend small-solute clearance targets (total weekly Kt/V urea) as the primary measure of adequacy of dialysis. It should be noted that residual kidney function is included in the total urea clearance for the PD patient; this is no longer typically done in the in-center HD population. Targets for PD adequacy are shown in Table 12.44.

However, recent practice recommendations for dialysis adequacy in PD also place far greater emphasis on the principles of a patient-centered approach with shared decision-making,[230] and decreased emphasis on a specific target for small-solute clearance.[231] Increased emphasis is also being given to

TABLE 12.44 ■ Criteria for Peritoneal Dialysis Adequacy

Peritoneal Dialysis Adequacy

Removal of toxins (dialysis dose) can be estimated by using:
1. CrCl ≥60 L per week per 1.73 m^2 body surface area (calculate using serum and dialysate creatinine measurements from a 24-hr collection of dialysate) OR
2. Weekly Kt/V urea ≥1.7–2.0 (either just dialysis clearance or a combination of dialysis clearance and residual kidney function). Calculate from http://www.kt-v.net using addition of residual renal function if UO is >100 mL/day. To calculate weekly Kt/V for peritoneal dialysis:

K = clearance of the urea (not creatinine)—measured by timed urine or dialysate collection
t = 10080 min (per week)
V = 0.6 (for males) or 0.5 (for females) × body weight in kg

CrCl, Creatinine clearance; *UO*, urine output.

regular assessment of fluid status and avoidance of fluid overload. PD prescriptions may therefore need to be highly individualized. The current Kt/V target of 1.7 remains the standard, however.

Other standard targets for high-quality PD would include management of HTN and fluid overload, control of metabolic acidemia ($HCO_3 \geq 24$ mEq/L), and maintenance of serum levels of albumin, sodium, potassium, calcium, phosphate, and magnesium as close to normal as possible.

Nutritional status is known to have a positive impact on the treatment outcomes of patients dependent upon PD,[232] although nutritional intake and status may be challenging to assess. Inadequate protein intake may result in protein malnutrition and protein-energy wasting, a condition diagnosed by low dietary protein intake, hypoalbuminemia, unintentional weight loss, and muscle wasting. An important complication of malnutrition in PD patients includes increased susceptibility to infection. Protein is lost into the peritoneal dialysate (averaging 6–7 g/day), and peritoneal protein clearance may be a marker for inflammation, endothelial dysfunction, and mortality.[233] Daily nutritional recommendations for the PD patient are based on international society guidelines as follows: protein 1.2 to 1.4 g/kg body weight, sodium 2 to 3 g, calcium 1000 to 1200 mg, phosphorus 1.2 to 4.0 g, and no potassium restriction.[232]

12.24 Urgent-Start Peritoneal Dialysis

Unfortunately, over half of new ESKD patients are lacking a dialysis plan at the time of dialysis initiation, with little progress in the past two decades. "Urgent-start" dialysis refers to the urgent initiation of dialysis in an ESKD patient with no preestablished functional vascular access for HD and no catheter in place for PD. Urgent-start PD in unplanned ESKD patients refers to the initiation of PD much earlier (24–72 hr after PD catheter placement) than is done with conventional PD.[234] Urgent-start PD is available in many centers for late-referred patients in urgent need of dialysis but with no modality plan, who are considered otherwise to be good PD candidates. Barriers to urgent-start PD have been cited as contributing to the relatively low utilization of PD overall. It involves prompt patient education, timely catheter placement, and provision of PD with lower dwell volumes (1 L) in the recumbent position, until the patient can be trained to perform dialysis at home. Compared with non-urgent–start PD, urgent-start PD appears to be associated with similar risks of infection, hospitalization, and short-term technique and patient survival, and a slight increase in peritoneal fluid leaks not associated with adverse outcomes.[234] Data from experienced urgent-start programs indicate a minor increased risk of mechanical complications such as dialysate leaks, but no impact on technical survival compared to conventional PD.[235] Comparisons of PD and HD in urgent-start patients are limited, but PD is at least as good, and is associated with a lower risk of bacteremia.[236]

A key feature is the timely placement of the PD catheter, either by interventional radiology or surgery. A structured urgent-start program (Table 12.45.) is required to ensure implementation once the catheter is placed. It provides an alternative to urgent initiation of HD using a central venous dialysis catheter.[236]

12.25 Complications of Peritoneal Dialysis

Complications of acute/chronic PD include weight gain, formation of hernias, leakage of dialysis fluid into the subcutaneous tissue, catheter exit site or pleura, abdominal pain, worsening blood sugars, and low potassium levels. A common worrisome complication is the appearance of turbid PD fluid, likely related to peritonitis (Table 12.46).

12.25.1 PD PERITONITIS

PD-associated peritonitis is associated with substantial morbidity, hospitalizations, transition to HD, and mortality risk.[237] The evaluation of possible peritonitis is shown in Figure 12.15.

TABLE 12.45 ■ Features of Urgent Start Peritoneal Dialysis

A. Patient education about dialysis options by the nephrologist/team
B. Evaluation of candidate patient:
  • Does not need emergency dialysis
  • Functional status/trainability determined by nephrologist
  • No history of abdominal surgeries that would complicate PD
  • No psychiatric or memory problems
  • Adequate visual/hearing capability
  • Satisfactory home assessment
  • Family support is helpful for certain patients
C. Timely catheter placement by surgeon or interventional radiology
D. Clinical course:
  • Break-in period of less than 2 weeks
    ◦ Dwell in recumbent position
    ◦ Dwell volume limited to maximum of 1 L
  • Dextrose concentration determined by ultrafiltration need

PD, Peritoneal dialysis.
Adapted from Htay H, Johnson DW, Craig JC, et al. Urgent-start peritoneal dialysis versus conventional-start peritoneal dialysis for people with chronic kidney disease. *Cochrane Database Syst Rev*. 020 Dec 15;12(12): CD012913. doi:10.1002/14651858.CD012913.pub2.

TABLE 12.46 ■ Causes of Turbid PD Fluid

• Peritonitis (culture-positive or culture-negative)
• Hemoperitoneum (hemorrhage, ovulation, menses)
• Severe constipation
• Fibrin or other proteins
• Lipids (chylous ascites)
• Prolonged dwell time
• Pancreatitis
• Dihydropyridine calcium channel blockers
• Eosinophilic peritonitis (10%–30%); may be allergic reaction to PD solutions or tubing; IP antibiotics
• Specimen taken from "dry" abdomen

IP, intraperitoneal; *PD*, peritoneal dialysis.

The most common cause of peritonitis is "touch contamination" of the PD catheter connection leading to infection of the dwelled peritoneal fluid. In addition, an important clinical risk factor for peritonitis is use of high peritoneal glucose loads, perhaps by impairing host defenses or damaging the peritoneal membrane itself.[238]

Key measures to reduce PD-associated peritonitis include[230,239,240]:

■ prophylactic systemic antibiotics immediately before catheter insertion;
■ for CAPD treatment, a disconnect system with a "flush before fill" design;
■ adequate training of PD patients and their caregivers;
■ daily topical gentamicin 0.1% at exit site for reducing both Gram-positive and Gram-negative organisms (do not apply either to PD catheter itself) and coprescription of oral nystatin or fluconazole during treatment for PD peritonitis;
■ prompt treatment of exit-site infection;
■ antibiotic prophylaxis before dental procedures, colonoscopy, or invasive gynecological procedures; and
■ following an episode of peritonitis, retraining for PD patients.[241]

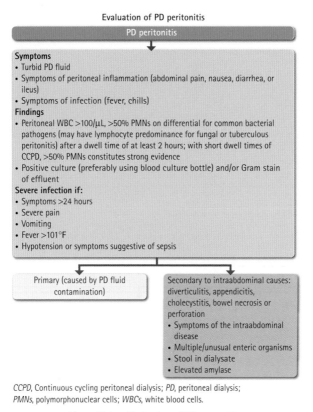

Evaluation of PD peritonitis

PD peritonitis

Symptoms
- Turbid PD fluid
- Symptoms of peritoneal inflammation (abdominal pain, nausea, diarrhea, or ileus)
- Symptoms of infection (fever, chills)

Findings
- Peritoneal WBC >100/μL, >50% PMNs on differential for common bacterial pathogens (may have lymphocyte predominance for fungal or tuberculous peritonitis) after a dwell time of at least 2 hours; with short dwell times of CCPD, >50% PMNs constitutes strong evidence
- Positive culture (preferably using blood culture bottle) and/or Gram stain of effluent

Severe infection if:
- Symptoms >24 hours
- Severe pain
- Vomiting
- Fever >101°F
- Hypotension or symptoms suggestive of sepsis

Primary (caused by PD fluid contamination)	Secondary to intraabdominal causes: diverticulitis, appendicitis, cholecystitis, bowel necrosis or perforation
	• Symptoms of the intraabdominal disease • Multiple/unusual enteric organisms • Stool in dialysate • Elevated amylase

CCPD, Continuous cycling peritoneal dialysis; *PD*, peritoneal dialysis; *PMNs*, polymorphonuclear cells; *WBCs*, white blood cells.

Figure 12.15 Evaluation of PD peritonitis.

Whenever peritonitis is suspected, the PD effluent should be tested for cell count, differential, Gram stain, and culture. Diagnosis of peritonitis relies upon: (1) clinical features consistent with peritonitis, such as abdominal pain and/or a cloudy dialysis effluent; (2) a dialysis effluent total white cell count >100/μL, along with >50% polymorphonuclear WBCs (sample taken after a dwell time of at least 2 hr); and (3) a positive dialysis effluent culture.

Note that the WBC count in the effluent may depend on the time PD fluid has been in the abdomen. For CCPD patients with a short dwell time, more reliance should be placed on the percentage of PMNs. Patients with abdominal pain in the absence of a PD dwell may have no fluid to drain, in which case 1 L of PD solution should be instilled, dwelled for 2 hours, and then drained for sampling/testing. A blood culture bottle is the preferred technique for bacterial culture.

Once culture and sensitivity results are known, antibiotic selection should be narrowed accordingly.

Fungal peritonitis is a relatively rare but serious complication in PD patients. Risk factors include preceding bacterial peritonitis and exposure to antimicrobial agents. Candida species are the most frequent cause.[242] Several routes of contamination causing infectious peritonitis should be considered, including touch contamination, exit-site/tunnel infection, GI infection, and hematogenous infection. Mortality is unusual, the most common cause being fungal infection. Management recommendations are indicated in Figure 12.16.[240]

In some cases, antibiotics for suspected and mild peritonitis cases can be initially administered at home, pending subsequent culture results of dialysate effluent. There is no widely accepted regimen. Recommendations are shown in Table 12.47. [240,243]

Evaluation and management recommendations for PD peritonitis

- Send cell count and differential, culture, and Gram stain on initial drainage; note that labs may only report neutrophil count and no total WBC, or may report all WBCs so that they must be added to determine total WBC count in order to establish a diagnosis (along with % PMNs) of peritonitis
- Start empiric antibiotics after sample is obtained:
  - Cefazolin or cephalothin 15 mg/kg of body weight or 1 g/2–3-L bag QD (in the long dwell) AND EITHER
  - Ceftazidime 10–15 mg/kg of body weight or 1 g/2–3-L bag QD (in the long dwell) OR
  - Aminoglycoside (not recommended if residual urine output >100 mL/day): tobramycin or gentamicin, 0.6 mg/kg body weight in only 1 exchange per day or amikacin 2.0 mg/kg body weight, in only 1 exchange per day (or gentamicin 3 mg/kg IV)
  - Or oral quinolone (500 mg levofloxacin ×1, then 250 mg QD for 2 weeks or ciprofloxacin 750 mg BID)
  - If secondary to an intraabdominal bowel cause, treat with metronidazole plus vancomycin, in combination with ceftazidime or an aminoglycoside
  - Note that antibiotic-containing PD solution should be allowed to dwell for at least 6 hours
  - If effluent is bloody or has fibrin strands, add heparin 500 units/L IP
  - Vancomycin and gentamicin, if used in combination, should be injected into different PD dwells
  - Concurrent prophylactic antifungal oral nystatin or fluconazole may be indicated to prevent secondary fungal peritonitis related to enteric fungal overgrowth and reduced defense due to peritonitis
  - Repeat PD fluid cell count and culture after 3 days
  - Refer patient to the ER for symptoms of severe infection
  - IV antibiotics are appropriate if patient has features of systemic sepsis; otherwise, IP route is preferred.
  - Note that vancomycin may be preferable if program has a high rate of MRSA or patient has a prior history of MRSA
  - Gram-positive cocci should be treated for 2 weeks (*Staphylococcus aureus* and Enterococci for 3 weeks); Gram-negative rods for 3 weeks

↓

Culture results return in 24–48 hours

↓

Culture positive:

- Gram (+) (40%–60%)
  - Enterococci: IP vancomycin for *3 weeks; add* IP aminoglycoside for *severe cases*
  - MSSA: Cephalosporin IP + rifampin 600 mg PO *for 3 weeks*
  - MRSA: Vancomycin 15–30 mg/kg in 1 bag per day, repeat in 3–7 days to keep serum level >15 mcg/mL; treat 3 weeks
  - Coagulase-negative *S. aureus*: Assume methicillin resistant, so IP vancomycin for 2 weeks
  - VRE: Removal of catheter may be necessary, daptomycin 4–6 mg/kg every 48 hr IV or oral linezolid 200–300 mg once daily
  - Other: Stop aminoglycoside, continue cephalosporin for *2 weeks*
- Gram (–) (15%–40%)
  - Single gram (–) non-*Xanthomonas*: Adjust ABx to sensitivity for *3 weeks*
  - Pseudomonas: IP aminoglycoside or oral ciprofloxacin + ceftazidime or cefepime for *3 weeks*, removal of catheter may be necessary
  - Multiple organisms/anaerobes: Add metronidazole 500 every 8 hr IV/PO *for 3 weeks*, consider evaluation for bowel perforation if not better in 72 hours
  - Note high failure rate with extended-spectrum beta-lactamase organisms

Culture negative (15%–20%)

- No improvement: Repeat culture, continue antibiotics *for 2 weeks*
- Improvement: Discontinue aminoglycoside, continue cephalosporin *for 2 weeks*

↓

- Often caused by coagulase-negative *S. aureus*
- Evaluate for other disease: TB, other mycobacterial, fungal, or parasitic peritonitis, eosinophilic peritonitis, intraabdominal disease, renal cell or ovarian cancer, leukemia, lymphoma
- Reculture can identify the cause in some patients

Fungi (2%–5%)

- Immediate catheter removal is often necessary
- Fluconazole 150–200 mg every other day IP or amphotericin 25 mg/day IV or amphotericin 25 mg/d IV and
- Flucytosine load 2000 mg PO, maintenance 1000 mg PO *for 4–6 weeks*
- Change to amphotericin if not better in 72 hours
- IP route not preferred over systemic treatment
- Aspergillus: Use caspofungin
- Non-albicans candida: Use caspofungin
- Filamentous fungi: Use posaconazole or voriconazole

ABx, antibiotics; *BID*, twice daily; *IP*, intraperitoneal injection; *MRSA*, methicillin-resistant *Staphylococcus aureus*; *MSSA*, methicillin-sensitive *Staphylococcus aureus*; *PD*, peritoneal dialysis; *PMNs*, polymorphonuclear neutrophils; *PO*, by mouth; *QD*, daily; *TB*, tuberculosis; *VRE*, vancomycin-resistant enterococci; *WBC*, white blood cell.

Figure 12.16 Evaluation and management recommendation for PD peritonitis. (Adapted in part from Li, PK, Szeto CC, Piraino B, et al. ISPD peritonitis recommendations: 2016 update on prevention and treatment. *Perit Dial Int*. 2016 Sep 10;36[5]:481–508. doi:10.3747/pdi.2016.00078.)

TABLE 12.47 ■ **"After-Hours" Initial Treatment of Suspected Peritonitis**

1. Only for mild episodes (mild pain, low-grade fever, no hypotension, duration <24 hr, able to drain)
2. Patient to place cloudy effluent bag in refrigerator for culture
3. Cephalexin 500 mg orally every 12 hr with initial dose of 1000 mg OR Cefdinir 300 mg orally daily OR trimethoprim 160 mg/sulfamethoxazole 800 mg twice daily if allergic to cephalosporins
4. Report to regular dialysis facility next business day for evaluation with effluent bag

Adapted from Li P K-T, Szeto CC, Piraino B, et al. ISPD peritonitis recommendations: 2016 update on prevention and treatment. *Perit Dial Int.* 2016 Sep 10;36(5):481–508. doi:10.3747/pdi.2016.00078.

TABLE 12.48 ■ **Indications for Catheter Removal**

- Refractory peritonitis—failure of effluent to clear after 5 days of treatment
- Relapsing or recurrent peritonitis
- Refractory exit-site and tunnel infection
- Concomitant pseudomonal or staphylococcal aureus exit-site infection
- Unresponsive pseudomonas or fungal peritonitis
- Nontuberculous mycobacterial peritonitis
- Fecal peritonitis or other significant intraabdominal pathology
- Mechanical failure of catheter

In some cases, removal of the PD catheter is recommended (Table 12.48). Note that refractory peritonitis is now defined as failure of the effluent to clear after 5 days of appropriate antibiotics. Reinsertion of the catheter and resumption of PD should only be attempted after complete resolution of symptoms and a holiday period of at least 2 weeks after catheter removal.

12.25.2 PD TECHNIQUE FAILURE

One reason for relatively low PD utilization is attrition off of PD due to technique failure, related to either patient factors or dialysis center factors.[244] Technique failure rates have improved, decreasing to roughly 25% of patients treated per year in death-censored analyses. Smaller centers with less cumulative PD experience may have higher rates. Technique failure may take the form of inadequate solute clearance (weekly Kt/V urea of <1.7) or of ultrafiltration insufficiency Insufficient ultrafiltration may be suspected when the net ultrafiltration from a 4–hour PET using 4.25% dextrose is <400 mL, or with 2.5% dextrose <100 mL.[224] Icodextrin has been associated with improved technique survival, including in those with diabetes.[221] Causes of ultrafiltration failure are shown in Table 12.49.

Whether at home or in the hospital, the patient's PD catheter may require evaluation for catheter malfunction. Following are common types of catheter malfunction requiring assessment:

■ Mechanical failure of either dialysate inflow or outflow is not uncommon. Inflow failure is uncommon and may be due to obstruction within the catheter (fibrin strands or kinking of

TABLE 12.49 ■ **Causes of Ultrafiltration Failure**

- Peritonitis
- Adhesions/loculation
- Malpositioned catheter
- Poor peritoneal blood flow

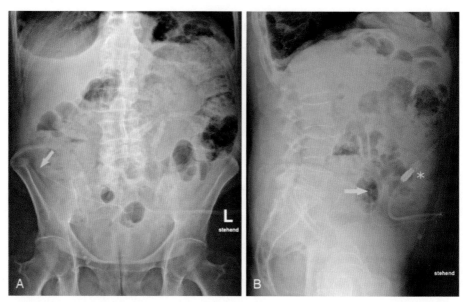

Figure 12.17 Location of peritoneal dialysis catheter on plain film of the abdomen. (A) Anterioposterior view demonstrates malposition of the catheter with its tip located in the mid-abdomen, close to the right iliac crest (arrow). (B) Lateral view depicts the external part of the catheter with the titanium adaptor (asterisk) and the intraabdominal portion turned up (arrow). The radio-opaque stripe is clearly visible and allows localization of the catheter. (From Windpessl M, Prischl FC, Prenner A, Vychytil A. Managing hospitalized peritoneal dialysis patients: ten practical points for the non-nephrologist. *Am J Med.* 2021 Jul;134[7]:833–839. doi:10.1016/j. amjmed.2021.02.007.)

the catheter) or outside the catheter (externally by a clamp inadvertently left closed) or internally (such as entrapment in omentum). Outflow failure is relatively common and may be defined as failure to drain the dwelling fluid within 45 minutes. It may be preceded by sluggish outflow, or may occur without warning.

■ The most common cause of catheter malfunction is constipation. Other causes are intraperitoneal adhesions, omental wrapping, catheter tip migration, luminal obstruction due to fibrin/clot, and catheter kinking. The latter two may be accompanied by two-way obstruction.

■ Evaluation should proceed from conservative to more aggressive interventions.
   a. Treat constipation aggressively.
   b. Rule out bladder distension causing extrinsic catheter compression.
   c. Evaluate catheter for location and kinking. On plain film, catheter location may be identified as a radiopaque stripe, preferentially located in the pelvic portion of the peritoneal cavity, as shown in Figure 12.17. Note that some cases may require a CT scan for visualization.
   d. Peritonitis should be ruled out.
   e. An empiric attempt to restore patency should be made, by a trained nurse using aseptic technique. Initially, attempt to repeatedly flush the catheter with 20 to 50 mL of heparinized 0.9% saline. If flushing is unsuccessful, fibrinolytic therapy with tPA may be attempted[218,245]; 8 mL of tPA (1 mg/mL) is slowly injected into the catheter. After a 1- to 2-hour dwell, attempt to drain PD fluid by gentle aspiration and flushing of the

catheter. If partially successful, this can be repeated. If flow is restored, 500 units of heparin should be added to each liter of PD fluid subsequently.

f. Laparoscopy to establish a diagnosis and provide a rescue procedure to salvage the catheter may ultimately be required.

g. When these steps have failed, catheter replacement may be done simultaneously with removal of the nonfunctioning peritoneal catheter.

12.25.3 ACID-BASE AND ELECTROLYTE DISTURBANCES IN PERITONEAL DIALYSIS

Multiple abnormalities in acid-base balance and electrolytes may occur in the patient treated with PD, and may be associated with adverse outcomes.[246] They sometimes provide limitations to the use of PD and may be associated with morbidity and even mortality.[247–249] Common laboratory abnormalities are shown in Table 12.50.

12.25.4 HEMOPERITONEUM

New onset of bloody peritoneal fluid is relatively uncommon and has multiple etiologies. Causes of intraperitoneal hemorrhage may be divided based on the severity and the underlying cause (Figure 12.18). In some cases, the cause is uncertain.[250] The diagnostic approach includes peritoneal fluid analysis and culture, coagulation studies, abdominal US, CT, diagnostic paracentesis, and laparoscopy/laparotomy. The method of management depends on the source of blood loss.[251]

12.25.5 OTHER COMPLICATIONS OF PD

With the decline in PD peritonitis rates, other complications have become relatively more common (Table 12.51). They may account for cases of PD technique failure.[252] Some require surgical management.

TABLE 12.50 ■ **Laboratory Disturbances in the PD Patient**

	Mechanism	Correction
Hypernatremia	Hypertonic dialysate ⇒ water shift into peritoneal space (removing water in excess of Na)	Water orally or D5W IV or lower glucose or Na level in dialysate
Hyponatremia	Low Na intake, excessive thirst, renal or stool losses, inadequate UF	Salt intake must be proportional to volume loss induced by dialysis, increase hypertonic dialysate if water overload
Hyperkalemia	High K^+ intake with low renal excretion and PD clearance, extracellular shift of K^+ due to low insulin or drugs	Higher dialysis clearance, standard treatment of acute hyperkalemia
Hypokalemia	Excessive K^+ clearance by PD, occurs in 60% of ESKD patients on PD	10%–30% of patients need K^+ supplement
Lactic acidosis	Conversion of lactate to bicarbonate can be affected in sepsis or by metformin	Replace lactate buffer with bicarbonate in dialysate

ESKD, End-stage kidney disease; *PD*, peritoneal dialysis; *UF*, ultrafiltration.

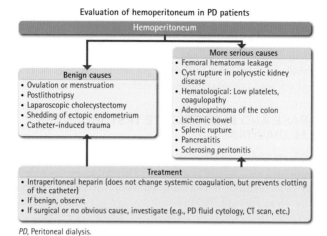

Figure 12.18   Evaluation of hemoperitoneum in PD patient.

TABLE 12.51 ■ Other Complications in the PD Patient

Problem	Diagnosis	Treatment
Hernia (↑ intraab-dominal pressure)	Clinical exam or CT scan	Surgical repair; corsets; dialysis with lower intraabdominal pressure (APD, eliminate daytime dwell or decrease volume)
Genital edema (<10% CAPD patients): tracking of PD fluid to scrotum/labia	Clinical exam, decreased PD fluid effluent return, US/CT scan	Stop PD and use temporary HD; low-volume APD at bed rest; further treatment depends on source of leak
Abdominal wall leak	Clinical exam, decreased PD fluid effluent return, US/CT scan	Stop PD, or convert to low-volume APD at bed rest; avoid sitting position; if severe, convert to temporary HD; consider catheter replacement or injecting fibrin glue (1 mL of a solution of fibrinogen and thrombin)
Hydrothorax/pleural effusion (incidence <5%)	Dyspnea, no improvement with hypertonic exchange, decreased PD fluid effluent return, diagnostic CXR with pleural effusion, thoracentesis with pleural fluid analysis showing high glucose, scan with isotope in abdomen	Stop PD and use temporary HD; thoracentesis; low-volume PD (after 2 weeks of HD may return to PD); pleurodesis (fibrin glue, autologous blood, talc, tetracycline); surgical repair
Sclerosing encapsulating peritonitis	Recurrent abdominal pain with fills, re-peated peritonitis predisposes to it, may cause bowel obstruction, or he-moperitoneum, decreased solute and water transport, characteristic appearance with CT; rarely, reported with use of icodextrin	Careful attention to nutrition and bowel function; laparoscopy; surgical intervention; antiinflammatory or im-munosuppressive meds (controver-sial); tamoxifen

TABLE 12.51 ■ **Other Complications in the PD Patient** (Continued)

Problem	Diagnosis	Treatment
Glucose intolerance	Hemoglobin A1c	Minimize use of high-dextrose concentration PD solutions; use of icodextrin for glucose-sparing
Pneumoperitoneum	Radiology imaging	Consider benign incidental cause, allowing air entry into PD catheter; assess for pathological abdominal cause (i.e., bowel perforation)

APD, ambulatory peritoneal dialysis; *CAPD*, continuous ambulatory peritoneal dialysis; *CXR*, chest X-ray; *HD*, hemodialysis; *PD*, peritoneal dialysis; *US*, ultrasound.

12.26 ESKD Peritoneal Dialysis Outcomes

PD outcomes in ESKD patients from randomized controlled trials are sparse, measured inconsistently, and limited by surrogate endpoints that have not been validated.[253] High risk of infections, inadequate clearance of small solutes, and eventual ultrafiltration failure were the basis for past concerns that PD was an inferior modality compared to HD. However, virtually all recent studies indicate that PD and in-center HD have similar short (1–2 years) or medium-term (up to 5 years) outcomes.[254] Metabolic factors potentially exacerbated by glucose-based dialysate solutions include dyslipidemia, insulin resistance/metabolic syndrome, and weight gain, but the effect on overall outcomes is unclear. PD is associated with better preservation of residual kidney function, which is associated with improved survival.[255]

Improvement in patient-reported outcomes is especially important. Hard outcomes such as mortality and technique failure are underreported in trials, and patient-important outcomes are even more limited. The Standardized Outcomes in Nephrology-Peritoneal Dialysis (SONG-PD) and other initiatives are seeking to validate relevant, meaningful PD outcomes in future trials with a goal of improving shared decision-making[256] (i.e., outcomes including PD-related infection, cardiovascular disease, mortality, technique survival, and quality of life).

Medication Management in ESKD

Both the effectiveness and the toxicity of drugs are commonly related to their concentrations in the body. Kidney dysfunction influences the pharmacokinetic parameters of at least 50% of drugs, and is also important in drug pharmacodynamics (the biochemical and physiological effects of the agent). Not only renal excretion, but also drug bioavailability and absorption, protein binding, and metabolism may be altered with impaired kidney function.

Changes in pharmacokinetics in ESKD can predispose the patient to either over- or underdosing. Dose-related drug toxicity or therapeutic failure may result.[257] For example, when the plasma half-life of a drug is prolonged in the setting of ESKD, the time to reach the steady-state concentration may increase proportionally, so administration of a loading dose may achieve therapeutic levels more quickly.[257]

The required change in dosing regimen for drugs in ESKD can in some cases be established through the application of pharmacokinetic principles.[258] In this case, drugs that are largely eliminated by the kidneys with normal renal function commonly require a dose adjustment (either by decreased dose [with more consistent but possibly toxic levels] or increased interval [with risk of subtherapeutic trough levels]) in patients with impaired kidney function or dialysis dependence. In general, dosage reduction is indicated when over one-third of the drug or active metabolite appears unchanged in the urine, although a normal loading dose may be given reven in CKD or ESKD patients. Drug elimination tends to correlate with GFR, although in many cases proximal tubular secretion is the primary mechanism of drug elimination.

Clearance of drugs and pharmacokinetics during HD are complex. Both dialysis properties (Table 12.52) and drug properties (Table 12.53) affect dosing regimens for many drugs in ESKD patients.

Attributes that would reduce the likelihood of clearance through dialysis include large molecular weight, large volume of distribution, high level of protein binding, and clearance through nonrenal mechanisms. It is important to estimate dialysis clearance of medications to adequately adjust the dose. That is especially true in drugs with a relatively narrow therapeutic window (e.g., lithium, chemotherapy, antibiotics). The complexity of the process has to do with multiple factors affecting drug clearance in dialysis; specifically, the characteristics of the dialyzer, dialysis procedure, dialysate, and properties of the drug itself. Clearance mechanisms may involve both diffusion and convection, and, rarely, adsorption to the dialysis membrane. Many drugs are small enough to be removed by dialysis so that the major determinant of drug removal is actually protein binding, since only unbound drug is removed. The term *sieving coefficient* describes how freely a solute crosses the dialysis membrane. Using these considerations, only very crude approximations of the clearance is possible in the absence of experimental data. Such experimental data are obtained for some, but not all, drugs (e.g., vancomycin[259]). Clearance of drugs by PD is generally less than with HD, but continues on a daily basis, making weekly drug dosing often comparable between the two modalities.[260]

Therefore, monitoring of drug levels is important, especially when the therapeutic target range is known.[261] During CRRT, for example, vancomycin levels are known to be frequently subtherapeutic.[259] Drug removal by dialysis may necessitate a supplemental dose following the procedure. For some specific drugs and toxins, dialysis is valuable in treating

---

TABLE 12.52 ■ Dialysis Properties That Affect Drug Clearance

- Dialyzer properties (pore size, surface area, type of membrane might affect binding)
- Dialysis procedure properties (blood flow rate, dialysate flow rate, ultrafiltration rate)
- Dialysate properties (solute concentration, pH, temperature)
- Duration of dialysis treatment

TABLE 12.53 ■ Drug Properties That Affect Dialytic Clearance

- Molecular size (Da)
  - <1000 Da—small molecules—diffusion-dependent transport. Most drugs are <500 Da.
  - 1000–2000 Da—only convective transport. Example: vancomycin (1448 Da).
  - >2000 Da—partially reflected by membrane even during UF, so clearance is low.
- Increased protein binding reduces clearance; heparin increases free fraction of many drugs (free fraction = 1-Protein-bound fraction). Kidney failure tends to decrease protein binding of drugs.
- VOD—the greater the VOD, the less the dialyzability. An estimate of all the compartments in which the drug may be found. VOD increased with lipid solubility and low plasma protein binding.
  - 1 L/kg BW—distribution volume—likely removed by dialysis.
  - 1–2 L/kg BW—distribution volume—marginal clearance by dialysis.
  - >2 L/kg BW—unlikely to be effectively removed by dialysis.
  - Multicompartmental distribution leads to dramatic rebound after dialysis.
- Molecular charge decreases dialyzability.
- Water or lipid solubility: poor dialyzability of lipid-soluble compounds.
- Dialyzer membrane binding increases clearance of the compound.

BW, Body weight; *UF*, ultrafiltration; *VOD*, volume of distribution.

TABLE 12.54 ■ **Reference Sources for Dosing Adjustments in Patients With ESKD**

MICROMEDEX Healthcare Series	www.micromedexsolutions.com
UPTODATE	www.utdol.com/online/index.do
EPOCRATES	www.epocrates.com
National Kidney Disease Education Program	www.nkdep.nih.gov
FDA MedWatch	http://fda.gov/medwatch
The Medical Letter on Drugs and Therapeutics	http://secure.medicalletter.org
Drug Prescribing in Renal Failure: Dosing Guidelines for Adults, 5th Edition	www.acponline.org

ESKD, End-stage kidney disease.

overdoses/intoxications, particularly IHD, which may exceed the clearance by normal kidney function in some cases.

Recent guidelines have addressed vancomycin dosing in dialysis patients, with important caveats.[262] Instead of trough-only dosing (based on the premise that the trough serum level is an adequate efficacy target), new recommendations make use of the serum concentration-time curve/minimum inhibitory concentration ratio. However, data justifying a specified area under the serum concentration curve (AUC)/minimum inhibitory concentration (MIC) ratio in the dialysis patient are lacking, and the approach presents important logistical issues. It is well recognized that numerous medications require dosage adjustment, or even cessation, in patients with renal failure, so the use of drug references is essential.

Because of the panoply of medications used in the management of the ESKD patient, it is important to have available reference sources to guide such decision-making. Several are listed in Table 12.54.

12.27 Extracorporeal Treatments for Intoxication

About 20% of reported poison exposures are intentional, and they are far more serious than unintentional exposures. The Extracorporeal Treatments In Poisoning (EXTRIP) workgroup has developed consensus guidelines on the role of extracorporeal treatment in patients suffering from accidental or intentional intoxications.[263] Additional considerations are supportive care, antidotes (such as naloxone for acute opioid intoxication), and corporeal elimination by activated charcoal or urine alkalinization. Over 50 poison control centers in the United States provide telephone or online guidance for human poison exposures.

When indicated, rapid introduction of effective dialysis is critical in improving outcomes. The major determinants of the benefit of extracorporeal treatments include the toxin's molecular weight, protein binding, volume of distribution, and endogenous clearance.[264] The utility of extracorporeal modalities in poisoning is shown in Table 12.55.[265]

Removal by dialysis is most efficient for agents with a low volume of distribution, limited protein binding, and low molecular weight. In the majority of indications, IHD is preferred. If dialysis is used to treat an acute intoxication and AKI is not present, replacement of potassium and phosphorus will likely be necessary.

The role for charcoal hemoperfusion has been markedly reduced, particularly when drug removal can be achieved by dialysis. A list of when extracorporeal therapy for various toxins is advised can be found at https://www.extrip-workgroup.org/recommendations.

TABLE 12.55 ■ **Role of Extracorporeal Modalities in Poisoning**

Modality	Toxin Molecular Mass (Da)	Toxin VOD (L/kg)	Protein Binding of Toxin	Examples of Toxins Amenable to Therapy	Primary Limitations of Therapy
Hemodialysis	Up to 10,000–15,000	≤1.5–2	≤80%	Salicylates, toxic alcohols, lithium, metformin	Hemodynamic stability
HCO filter HD	Up to 50,000	≤1.5–2	≤80%	Small-peptide therapeutics; any therapy amenable to HD	Limited availability Limited role in poisoning
CRRT	Up to 15,000–25,000	≤1.5–2	≤80%	Lithium	Slow toxin clearance (except for toxins with slow redistribution)
Hemoperfusion	Unclear, but high	≤1 L/kg	Any	Valproic acid, carbamazepine	Limited availability Clotting Hypocalcemia
Plasma exchange	No limit	≤1 L/kg	Any	Monoclonal antibodies, arsine	Limited availability Very slow clearance

HCO, High-molecular-mass cutoff; *HD*, hemodialysis; *CRRT*, continuous renal replacement therapy; *VOD*, volume of distribution
Adapted from King JD, Kern MH, Jaar BG. Extracorporeal removal of poisons and toxins. *Clin J Am Soc Nephrol.* 2019 Sep 6;14(9):1408–1415. doi:10.2215/CJN.02560319.

If the intoxicant has a large volume of distribution, HD can be used to reduce the initial intravascular burden of the agent. CRRT can be especially useful for intoxications for drugs with pharmacokinetics that lead to a "rebound" increase in blood levels when rapidly removed by HD, such as lithium and N-acetyl procainamide. CRRT can avoid the rebound that follows discontinuation of dialysis, while continuing the drug removal process.

Lithium remains one of the poisons where extracorporeal removal is most often needed. Dialysis is recommended when kidney function is impaired and the serum Li+ level is >4.0 mEq/L, or in the presence of decreased consciousness, seizures, or life-threatening dysrhythmias regardless of the serum level.[266] While CRRT may be a useful alternative, HD is the most effective way to rapidly reduce toxic serum levels and brain exposure in poisoned patients.

For metformin-associated lactic acidosis, HD is recommended in cases of marked serum lactate elevation, severe acidemia, and decreased level of consciousness.[267] Alternatively, SLED has been shown to improve outcomes.

12.28 Therapeutic Apheresis

The nephrology service may be consulted to determine the value of therapeutic apheresis (TA), or in some programs be asked to perform TA for various indications.[268] TA is a process that removes a circulating pathogenic solute substance from the plasma and replaces it with allogeneic plasma (therapeutic plasma exchange) or with albumin. Examples may include autoantibodies, paraproteins, Ag-Ab complexes, nonimmunological proteins, endotoxin, or exogenous toxins. The nephrologist may be involved in patient consultation, or in some cases may manage the TA process itself.[69] The 2019 *Journal of Clinical Apheresis* guidelines address several diseases managed by the nephrologist and provide ratings of clinical efficacy of TA.[269]

TABLE 12.56 ■ **Potential Renal Indications for Therapeutic Apheresis**

1. Anti-GBM diseases (dialysis independence or diffuse alveolar hemorrhage)
2. Thrombotic thrombocytopenic purpura
3. Kidney transplant antibody-mediated rejection
4. Kidney transplant desensitization (ABO incompatible)
5. Symptomatic, severe cryoglobulinemia
6. Prevention of recurrent focal segmental glomerulosclerosis in transplant
7. HUS—Factor H antibodies
8. Drug-associated thrombotic microangiopathy—Ticlopidine, quinine, quetiapine, and gemcitabine, but effect of TA in drug-associated TMA is questionable.[a]

[a]George JN, Nester CM. Syndromes of thrombotic microangiopathy. *N Engl J Med*. 2014 Aug 14;371(7): 654–666. doi:10.1056/NEJMra1312353.
GBM, Glomerular basement membrane; *HUS*, hemolytic uremic syndrome; *TA*, therapeutic apheresis; *TMA*, thrombotic microangiopathy.
Adapted from Williams ME, Balogan RA. Principles of separation: indications and therapeutic targets for plasma exchange. *Clin J Am Soc Nephrol*. 2014 Jan;9(1):181–190. doi:10.2215/CJN.04680513.

Plasma separation may be achieved through either centrifugation or a filter membrane. Nephrologists are more likely to be familiar with membrane-based filter technology, which may be adapted to conventional HD or hemofiltration. The TA membrane's pores are large enough to allow removal of large circulating molecules while retaining cellular components.[268] A typical TA schedule is every other day, with a volume exchange of 1.0 to 1.5 plasma volumes. In anti-glomerular basement membrane (anti-GBM) disease, daily treatment is required. Albumin is the most common nonplasma replacement fluid and has a superior side-effect profile. Allogeneic plasma may be needed to provide proteins or other factors, such as a source of ADAMTS13 in thrombotic thrombocytopenic purpura (TTP).

Potential renal indications for therapeutic apheresis are shown in Table 12.56. [69,269-270]

However, note that while the benefit of TA in antineutrophilic cytoplasmic autoantibody (ANCA) vasculitis was suggested by the MEPEX trial (if serum Cr >5.7 mg/dL) and by a subsequent meta-analysis, the recent PEVIXAS randomized trial showed no renal benefit over steroids, and TA was also not beneficial for pulmonary hemorrhage.[271] A recent report suggested a role for TA in patients with septic shock/multiple organ failure.[272]

References

1. Mehrotra R. Choice of dialysis modality. *Kidney Int*. 2011;80(9):909–911. doi:10.1038/ki.2011.262.
2. Holley JL. We offer renal replacement therapy to patients who are not benefitted by it. *Semin Dial*. 2016;29(4):306–308. doi:10.1111/sdi.12492.
3. Da Silva-Gane M, Wellsted D, Greenshields H, Norton S, Chandna SM, Farrington K. Quality of life and survival in patients with advanced chronic kidney failure managed conservatively or by dialysis. *Clin J Am Soc Nephrol*. 2012;7(12):2002–2009. doi:10.2215/CJN.01130112.
4. Moss AH. Ethical principles and processes guiding dialysis decision-making. *Clin J Am Soc Nephrol*. 2011;6(9):2313–2317. doi:10.2215/CJN.03960411.
5. Granado R C-D, Mehta RL. Withholding and withdrawing renal support in acute kidney injury. *Semin Dial*. 2011;24(2):208–214. doi:10.1111/j.1525-139X.2011.00832.x.
6. Patel SS, Holley JL. Withholding and withdrawing dialysis in the intensive care unit: benefits derived from consulting the Renal Physicians Association/American Society of Nephrology clinical practice guideline, shared decision-making in the appropriate initiation of and withdrawal from dialysis. *Clin J Am Soc Nephrol*. 2008;3(2):587–593. doi:10.2215/CJN.04040907.

7. Nash DM, Przech S, Wald R, O'Reilly D. Systematic review and meta-analysis of renal replacement therapy modalities for acute kidney injury in the intensive care unit. *J Crit Care*. 2017;41:138–144. doi:10.1016/j.jcrc.2017.05.002.

8. Schefold JC, von Haehling S, Pschowski R, et al. The effect of continuous versus intermittent renal replacement therapy on the outcome of critically ill patients with acute renal failure (CONVINT): a prospective randomized controlled trial. *Crit Care*. 2014;18(1):R11. doi:10.1186/cc13188.

9. Liang KV et al. Modality of RRT and recovery of kidney function after AKI in patients surviving to hospital discharge. *Clin J Am Soc Nephrol*. 2016;11(1):30–38. doi:10.2215/CJN.01290215.

10. Cullis B, Al-Hwiesh A, Kilonzo K, et al. ISPD guidelines for peritoneal dialysis in acute kidney injury: 2020 update (adults). *Perit Dial Int*. 2021;41(1):15–31. doi:10.1177/0896860820970834.

11. Gabriel DP, Caramori JT, Martim LE, Barretti P, Balbi AL. High volume peritoneal dialysis vs daily hemodialysis: a randomized, controlled trial in patients with acute kidney injury. *Kidney Int Suppl*. 2008;(108):S87–S93. doi:10.1038/sj.ki.5002608.

12. Al-Hwiesh A, Abdul-Rahman I, Finkelstein F, et al. Acute kidney injury in critically ill patients: a prospective randomized study of tidal peritoneal dialysis versus continuous renal replacement therapy. *Ther Apher Dial*. 2018;22(4):371–379. doi:10.1111/1744-9987.12660.

13. Granado R C-D, Mehta RL. Withholding and withdrawing renal support in acute kidney injury. *Semin Dial*. 2011;24(2):208–214. doi:10.1111/j.1525-139X.2011.00832.x.

14. Patel SS, Holley JL. Withholding and withdrawing dialysis in the intensive care unit: benefits derived from consulting the renal physicians association/American Society of Nephrology clinical practice guideline, shared decision-making in the appropriate initiation of and withdrawal from dialysis. *Clin J Am Soc Nephrol*. 2008;3(2):587–593. doi:10.2215/CJN.04040907.

15. Zarbock A, Mehta RL. Timing of kidney replacement therapy in acute kidney injury. *Clin J Am Soc Nephrol*. 2019;14(1):147–149. doi:10.2215/CJN.08810718.

16. Sohaney R, Yessayan LT, Heung M. Towards consensus in timing of kidney replacement therapy for acute kidney injury. *Am J Kidney Dis*. 2021;77(4):542–545. doi:10.1053/j.ajkd.2020.08.004.

17. Gaudry S, Hajage D, Schortgen F, et al. Initiation strategies for renal-replacement therapy in the intensive care unit. *N Engl J Med*. 2016;375(2):122–133. doi:10.1056/NEJMoa1603017.

18. STARRT-AKI Investigators, Canadian Critical Care Trials Group, Australian and New Zealand Intensive Care Society Clinical Trials Group, et al. Timing of initiation of renal-replacement therapy in acute kidney injury. *N Engl J Med*. 2020;383(3):240–251. doi:10.1056/NEJMoa2000741.

19. Gaudry S, Hajage D, Martin-Lefevre L, et al. Comparison of two delayed strategies for renal replacement therapy initiation for severe acute kidney injury (AKIKI-2): a multicentre, open-label, randomized, controlled trial. *Lancet*. 2021;397(10281):1293–1300. doi:10.1016/S0140-6736(21)00350-0.

20. Zarbock A, Kellum JA, Schmidt C, et al. Effect of early vs delayed initiation of renal replacement therapy on mortality in critically ill patients with acute kidney injury: the ELAIN randomized clinical trial. *JAMA*. 2016;315(20):2190–2199. doi:10.1001/jama.2016.5828.

21. Shiao C-C, Wu V-C, Li WY, et al. Late initiation of renal replacement therapy is associated with worse outcomes in acute kidney injury after major abdominal surgery. *Crit Care*. 2009;13(5):R171. doi:10.1186/cc8147.

22. Gaudry S, Hajage D, Benichou N, et al. Delayed versus early initiation of renal replacement therapy for severe acute kidney injury: a systematic review and individual patient data meta-analysis of randomized clinical trials. *Lancet*. 2020;395(10235):1506–1515. doi:10.1016/S0140-6736(20)30531-6

23. Viallet N, Brunot V, Kuster N, et al. Daily urinary creatinine predicts the weaning of renal replacement therapy in ICU acute kidney injury patients. *Ann Intensive Care*. 2016;6(1):71. doi:10.1186/s13613-016-0176-y.

24. KDIGO Clinical Practice Guideline for Acute Kidney Injury. *Kidney Internat. Suppl*. 2012;2(1):1–138. https://kdigo.org/wp-content/uploads/2016/10/KDIGO-2012-AKI-Guideline-English.pdf.

25. The VA/NIH Acute Renal Failure Trial Network, Palevsky PM, Hongyuan Zhang J, et al. Intensity of renal support in critically ill patients with acute kidney injury. *N Engl J Med*. 2008;359(1):7–20. doi:10.1056/NEJMoa0802639.

26. Liang KV, Zhang JH, Palevsky PM. Urea reduction ratio may be a simpler approach for measurement of adequacy of intermittent hemodialysis in acute kidney injury. *BMC Nephrol*. 2019;20(1):82. doi:10.1186/s12882-019-1272-7.

27. Macedo E, Mehta RL. Continuous dialysis therapies: core curriculum 2016. *Am J Kidney Dis*. 2016; 68(4):645–657. doi:10.1053/j.ajkd.2016.03.427.

28. Tolwani A. Continuous renal-replacement therapy for acute kidney injury. *N Engl J Med*. 2012; 367(26):2505–2514. doi:10.1056/NEJMct1206045.

29. Ghoshal S, Parikh A. Dialysis-associated neurovascular injury (DANI) in acute brain injury. Practical considerations for intermittent dialysis in the Neuro-ICU. *Clin J Am Soc Nephrol*. 2021;16(7): 1110–1112. doi:10.2215/CJN.15000920.

30. Rosner MH, Connor MJ Jr. Management of severe hyponatremia with continuous renal replacement therapies. *Clin J Am Soc Nephrol*. 2018;13(5):787–789. doi:10.2215/CJN.13281117.

31. Neyra JA, Yessayan L, Thompson Bastin ML, Wille KM, Tolwani AJ. How to prescribe and troubleshoot continuous renal replacement therapy: a case-based review. *Kidney360*. 2020;2(2):371–384. doi:10.34067/KID.0004912020.

32. Ting S, Chua H-R, Cove ME. Euglycemic ketosis during continuous kidney replacement therapy with glucose-free solution: a report of 8 cases. *Am J Kidney Dis*. 2021;78(2):305–308. doi:10.1053/j.ajkd. 2020.10.014.

33. Hatamizadeh P, Tolwani A, Palevsky P. Revisiting filtration fraction as an index of the risk of hemofilter clotting in continuous venovenous hemofiltration. *Clin J Am Soc Nephrol*. 2020;15(11):1660–1662. doi:10.2215/CJN.02410220.

34. Thompson AJ. Drug dosing during continuous renal replacement therapies. *J Pediatr Pharmacol Ther*. 2008;13(2):99–113. doi:10.5863/1551-6776-13.2.99.

35. Zarbock A, Küllmar M, Kindgen-Milles D, et al. Effect of regional citrate anticoagulation vs systemic heparin anticoagulation during continuous kidney replacement therapy on dialysis filter life span and mortality among critically ill patients with acute kidney injury: a randomized clinical trial. *JAMA*. 2020;324(16):1629–1639. doi:10.1001/jama.2020.18618.

36. Szamosvalvi B, Yessayan LT, Heung M. Citrate anticoagulation for continuous kidney replacement therapy: an embarrassment of RICH-es. *Am J Kidney Dis*. 2021;78(1):146–150. doi:10.1053/j.ajkd.2021.01.005.

37. Cervantes CE, Menez S, Hanouneh M. CKRT clotting and cerebrovascular accident in a critically ill patient. *Kidney360*. 2020;1(7):718–719. doi:10.34067/KID.0003112020.

38. Dickie H, Tovey L, Berry W, Ostermann M. Revised algorithm for heparin anticoagulation during continuous renal replacement therapy. *Crit Care*. 2015;19:376. doi:10.1186/s13054-015-1099-y.

39. Mottes TA, Goldstein SL, Basu RK. Process based quality improvement using a continuous renal replacement therapy dashboard. *BMC Nephrol*. 2019;20(1):17. doi:10.1186/s12882-018-1195-8.

40. Gautam SC, Srialluri N, Jaar BG. Strategies for continuous renal replacement therapy de-escalation. *Kidney 360*. 2021;2(7):1166–1169. doi:10.34067/KID.0000912021

41. Ricci Z, Romagnoli S, Ronco C. Acute kidney injury: to dialyse or to filter? *Nephrol Dial Transplant*. 2020;35(1):44–46. doi:10.1093/ndt/gfz022.

42. Yoshida T, Komaru Y, Matsuura R, et al. Findings from two large randomized controlled trials on renal replacement therapy in acute kidney injury. *Ren Replace Ther*. 2016;2:13–20. doi:10.1186/s41100-016-0027-1.

43. Bellomo R, Cass A, Cole L, et al. Intensity of continuous renal-replacement therapy in critically ill patients. *N Engl J Med*. 2009;361(17):1627–1638. doi:10.1056/NEJMoa0902413.

44. Jun M, Lambers Heerspink HJ, Ninomiya T, et al. Intensities of renal replacement therapy in acute kidney injury: a systematic review and meta-analysis. *Clin J Am Soc Nephrol*. 2010;5(6):956–963. doi:10.2215/CJN.09111209.

45. Kovacs B, Sullivan KJ, Hiremath S, Patel RV. Effect of sustained low efficient dialysis versus continuous renal replacement therapy on renal recovery after acute kidney injury in the intensive care unit: a systematic review and meta-analysis. *Nephrology (Carlton)*. 2017;22(5):343–353. doi:10.1111/nep.13009.

46. Zhang L, Yang J, Eastwood GM, Zhu G, Tanaka A, Bellomo R. Extended daily dialysis versus continuous renal replacement therapy for acute kidney injury: a meta-analysis. *Am J Kidney Dis*. 2015;66(2):322–330. doi:10.1053/j.ajkd.2015.02.328.

47. Chionh CY, Ronco C, Finkelstein FO, Soni SS, Cruz DN. Acute peritoneal dialysis: what is the "adequate" dose for acute kidney injury? *Nephrol Dial Transplant*. 2010;25(10):3155–3160. doi:10.1093/ndt/gfq178.

48. Cullis B, Al-Hwiesh A, Kilonzo K, et al. ISPD guidelines for peritoneal dialysis in acute kidney injury: 2020 update (adults). *Perit Dial Int*. 2021;41(1):15–31. doi:10.1177/0896860820970834.

49. Srivatana V, Aggarwal V, Finkelstein FO, Naljayan M, Crabtree JH, Perl J. Peritoneal dialysis for acute kidney injury treatment in the United States: brought to you by the COVID-19 pandemic. *Kidney360*. 2020;1(5):410–415. doi:10.34067/KID.0002152020.

50. Chen W, Caplin N, El Shamy O, et al. NYC-PD Consortium. Use of peritoneal dialysis for acute kidney injury during the COVID-19 pandemic in New York City: a multicenter observational study. *Kidney Int.* 2021;100(1):2–5. doi:10.1016/j.kint.2021.04.017.

51. Rastogi A, Lerma EV. Anemia management for home dialysis including the new US public policy initiative. *Kidney Int Suppl (2011).* 2021;11(1):59–69. doi:10.1016/j.kisu.2020.12.005.

52. Chertow GM, Levin NW, Beck GJ, et al. Long-term effects of frequent in-center hemodialysis. *J Am Soc Nephrol.* 2016;27(6):1830–1836. doi:10.1681/ASN.2015040426.

53. Tentori F, Zhang J, Li Y, et al. Longer dialysis session length is associated with better intermediate outcomes and survival among patients on in-center three times per week hemodialysis: results from the Dialysis Outcomes and Practice Patterns Study (DOPPS). *Nephrol Dial Transplant.* 2012;27(11): 4180–4188. doi:10.1093/ndt/gfs021.

54. Kalim S, Wald R, Yan AT, et al. Extended duration nocturnal hemodialysis and changes in plasms metabolite profiles. *Clin J Am Soc Nephrol.* 2018;13(3):436–444. doi:10.2215/CJN.08790817.

55. Chazot C, Ok E, Lacson E Jr, Kerr PG, Jean G, Misra M. Thrice-weekly nocturnal hemodialysis: the overlooked alternative to improve patient outcomes. *Nephrol Dial Transplant.* 2013;28(10):2447–2455. doi:10.1093/ndt/gft078.

56. Foley RN, Gilbertson DT, Murray T, Collins, AJ. Long interdialytic interval and mortality among patients receiving hemodialysis. *N Engl J Med.* 2011;365(12):1099–1107. doi:10.1056/NEJMoa1103313.

57. McIntyre CW, Rosansky SJ. Starting dialysis is dangerous: how do we balance the risk? *Kidney Int.* 2012;82(4):382–387. doi:10.1038/ki.2012.133.

58. Cooper BA, Branley P, Bulfone L, et al. A randomized, controlled trial of early versus late initiation of dialysis. *N Engl J Med.* 2010;363(7):609–619. doi:10.1056/NEJMoa1000552.

59. Wright D, Klausner B, Baird ME, et al. Timing of dialysis initiation and survival in ESRD. *Clin J Am Soc Nephrol.* 2010;5(10):1828–1835. doi:10.2215/CJN.06230909.

60. Chan CT, Blankestijn PJ, Dember LM, et al. Dialysis initiation, modality choice, access, and prescription: conclusions from a Kidney Disease: Improving Global Outcomes (KDIGO) controversies conference. *Kidney Int.* 2019;96(1):37–47. doi:10.1016/j.kint.2019.01.017.

61. Moss AH. Ethical principles and processes guiding dialysis decision-making. *Clin J Am Soc Nephrol.* 2011;6(9):2313–2317. doi:10.2215/CJN.03960411.

62. Kalantar-Zadeh K, Wightman A, Liao S. Ensuring choice for people with kidney failure—dialysis, supportive care, and hope. *N Engl J Med.* 2020;383(2):99–101. doi:10.1056/NEJMp2001794.

63. Brennan F, Stewart C, Burgess H, et al. Time to improve informed consent for dialysis: an international perspective. *Clin J Am Soc Nephrol.* 2017;12(6):1001–1009. doi:10.2215/CJN.09740916.

64. Brown MA, Collett GK, Josland EA, Foote C, Li Q, Brennan FP. CKD in elderly patients managed without dialysis: survival, symptoms, and quality of life. *Clin J Am Soc Nephrol.* 2015;10(2):260–268. doi:10.2215/CJN.03330414.

65. Murtagh FEM, Burns A, Moranne O, Morton RL, Naicker S. Supportive care: comprehensive conservative care in end-stage kidney disease. *Clin J Am Soc Nephrol.* 2016;11(10):1909–1914. doi:10.2215/CJN.04840516.

66. Kalantar-Zadeh K, Jafar TH, Nitsch D, Neuen BL, Perkovic V. Chronic kidney disease. *Lancet.* 2021; 398(10302):786–802. doi:10.1016/S0140-6736(21)00519-5.

67. Ward RA, Ronco C. Dialyzer and machine technologies: application of recent advances to clinical practice. *Blood Purif.* 2006;24(1):6–10. doi:10.1159/000089429.

68. Storr M, Ward RA. Membrane innovation: closer to native kidneys. *Nephrol Dial Transplant.* 2018; 33(suppl_3):iii22–iii27. doi:10.1093/ndt/gfy228.

69. Williams ME, Balogun RA. Principles of separation: indications and therapeutic targets for plasma exchange. *Clin J Am Soc Nephrol.* 2014;9(1):181–190. doi:10.2215/CJN.04680513.

70. Weiner DE, Falzon L, Skoufos L, et al. Efficacy and safety of expanded hemodialysis with the Theranova 400 Dialyzer: a randomized controlled trial. *Clin J Am Soc Nephrol.* 2020;15(9):1310–1319. doi:10.2215/ CJN.01210120.

71. Cozzolino M, Magagnoli L, Ciceri P, Conte F, Galassi A. Effects of a medium cut-off (Theranova) dialyser on haemodialysis patients: a prospective, cross-over study. *Clin Kidney J.* 2019;14(1):382–389. doi:10.1093/ckj/sfz155.

72. Kokubo K, Kurihara Y, Kobayashi K, Tsukao H, Kobayashi H. Evaluation of the biocompatibility of dialysis membranes. *Blood Purif.* 2015;40(4):293–297. doi:10.1159/000441576.

73. Lok CE, Huber TS, Lee T, et al. KDOQI clinical practice guideline for vascular access: 2019 update. *Am J Kidney Dis.* 2020;75(4 suppl 2):S1–S164. doi:10.1053/j.ajkd.2019.12.001.

74. Lok CE. Fistula first initiative: advantages and pitfalls. *Clin J Am Soc Nephrol.* 2007;2(5):1043–1053. doi:10.2215/CJN.01080307.
75. DeSilva RN, Patibandla BK, Vin Y, et al. Fistula first is not always the best strategy for the elderly. *J Am Soc Nephrol.* 2013;24(8):1297–1304. doi:10.1681/ASN.2012060632.
76. Brown RS, Patibandla BK, Goldfarb-Rumyantzev AS. The survival benefit of "fistula first, catheter last" in hemodialysis is primarily due to patient factors. *J Am Soc Nephrol.* 2017;28(2):645–652. doi:10.1681/ASN.2016010019.
77. Shah S, Chan MR, Lee T. Perspectives in individualizing solutions for dialysis access. *Adv Chronic Kidney Dis.* 2020;27(3):183–190. doi:10.1053/j.ackd.2020.03.004.
78. Brown RS. Barriers to optimal vascular access for hemodialysis. *Semin Dial.* 2020;33(6):457–463. doi:10.1111/sdi.12922.
79. Pisoni RL, Zepel L, Zhao J, et al. International comparisons of native arteriovenous fistula patency and time to becoming catheter-free: findings from the Dialysis Outcomes and Practice Patterns Study (DOPPS). *Am J Kidney Dis.* 2021;77(2):245–254. doi:10.1053/j.ajkd.2020.06.020.
80. Koirala N, Anvari E, McLennan G. Monitoring and surveillance of hemodialysis access. *Semin Intervent Radiol.* 2016;33(1):25–30. doi:10.1055/s-0036-1572548.
81. Boubes K, Shaikh A, Alsauskas Z, Dwyer A. New directions in ensuring catheter safety. *Adv Chronic Kidney Dis.* 2020;27(3):228–235. doi:10.1053/j.ackd.2020.02.004.
82. Vascular Access Work Group. Clinical practice guidelines for vascular access. *Am J Kidney Dis.* 2006;48 suppl 1:S248–S273. doi:10.1053/j.ajkd.2006.04.040.
83. Ravani P, Palmer SC, Oliver MJ, et al. Associations between hemodialysis access type and clinical outcomes: a systematic review. *J Am Soc Nephrol.* 2013;24(3):465–473. doi:10.1681/ASN.2012070643.
84. Allon M. Treatment guidelines for dialysis catheter-related bacteremia: an update. *Am J Kidney Dis.* 2009;54(1):13–17. doi:10.1053/j.ajkd.2009.04.006.
85. Ouseph R, Ward RA. Anticoagulation for intermittent hemodialysis. *Semin Dial.* 2000;13(3):181–187. doi:10.1046/j.1525-139x.2000.00052.x.
86. Jain N, Reilly RF. Clinical pharmacology of oral anticoagulants in patients with kidney disease. *Clin J Am Soc Nephrol.* 2019;14(2):278–287. doi:10.2215/CJN.02170218.
87. Randhawa MS, Vishwanath R, Rai MP, et al. Association between use of warfarin for atrial fibrillation and outcomes among patients with end-stage renal disease: a systematic review and meta-analysis. *JAMA Netw Open.* 2020;3(4):e202175. doi:10.1001/jamanetworkopen.2020.2175.
88. Feldberg J, Patel P, Farrell A, et al. A systematic review of direct oral anticoagulant use in chronic kidney disease and dialysis patients with atrial fibrillation. *Nephrol Dial Transplant.* 2019;34(2):265–277. doi:10.1093/ndt/gfy031.
89. DeVriese AS, Caluwé R, Van Der Meersch H, De Boeck K, De Bacquer D. Safety and efficacy of vitamin K antagonists versus rivaroxaban in hemodialysis patients with atrial fibrillation: a multicenter randomized controlled trial. *J Am Soc Nephrol.* 2021;32(6):1474–1483. doi:10.1681/ASN.2020111566.
90. Greenberg KI, Choi MJ. Hemodialysis emergencies: core curriculum 2021. *Am J Kidney Dis.* 2021;77(5):796–809. doi:10.1053/j.ajkd.2020.11.024.
91. Saha M, Allon M. Diagnosis, treatment, and prevention of hemodialysis emergencies. *Clin J Am Soc Nephrol.* 2017;12(2):357–369. doi:10.2215/CJN.05260516.
92. Dalia T, Tuffaha AM. Dialysis disequilibrium syndrome leading to sudden brain death in a chronic hemodialysis patient. *Hemodial Int.* 2018;22(3):E39–E44. doi:10.1111/hdi.12635.
93. Samanta R, Chan C, Chauhan VS. Arrhythmias and sudden cardiac death in end stage renal disease: epidemiology, risk factors, and management. *Can J Cardiol.* 2019;35(9):1228–1240. doi:10.1016/j.cjca.2019.05.005.
94. Loutradis C, Sarafidis PA, Papadopoulos CE, Papagianni A, Zoccali C. The ebb and flow of echocardiographic cardiac function parameters in relationship to hemodialysis treatment in patients with ESRD. *J Am Soc Nephrol.* 2018;29(5):1372–1381. doi:10.1681/ASN.2017101102.
95. Sarafidis PA, Persu A, Agarwal R, et al. Hypertension in dialysis patients: a consensus document by the European Renal and Cardiovascular Medicine (EURECA-m) working group of the European Renal Association—European Dialysis and Transplant Association (ERA-EDTA) and the Hypertension and the Kidney Working Group of the European Society of Hypertension. *Nephrol Dial Transplant.* 2017;32(4):620–640. doi:10.1093/ndt/gfw433.
96. Denker MG, Cohen DL. Antihypertensive medications in end-stage renal disease. *Semin Dial.* 2015;28(4):330–336. doi:10.1111/sdi.12369.

97. Zoccali C, Torino C, Tripepi R, et al. Pulmonary congestion predicts cardiac events and mortality in ESRD. *J Am Soc Nephrol*. 2013;24(4):639–646. doi:10.1681/ASN.2012100990.

98. Flythe JE, Kimmel SE, Brunelli SM. Rapid fluid removal during dialysis is associated with cardiovascular morbidity and mortality. *Kidney Int*. 2011;79(2):250–257. doi:10.1038/ki.2010.383.

99. Zhou H, Sim JJ, Shi J, et al. Beta-blocker use and risk of mortality in heart failure patients initiating maintenance dialysis. *Am J Kidney Dis*. 2021;77(5):704–712. doi:10.1053/j.ajkd.2020.07.023.

100. Navaneethan SD, Wehbe E, Heresi GA, et al. Presence and outcomes of kidney disease in patients with pulmonary hypertension. *Clin J Am Soc Nephrol*. 2014;9(5):855–863. doi:10.2215/CJN.10191013.

101. Bansal S, Prasad A, Linas S. Right heart failure—unrecognized cause of cardiorenal syndrome. *J Am Soc Nephrol*. 2018;29(7):1795–1798. doi:10.1681/ASN.2018020224.

102. Sise ME, Courtwright AM, Channick RN. Pulmonary hypertension in patients with chronic and end-stage kidney disease. *Kidney Int*. 2013;84(4):682–692. doi:10.1038/ki.2013.186.

103. Seong EY, Liu S, Song SH, et al. Intradialytic hypotension and newly recognized peripheral artery disease in patients receiving hemodialysis. *Am J Kidney Dis*. 2021;77(5):730–738. doi:10.1053/j.ajkd.2020.10.012.

104. Okamoto S, Iida O, Mano T. Current perspective on hemodialysis patients with peripheral artery disease. *Ann Vasc Dis*. 2017;10(2):88–91. doi:10.3400/avd.ra.17-00034.

105. Reeves PB, McCausland FR. Mechanisms, clinical implications, and treatment of intradialytic hypotension. *Clin J Am Soc Nephrol*. 2018;13(8):1297–1303. doi:10.2215/CJN.12141017.

106. McIntyre CW, Salerno FR. Diagnosis and treatment of intradialytic hypotension in maintenance hemodialysis patients. *Clin J Am Soc Nephrol*. 2018;13(3):486–489. doi:10.2215/CJN.11131017.

107. Kuipers J, Verboom LM, Ipema KJR, et al. The prevalence of intradialytic hypotension in patients on conventional hemodialysis: a systematic review with meta-analysis. *Am J Nephrol*. 2019;49(6):497–506. doi:10.1159/000500877.

108. Flythe JE, Xue H, Lynch KE, Curhan GC, Brunelli SM. Association of mortality risk with various definitions of intradialytic hypotension. *J Am Soc Nephrol*. 2015;26(3):724–734. doi:10.1681/ASN.2014020222.

109. Kanbay M, Ertuglu LA, Afsar B, et al. An update review of intradialytic hypotension: concept, risk factors, clinical implications and management. *Clin Kidney J*. 2020;13(6):981–993. doi:10.1093/ckj/sfaa078.

110. McIntyre CW, Burton JO, Selby NM, et al. Hemodialysis-induced cardiac dysfunction is associated with an acute reduction in global and segmental myocardial blood flow. *Clin J Am Soc Nephrol*. 2008;3(1):19–26. doi:10.2215/CJN.03170707.

111. Hryciw N, Joannidis M, Hiremath S, Callum J, Clark EG. Intravenous albumin for mitigating hypotension and augmenting ultrafiltration during kidney replacement therapy. *Clin J Am Soc Nephrol*. 2021;16(5):820–828. doi:10.2215/CJN.09670620.

112. Karaboyas A, Morgenstern H, Waechter S, et al. Low hemoglobin at hemodialysis initiation: an international study of anemia management and mortality in the early dialysis period. *Clin Kidney J*. 2019;13(3):425–433. doi: 10.1093/ckj/sfz065.

113. Kliger AS, Foley RN, Goldfarb DS, et al. KDOQI US commentary on the 2012 KDIGO clinical practice guideline for anemia in CKD. *Am J Kidney Dis*. 2013;62(5):849–859. doi:10.1053/j.ajkd.2013.06.008.

114. Besarab A, Bolton WK, Browne JK, et al. The effects of normal as compared with low hematocrit values in patients with cardiac disease who are receiving hemodialysis and epoetin. *N Engl J Med*. 1998;339(9):584–590. doi:10.1056/NEJM199808273390903.

115. Fishbane S, Spinowitz BS, Wisemandle WA, Martin NE. Randomized controlled trial of subcutaneous epoetin alfa-epbx versus epoetin alfa in end-stage renal disease. *Kidney Int Rep*. 2019;4(9):1235–1247. doi:10.1016/j.ekir.2019.05.010.

116. Fishbane S, Singh B, Kumbhat S, Wisemandle WA, Martin NE. Intravenous epoetin alfa-epbx versus epoetin alfa for treatment of anemia in end-stage kidney disease. *Clin J Am Soc Nephrol*. 2018;13(8):1204–1214. doi:10.2215/CJN.11631017.

117. Sinha SD, Bandi VK, Bheemareddy BR, et al. Efficacy, tolerability and safety of darbepoetin alfa injection for the treatment of anemia associated with chronic kidney disease (CKD) undergoing dialysis: a randomized, phase III trial. *BMC Nephrol*. 2019;20(1):90. doi:10.1186/s12882-019-1209-1.

118. Chen N, Hao C, Liu B-C, et al. Roxadustat treatment for anemia in patients undergoing long-term dialysis. *N Engl J Med*. 2019;381(11):1011–1022. doi:10.1056/NEJMoa1901713.

119. Akizawa T, Iwasaki M, Yamaguchi Y, Majikawa Y, Reusch M. Phase 3, randomized, double-blind, active-comparator (darbepoetin alfa) study of oral roxadustat in CKD patients with anemia on hemodialysis in Japan. *J Am Soc Nephrol*. 2020;31(7):1628–1639. doi:10.1681/ASN.2019060623.

120. Singh AK, Carroll K, Perkovic V, et al. Daprodustat for the treatment of anemia in patients undergoing dialysis. *N Engl J Med*. 2021;385(25):2325–2335. doi:10.1056/NEJMoa2113379.

121. Saglimbene VM, Palmer SC, Ruospo M, Natale P, Craig JC, Strippoli GFM. Continuous erythropoiesis receptor activator (CERA) for the anaemia of chronic kidney disease. *Cochrane Database Syst Rev*. 2017;8(8):CD009904. doi:10.1002/14651858.CD009904.pub2.

122. Asirvatham JR, Moses V, Bjornson L. Errors in potassium measurement: a laboratory perspective for the clinician. *N Am J Med Sci*. 2013;5(4):255–259. doi:10.4103/1947-2714.110426.

123. Karaboyas A, Robinson BM, James G, et al. Hyperkalemia excursions are associated with an increased risk of mortality and hospitalizations in hemodialysis patients. *Clin Kidney J*. 2020;14(7):1760–1769. doi:10.1093/ckj/sfaa208.

124. Quach K, Lvtvyn L, Baigent C, et al. The safety and efficacy of mineralocorticoid receptor antagonists in patients who require dialysis: a systematic review and meta-analysis. *Am J Kidney Dis*. 2016;68(4): 591–598. doi:10.1053/j.ajkd.2016.04.011.

125. Lee R, Yin M, He Z, Gurm H, Heung M. Dialysis paradox: impact of aldosterone antagonism on survival in patients with HF and ESRD. *J Am Coll Cardiol*. 2019;73(9_suppl_1):924. doi:10.1016/S0735-1097(19)31531-1.

126. Charytan DM, Himmelfarb J, Ikizler TA, et al. Safety and cardiovascular efficacy of spironolactone in dialysis-dependent ESRD (Spin-D): a randomized, placebo-controlled, multiple dosage trial. *Kidney Int*. 2019;95(4):973–982. doi:10.1016/j.kint.2018.08.034.

127. Wong SWS, Zhang G, Norman P, Welihinda H, Thiwanka Wijeratne D. Polysulfonate resins in hyperkalemia: a systematic review. *Can J Kidney Health Dis*. 2020;7:2054358120965838. doi:10.1177/2054358120965838.

128. Shrestha DB, Budhathoki P, Sedhai YR, et al. Patiromer and sodium zirconium cyclosilicate in treatment of hyperkalemia: a systematic review and meta-analysis. *Curr Ther Res Clin Exp*. 2021;95:100635. doi:10.1016/j.curtheres.2021.100635.

129. Bushinsky DA, Williams GH, Pitt B, et al. Patiromer induces rapid and sustained potassium lowering in patients with chronic kidney disease. *Kidney Int*. 2015;88(6):1427–1433. doi:10.1038/ki.2015.270.

130. Kidney Disease: Improving Global Outcomes CKD-MBD Working Group. KDIGO 2017 clinical practice guideline update for the diagnosis, evaluation, prevention, and treatment of chronic kidney disease-mineral and bone disorder (CKD-MBD). *Kidney Int Suppl (2011)*. 2017;7(1):1–59. doi:10.1016/j.kisu.2017.04.001.

131. Cunningham J, Danese M, Olson K, Klassen P, Chertow GM. Effects of the calcimimetic cinacalcet HCl on cardiovascular disease, fracture, and health-related quality of life in secondary hyperparathyroidism. *Kidney Int*. 2005;68(4):1793–1800. doi:10.1111/j.1523-1755.2005.00596.x.

132. EVOLVE Trial Investigators. Effect of cinacalcet on cardiovascular disease in patients undergoing dialysis. *N Engl J Med*. 2012;367(26):2482–2494. doi:10.1056/NEJMoa1205624.

133. Moe SM, Abdalla S, Chertow GM, et al. Effects of cinacalcet on fracture events in patients receiving hemodialysis: the EVOLVE Study. *J Am Soc Nephrol*. 2015;26(6):1466–1475. doi:10.1681/ASN.2014040414.

134. Block GA, Bushinsky DA, Sunfa Cheng S, et al. Effect of etelcalcitide versus cinacalcet on serum hormone in patients receiving hemodialysis with secondary hyperparathyroidism: a randomized clinical trial. *JAMA*. 2017;317(2):156–164. doi:10.1001/jama.2016.19468.

135. Parikh C, Gutgarts V, Eisenberg E, Melamed ML. Vitamin D and clinical outcomes in dialysis. *Semin Dial*. 2015;28(6):604–609. doi:10.1111/sdi.12446.

136. Zheng Z, Shi H, Jia J, Li D, Lin S. Vitamin D supplementation and mortality risk in chronic kidney disease: a meta-analysis of 20 observational studies. *BMC Nephrol*. 2013;14:199. doi:10.1186/1471-2369-14-199.

137. Isakova T, Nickolas TL, Denburg M, et al. KDOQI US commentary on the 2017 KDIGO Clinical Practice Guideline Update for the Diagnosis, Evaluation, Prevention, and Treatment of Chronic Kidney Disease—Mineral and Bone Disorder. *Am J Kidney Dis*.;70(6):737–751. doi:10.1053/j.ajkd.2017.07.019.

138. Isaka Y, Hamano T, Fujii H, et al. Optimal phosphate control related to coronary artery calcification in dialysis patients. *J Am Soc Nephrol*. 2021;32(3):723–735. doi:10.1681/ASN.2020050598.

139. Hutchison AJ. Oral phosphate binders. *Kidney Int*. 2009;75(9):906–914. doi:10.1038/ki.2009.60.

140. Isakova T, Gutiérrez OM, Chang Y, et al. Phosphorus binders and survival on hemodialysis. *J Am Soc Nephrol.* 2009;20(2):388–396. doi:10.1681/ASN.2008060609.

141. Chan S, Au K, Francis RS, Mudge DW, Johnson DW, Pillans PI. Phosphate binders in patients with chronic kidney disease. *Aust Prescr.* 2017;40(1):10–14. doi:10.18773/austprescr.2017.002.

142. Spoendlin J, Paik JM, Tsacogianis T, Kim SC, Schneeweiss S, Desai RJ. Cardiovascular outcomes of calcium-free vs calcium-based phosphate binders in patients 65 years or older with end-stage renal disease requiring hemodialysis. *JAMA Intern Med.* 2019;179(6):741–749. doi:10.1001/jamainternmed.2019.0045.

143. Gutekunst L. An update on phosphate binders: a dietician's perspective. *J Ren Nutr.* 2016;26(4):209–218. doi:10.1053/j.jrn.2016.01.009.

144. Lopes MB, Karaboyas A, Bieber B, et al. Impact of longer term phosphorus control on cardiovascular mortality in hemodialysis patients using an area under the curve approach: results from the DOPPS. *Nephrol Dial Transplant.* 2020;35(10):1794–1801. doi:10.1093/ndt/gfaa054.

145. Edmonston DL, Isakova T, Dember LM, et al. Design and rationale of HiLo: a pragmatic, randomized trial of phosphate management for patients receiving maintenance hemodialysis. *Am J Kidney Dis.* 2021;77(6):920–930.e1. doi:10.1053/j.ajkd.2020.10.008.

146. Kodumudi V, Jeha GM, Mydlo N, Kaye AD. Management of cutaneous calciphylaxis. *Adv Ther.* 2020;37(12):4797–4807. doi:10.1007/s12325-020-01504-w.

147. Sprague SM. Painful skin ulcers in a hemodialysis patient. *Clin J Am Soc Nephrol.* 2014;9(1):166–173. doi:10.2215/CJN.00320113.

148. Yu WY-H, Bhutani T, Kornik R, et al. Warfarin-associated nonuremic calciphylaxis. *JAMA Dermatol.* 2017;153(3):309–314. doi:10.1001/jamadermatol.2016.4821.

149. Singh RP, Derendorf H, Ross EA. Simulation-based sodium thiosulfate dosing strategies for the treatment or calciphylaxis. *Clin J Am Soc Nephrol.* 2011;6(5):1155–1159. doi:10.2215/CJN.09671010.

150. Coelho S. Is the management of diabetes different in dialysis patients? *Semin Dial.* 2018;31(4):367–376. doi:10.1111/sdi.12698.

151. DeBoer I, Caramori ML, Chan JCN, et al. Executive summary of the 2020 KDIGO diabetes management in CKD guideline: evidence-based advances in monitoring and treatment. *Kidney Int.* 2020;98(4):839–848. doi:10.1016/j.kint.2020.06.024.

152. Chen TK, Sperati CJ, Thavarajah S, Grams ME. Reducing kidney function decline in patients with CKD: core curriculum 2021. *Am J Kidney Dis.* 2021;77(6):969–983. doi:10.1053/j.ajkd.2020.12.022.

153. Hill CJ, Maxwell AP, Cardwell CR, et al. Glycated hemoglobin and risk of death in diabetic patients treated with hemodialysis: a meta-analysis. *Am J Kidney Dis.* 2014;63(1):84–94. doi:10.1053/j.ajkd.2013.06.020.

154. Presswala L, Hong S, Harris Y, et al. Continuous glucose monitoring and glycemic control in patients with type 2 diabetes mellitus and CKD. *Kidney Med.* 2019;1(5):281–287. doi:10.1016/j.xkme.2019.07.006.

155. Williams ME, Lacson E Jr, Wang W, Lazarus JM, Hakim R. Glycemic control and extended hemodialysis survival in patients with diabetes mellitus: comparative results of traditional and time-dependent Cox model analyses. *Clin J Am Soc Nephrol.* 2010;5(9):1595–1601. doi:10.2215/CJN.09301209.

156. Hoshino J, Larkina M, Karaboyas A, et al. Unique hemoglobin A1c level distribution and its relationship with mortality in diabetic hemodialysis patients. *Kidney Int.* 2017;92(2):497–503. doi:10.1016/j.kint.2017.02.008.

157. Ricks J, Molnar MZ, Kovesdy CP, et al. Glycemic control and cardiovascular mortality in hemodialysis patients with diabetes: a 6-year cohort study. *Diabetes.* 2012;61(3):708–715. doi:10.2337/db11-1015.

158. Hoshino J, Hamano T, Abe M, et al. Glycated albumin versus hemoglobin A1c and mortality in diabetic hemodialysis patients: a cohort study. *Nephrol Dial Transplant.* 2018;33(7):1150–1158. doi:10.1093/ndt/gfy014.

159. American Diabetes Association. Pharmacological approaches to glycemic treatment: standards of medical care in diabetes—2021. *Diabetes Care.* 2021;44(suppl 1):S111–S124. doi:10.2337/dc21-S009.

160. Garg R, Williams M. Diabetes management in the kidney patient. *Med Clin North Am.* 2013;97(1):135–156. doi:10.1016/j.mcna.2012.11.001.

161. Bally L, Gubler P, Thabit H, et al. Fully closed-loop insulin delivery improves glucose control of inpatients with type 2 diabetes receiving hemodialysis. *Kidney Int.* 2019;96(3):593–596. doi:10.1016/j.kint.2019.03.006.

162. Hong S, Presswala L, Harris YT, et al. Hypoglycemia in patients with type 2 diabetes mellitus and chronic kidney disease: a prospective observational study. *Kidney360.* 2020;1(9):897–903. doi:10.34067/KID.0001272020.

163. Abe M, Kalantar-Zadeh K. Haemodialysis-induced hypoglycaemia and glycaemic disarrays. *Nat Rev Nephrol*. 2015;11(5):302–313. doi:10.1038/nrneph.2015.38.

164. Bansal AD, Hill CE, Berns JS. Use of antiepileptic drugs in patients with chronic kidney disease in end-stage renal disease. *Semin Dial*. 2015;28(4):404–412. doi:10.1111/sdi.12385.

165. Cohen SD, Kimmel PL, Neff R, Agodoa L, Abbott KC. Association of incident gout and mortality in dialysis patients. *J Am Soc Nephrol*. 2008;19(11):2204–2210. doi:10.1681/ASN.2007111256.

166. Vargas-Santos AB, Neogi T. Management of gout and hyperuricemia in CKD. *Am J Kidney Dis*. 2017;70(3):422–439. doi:10.1053/j.ajkd.2017.01.055.

167. Schlesinger N, Lipsky PE. Pegloticase treatment of chronic refractory gout: update on efficacy and safety. *Semin Arthritis Rheum*. 2020;50(3S):S31–S38. doi:10.1016/j.semarthrit.2020.04.011.

168. Alakel N, Middeke JM, Schetelig J, Bornhäuser M. Prevention and treatment of tumor lysis syndrome, and the efficacy and role of rasburicase. *Onco Targets Ther*. 2017;10:597–605. doi:10.2147/OTT. S103864.

169. Rosner MH. Cancer screening in patients undergoing maintenance dialysis: who, what, and when. *Am J Kidney Dis*. 2020;76(4):558–566. doi:10.1053/j.ajkd.2019.12.018.

170. Farivar-Mohseni H, Perlmutter AE, Wilson S, Shingleton WB, Bigler SA, Fowler JE Jr. Renal cell carcinoma and end stage renal disease. *J Urol*. 2006;175(6):2018–2020; discussion 2021. doi:10.1016/S0022-5347(06)00340-5.

171. De Meester J, De Bacquer D, Naesens M, et al. Incidence, characteristics, and outcome of COVID-19 in adults on kidney replacement therapy: a regionwide registry study. *J Am Soc Nephrol*. 2021;32(2):385–396. doi:10.1681/ASN.2020060875.

172. Jiang H-J, Tang H, Xiong F, et al. COVID-19 in peritoneal dialysis patients. *Clin J Am Soc Nephrol*. 2020;16(1):121–123. doi:10.2215/CJN.07200520.

173. Flythe JE, Assimon MM, Tugman MJ, et al. Characteristics and outcomes of individuals with pre-existing kidney disease and COVID-19 admitted to intensive care units in the United States. *Am J Kidney Dis*. 2021;77(2):190–203.e1. doi:10.1053/j.ajkd.2020.09.003.

174. Walker AG, Sibbel S, Wade C, et al. SARS-CoV-2 antibody seroprevalence among maintenance dialysis patients in the United States. *Kidney Med*. 2021;3(2):216–222.e1. doi:10.1016/j.xkme.2021.01.002.

175. Tang H, Tian J-B, Dong J-W, et al. Serologic detection of SARS-CoV-2 infections in hemodialysis centers: a multicenter retrospective study in Wuhan, China. *Am J Kidney Dis*. 2020;76(4):490–499.e1. doi:10.1053/j.ajkd.2020.06.008.

176. Weinhandl ED, Wetmore JB, Peng Y, Liu J, Gilbertson DT, Johansen KL. Initial effects of COVID-19 on patients with ESKD. *J Am Soc Nephrol*. 2021;32(6):1444–1453. doi:10.1681/ASN.2021010009.

177. Yau K, Muller MP, Lin M, et al. COVID-19 outbreak in an urban hemodialysis unit. *Am J Kidney Dis*. 2020;76(5):690–695.e1. doi:10.1053/j.ajkd.2020.07.001.

178. Hsu CM, Weiner DE. COVID-19 in dialysis patients: outlasting and outsmarting a pandemic. *Kidney Int*. 2020;98(6):1402–1404. doi:10.1016/j.kint.2020.10.005.

179. Miller-Handley H, Luckett K, Govil A. Treatment options for coronavirus disease 2019 in patients with reduced or absent kidney function. *Adv Chronic Kidney Dis*. 2020;27(5):434–441. doi:10.1053/j.ackd.2020.09.001.

180. Adamsick ML, Gandhi RG, Bidell MR, et al. Remdesivir in patients with acute or chronic kidney disease and COVID-19. *J Am Soc Nephrol*. 2020;31(7):1384–1386. doi:10.1681/ASN.2020050589.

181. Shankaranarayanan D, Muthukumar T, Barbar T, et al. Anticoagulation strategies and filter life in COVID-19 patients receiving continuous renal replacement therapy: a single-center experience. *Clin J Am Soc Nephrol*. 2020;16(1):124–126. doi:10.2215/CJN.08430520.

182. Alfano G, Fontana F, Ferrari A, et al. Peritoneal dialysis in the time of coronavirus disease 2019. *Clin Kidney J*. 2020;13(3):265–268. doi:10.1093/ckj/sfaa093.

183. Windpessl M, Bruchfeld A, Anders H-J, et al. COVID-19 vaccines and kidney disease. *Nat Rev Nephrol*. 2021;17(5):291–293. doi:10.1038/s41581-021-00406-6.

184. Grupper A, Sharon N, Finn T, et al. Humoral response to the Pfizer BNT162b2 vaccine in patients undergoing maintenance hemodialysis. *Clin J Am Soc Nephrol*. 2021;16(7):1037–1042. doi:10.2215/CJN.03500321.

185. Cohen DE, Sibbel S, Marlowe G, et al. Antibody status, disease history, and incidence of SARS-CoV-2 infection among patients on chronic dialysis. *J Am Soc Nephrol*. 2021;32(8):1880–1886. doi:10.1681/ASN.2021030387.

186. Gelfand SL, Scherer JS, Koncicki HM. Kidney supportive care: core curriculum 2020. *Am J Kidney Dis.* 2020;75(5):793–806. doi:10.1053/j.ajkd.2019.10.016.

187. Sondergaard H. Fatigue while undergoing long-term hemodialysis. *Clin J Am Soc Nephrol.* 2020;15(11):1539–1540. doi:10.2215/CJN.14870920.

188. Gregg LP, Bossola M, Ostrosky-Frid M, Hedayati SS. Fatigue in CKD: epidemiology, pathophysiology, and treatment. *Clin J Am Soc Nephrol.* 2021;16(9):1445–1455. doi:10.2215/CJN.19891220.

189. Ju A, Teixeira-Pinto A, Tong A, et al. Validation of a core patient-reported outcome measure for fatigue in patients receiving hemodialysis: the SONG-HD Fatigue instrument. *Clin J Am Soc Nephrol.* 2020;15(11):1614–1621. doi:10.2215/CJN.05880420.

190. Moist L. Pain management in a patient with kidney failure. *Clin J Am Soc Nephrol.* 2020;15(11): 1657–1659. doi:10.2215/CJN.01440220.

191. Baker M, Perazella MA. NSAIDs in CKD: are they safe? *Am J Kidney Dis.* 2020;76(4):546–557. doi:10.1053/j.ajkd.2020.03.023.

192. Lu E, Schell JO, Koncicki HM. Opioid management in CKD. *Am J Kidney Dis.* 2021;77(5): 786–795. doi:10.1053/j.ajkd.2020.08.018.

193. Pisoni RL, Wikström B, Elder SJ, et al. Pruritus in hemodialysis patients: international results from the Dialysis Outcomes and Practice Patterns Study (DOPPS). *Nephrol Dial Transplant.* 2006;21(12): 3495–3505. doi:10.1093/ndt/gfl461.

194. Simonsen E, Komenda P, Lerner B, et al. Treatment of uremic pruritus: a systematic review. *Am J Kidney Dis.* 2017;70(5):638–655. doi:10.1053/j.ajkd.2017.05.018.

195. Fishbane S, Jamal A, Munera C, et al. A phase 3 trial of difelikefalin in hemodialysis patients with pruritus. *N Engl J Med.* 2020;382(3):222–232. doi:10.1056/NEJMoa1912770.

196. Friedli K, Guirguis A, Almond M, et al. Sertraline versus placebo in patients with major depressive disorder undergoing hemodialysis: a randomized, controlled feasibility trial. *Clin J Am Soc Nephrol.* 2017;12(2):280–286. doi:10.2215/CJN.02120216.

197. Zhao Y, Zhang Y, Yang Z, et al. Sleep disorders and cognitive impairment in peritoneal dialysis: a multicenter prospective cohort study. *Kidney Blood Press Res.* 2019;44(5):1115–1127. doi:10.1159/000502355.

198. Chan CT, Wallace E, Golper TA, et al. Exploring barriers and potential solutions in home dialysis: an NKF-KDOQI Conference Outcomes Report. *Am J Kidney Dis.* 2019;73(3):363–371. doi:10.1053/j.ajkd.2018.09.015.

199. Chan CT, Collins K, Ditschman EP, et al. Overcoming barriers for uptake and retention of home dialysis patients: an NKF KDOQI Home Dialysis Conference. *Am J Kidney Dis.* 2020;75(6):926–934. doi:10.1053/j.ajkd.2019.11.007.

200. Bonenkamp AA, van Eck van der Sluijs A, Hoekstra T, et al. Health-related quality of life in home dialysis patients compared to in-center hemodialysis patients: a systematic review and meta-analysis. *Kidney Med.* 2020;2(2):139–154. doi:10.1016/j.xkme.2019.11.005.

201. Chan CT, Collins K, Ditschman EP, et al. Overcoming barriers for uptake and continued use of home dialysis: an NKF-KDOQI conference report. *Am J Kidney Dis.* 2020;75(6):926–934. doi:10.1053/j.ajkd.2019.11.007.

202. Ashby D, Borman N, Burton J, et al. Renal Association clinical practice guideline on haemodialysis. *BMC Nephrol.* 2019;20(1):379. doi:10.1186/s12882-019-1527-3.

203. Rivara MB, Ravel V, Streja E, et al. Weekly standard Kt/V urea and clinical outcomes in home and in-center hemodialysis. *Clin J Am Soc Nephrol.* 2018;13(3):445–455. doi:10.2215/CJN.05680517.

204. Chertow GM, Levin NW, Beck GJ, et al. Long-term effects of frequent in-center hemodialysis. *J Am Soc Nephrol.* 2016;27(6):1830–1836. doi:10.1681/ASN.2015040426.

205. Culleton BF, Walsh M, Klarenbach SW, et al. Effect of frequent nocturnal hemodialysis versus conventional hemodialysis on left ventricular mass and quality of life: a randomized controlled trial. *JAMA.* 2007;298(11):1291–1299. doi:10.1001/jama.298.11.1291.

206. National Kidney Foundation. KDOQI clinical practice guideline for hemodialysis adequacy: 2015 update. *Am J Kidney Dis.* 2015;66(5):884–930. doi:10.1053/j.ajkd.2015.07.015.

207. Eknoyan G, Beck GJ, Cheung AK, et al. Effect of dialysis dose and membrane flux in maintenance hemodialysis. *N Engl J Med.* 2002;347(25):2010–2019. doi:10.1056/NEJMoa021583.

208. Cherukuri S, Bajo M, Colussi G, et al. Home hemodialysis treatment and outcomes: retrospective analysis of the Knowledge to Improve Home Dialysis Network in Europe (KIHDNEy) cohort. *BMC Nephrol.* 2018;19(1):262. doi:10.1186/s12882-018-1059-2.

209. Lowrie EG, Laird NM, Parker TF, Sargent JA. Effect of the hemodialysis prescription on patient morbidity: report from the National Cooperative Dialysis Study. *N Engl J Med.* 1981;305(20):1176–1181. doi:10.1056/NEJM198111123052003.

210. Gotch FA, Sargent JA. A mechanistic analysis of the National Cooperative Dialysis Study (NCDS). *Kidney Int.* 1985;28(3):526–534. doi:10.1038/ki.1985.160.

211. Steyaert S, Holvoet E, Nagler E, Malfait S, Van Biesen W. Reporting of "dialysis adequacy" as an outcome in randomized trials conducted in adults on haemodialysis. *PLoS One.* 2019;14(2):e0207045. doi:10.1371/journal.pone.0207045.

212. Perl J, Dember LM, Bargman JM, et al. The use of a multidimensional measure of dialysis adequacy—moving beyond small solute kinetics. *Clin J Am Soc Nephrol.* 2017;12(5):839–847. doi:10.2215/CJN.08460816.

213. Windpessl M, Prischl FC, Prenner A, Vychytil A. Managing hospitalized peritoneal dialysis patients: ten practical points for the non-nephrologist. *Am J Med.* 2021;134(7):833–839. doi:10.1016/j.amjmed.2021.02.007.

214. Sloan CE, Coffman CJ, Sanders LL, et al. Trends in peritoneal dialysis use in the United States after Medicare Payment Reform. *Clin J Am Soc Nephrol.* 2019;14(12):1763–1772. doi:10.2215/CJN.05910519.

215. Klomjit N, Kattah AG, Cheungpasitporn W. The cost-effectiveness of peritoneal dialysis is superior to hemodialysis: updated evidence from a more precise model. *Kidney Med.* 2020;3(1):15–17. doi:10.1016/j.xkme.2020.12.003.

216. Francois K, Ronco C, Bargman JM. Peritoneal dialysis for chronic congestive heart failure. *Blood Purif.* 2015;40(1):45–52. doi:10.1159/000430084.

217. Kazory A. Peritoneal dialysis for chronic cardiorenal syndrome: lessons learned from ultrafiltration trials. *World J Cardiol.* 2015;7(7):392–396. doi:10.4330/wjc.v7.i7.392.

218. Cullis B, Al-Hwiesh A, Kilonzo K, et al. ISPD guidelines for peritoneal dialysis in acute kidney injury: 2020 update (adults). *Perit Dial Int.* 2021;41(1):15–31. doi:10.1177/0896860820970834.

219. Crabtree JH, Shrestha BM, Chow K-M, et al. ISPD guidelines/recommendations: creating and maintaining optimal peritoneal dialysis access in the adult patient: 2019 update. *Perit Dial Int.* 2019;39(5):414–436. doi:10.3747/pdi.2018.00232.

220. Wolfson M, Piraino B, Hamburger RJ, Morton AR, Icodextrin Study Group. A randomized controlled trial to evaluate the efficacy and safety of icodextrin in peritoneal dialysis. *Am J Kidney Dis.* 2002;40(5):1055–1065. doi:10.1053/ajkd.2002.36344.

221. Takatori Y, Akagi S, Sugiyama H, et al. Icodextrin increases technique survival rate in peritoneal dialysis patients with diabetic nephropathy by improving body fluid management: a randomized controlled trial. *Clin J Am Soc Nephrol.* 2011;6(6):1337–1344. doi:10.2215/CJN.10041110.

222. Li PKT, Culleton BF, Ariza A, et al. Randomized, controlled trial of glucose-sparing peritoneal dialysis in diabetic patients. *J Am Soc Nephrol.* 2013;24(11):1889–1900. doi:10.1681/ASN.2012100987.

223. Teitelbaum I. Crafting the prescription for patients starting peritoneal dialysis. *Clin J Am Soc Nephrol.* 2018;13(3):483–485. doi:10.2215/CJN.10770917.

224. Morelle J, Stachowska-Pietka J, Öberg C, et al. ISPD recommendations for the evaluation of peritoneal membrane dysfunction in adults: classification, measurement, interpretation and rationale for intervention. *Perit Dial Int.* 2021;41(4):352–372. doi:10.1177/0896860820982218.

225. Mehrotra R, Ravel V, Streja E, et al. Peritoneal equilibration test and patient outcomes. *Clin J Am Soc Nephrol.* 2015;10(11):1990–2001. doi:10.2215/CJN.03470315.

226. Twardowski ZJ, Nolph KD, Khanna R, et al. Peritoneal equilibration test. *Perit Dial Bull.* 1987;7:138.

227. Mujais S, Vonesh E. Profiling of peritoneal ultrafiltration. *Kidney Int Suppl.* 2002;(81):S17–S22. doi:10.1046/j.1523-1755.62.s81.4.x.

228. NKF-DOQI clinical practice guidelines for peritoneal dialysis adequacy. National Kidney Foundation. *Am J Kidney Dis.* 1997;30(3 suppl 2):S67–S136. doi:10.1016/s0272-6386(97)70028-3.

229. Lo WK, Bargman JM, Burkart J, et al. Guideline on targets for solute and fluid removal in adult patients on chronic peritoneal dialysis. *Perit Dial Int.* 2006;26(5):520–522. doi:10.1177/089686080602600502.

230. Brown EA, Blake PG, Boudville N, et al. International Society for Peritoneal Dialysis practice recommendations: prescribing high-quality goal-directed peritoneal dialysis. *Perit Dial Int.* 2020;40(3):244–253. doi:10.1177/0896860819895364.

231. Teitelbaum I, Glickman J, Neu A, et al. KDOQI US commentary on the 2020 ISPD practice recommendations for prescribing high-quality goal-directed peritoneal dialysis. *Am J Kidney Dis.* 2021; 77(2):157–171. doi:10.1053/j.ajkd.2020.09.010.

232. Kiebalo T, Holotka J, Habura I, Pawlaczyk K. Nutritional status in peritoneal dialysis: nutritional guidelines, adequacy and the management of malnutrition. *Nutrients.* 2020;12(6):1715. doi:10.3390/nu 12061715.

233. Lu W, Pang WF, Jin L, et al. Peritoneal protein clearance predicts mortality in peritoneal dialysis patients. *Clin Exp Nephrol.* 2019;23(4):551–560. doi:10.1007/s10157-018-1677-9.

234. Ghaffari A. Urgent-start peritoneal dialysis: a quality improvement report. *Am J Kidney Dis.* 2012; 59(3):400–408. doi:10.1053/j.ajkd.2011.08.034.

235. Htay H, Johnson DW, Craig JC, et al. Urgent-start peritoneal dialysis versus conventional-start peritoneal dialysis for people with chronic kidney disease. *Cochrane Database Syst Rev.* 020;12(12):CD012913. doi:10.1002/14651858.CD012913.pub2.

236. Jin H, Fang W, Zhu M, et al. Urgent-start peritoneal dialysis and hemodialysis in ESRD patients: complications and outcomes. *PLoS One.* 2016;11(11):e0166181. doi:10.1371/journal.pone.0166181.

237. Al Sahlawi M, Bargman JM, Perl J. Peritoneal dialysis-associated peritonitis: suggestions for management and mistakes to avoid. *Kidney Med.* 2020;2(4):467–475. doi:10.1016/j.xkme.2020.04.010.

238. Uiterwijk H, Franssen CFM, Kuipers J, Westerhuis R, Nauta FL. Glucose exposure in peritoneal dialysis is a significant factor predicting peritonitis. *Am J Nephrol.* 2020;51(3):237–243. doi:10.1159/ 000506324.

239. Szeto C-C, Li P K-T. Peritoneal dialysis-associated peritonitis. *Clin J Am Soc Nephrol.* 2019;14(7): 1100–1105. doi:10.2215/CJN.14631218.

240. Li P K-T, Szeto CC, Piraino B, et al. ISPD peritonitis recommendations: 2016 update on prevention and treatment. *Perit Dial Int.* 2016;36(5):481–508. doi:10.3747/pdi.2016.00078.

241. Szeto CC. The new ISPD peritonitis guideline. *Renal Replacement Therapy.* 2018;4:7–12. doi:10.1186/ s41100-018-0150-2.

242. Auricchio S, Giovenzana ME, Pozzi M, et al. Fungal peritonitis in peritoneal dialysis: a 34-year single centre evaluation. *Clin Kidney J.* 2018;11(6):874–880. doi:10.1093/ckj/sfy045.

243. Schreiber MJ, Pegues DA, van Hout B, et al. Analysis of after-hours oral antibiotic protocol for the treatment of suspected peritonitis in peritoneal dialysis patients (Abstract). Poster Presentation at American Society of Nephrology Kidney Week 2018. DaVita Clinical Research. Accessed Month, day, year. https:// www.davitaclinicalresearch.com/publication/analysis-of-after-hours-oral-antibiotic-protocol-for-the-treatment-of-suspected-peritonitis-in-peritoneal-dialysis-patients.

244. Htay H, Cho Y, Pascoe EM, et al. Multicenter registry analysis of center characteristics associated with technique failure in patients on incident peritoneal dialysis. *Clin J Am Soc Nephrol.* 2017;12(7): 1090–1099. doi:10.2215/CJN.12321216.

245. Shani MM, Mukhtar KN, Boorgu R, Leehey DJ, Popli S, Ing TS. Tissue plasminogen activator can effectively declot peritoneal dialysis catheters (letter). *Am J Kidney Dis.* 2000;36(3):675. doi:10.1053/ ajkd.2000.16212.

246. Ravel VA, Streja E, Mehrotra R, et al. Serum sodium and mortality in a national peritoneal dialysis cohort. *Nephrol Dial Transplant.* 2017;32(7):1224–1233. doi:10.1093/ndt/gfw254.

247. Torlen K, Kalantar-Zadeh K, Molnar MZ, Vashistha T, Mehrotra R. Serum potassium and cause-specific mortality in a large peritoneal dialysis cohort. *Clin J Am Soc Nephrol.* 2012;7(8):1272–1284. doi:10.2215/CJN.00960112.

248. Uribarri J, Prabhakar S, Kahn T. Hyponatremia in peritoneal dialysis patients. *Clin Nephrol.* 2004;61(1):54–58. doi:10.5414/cnp61054.

249. Zanger R et al. Hyponatremia and hypokalemia in patients on peritoneal dialysis. *Semin Dial.* 2010;23(6):575–580. doi:10.1111/j.1525-139X.2010.00789.x.

250. Greenberg A, Bernardini J, Piraino BM, Johnston JR, Perlmutter JA. Hemoperitoneum complicating chronic peritoneal dialysis: a single-center experience and literature review. *Am J Kidney Dis.* 1992; 19(3):252–256. doi:10.1016/s0272-6386(13)80006-6.

251. Lew SQ. Hemoperitoneum: bloody peritoneal dialysate in ESRD patients receiving peritoneal dialysis. *Perit Dial Int.* 2007;27(3):226–233.

252. McCormick BB, Bargman JM. Noninfectious complications of peritoneal dialysis: implications for patient and technique survival. *J Am Soc Nephrol.* 2007;18(12):3023–3025. doi:10.1681/ASN.2007070796.

253. Teitelbaum I. Delivering high-quality peritoneal dialysis. What really matters? *Clin J Am Soc Nephrol.* 2020;15(11):1663–1665. doi:10.2215/CJN.02930320.

254. Mehrotra R, Devuyst O, Davies SJ, Johnson DW. The current state of peritoneal dialysis. *J Am Soc Nephrol.* 2016;27(11):3238–3252. doi:10.1681/ASN.2016010112.

255. Selby NM, Kazmi I. Peritoneal dialysis has optimal intradialytic hemodynamics and preserves residual renal function: why isn't it better than hemodialysis? *Semin Dial.* 2019;32(1):3–8. doi:10.1111/sdi.12752.

256. Manera KE, Johnson DW, Craig JC, et al. Establishing a core outcome set for peritoneal dialysis: report of the SONG-PD (Standardized Outcomes in Nephrology-Peritoneal Dialysis) Consensus Workshop. *Am J Kidney Dis.* 2020;75(3):404–412. doi:10.1053/j.ajkd.2019.09.017.

257. Roberts DM, Sevastos J, Carland JE, Stocker SL, Lea-Henry TN. Clinical pharmacokinetics in kidney disease: application to rational design of dosing regimens. *Clin J Am Soc Nephrol.* 2018;13(8):1254–1263. doi:10.2215/CJN.05150418.

258. Lea-Henry TN, Carland JE, Stocker SL, Sevastos J, Roberts DM. Clinical pharmacokinetics in kidney disease. Fundamental principles. *Clin J Am Soc Nephrol.* 2018;13(7):1085–1095. doi:10.2215/CJN.00340118.

259. Wilson FP, Berns JS. Vancomycin levels are frequently subtherapeutic during continuous venovenous hemodialysis. *Clin Nephrol.* 2012;77(4):329–331. doi:10.5414/cn106993.

260. Hirata S, Kadowaki D. Appropriate drug dosing in patients receiving peritoneal dialysis. *Contrib Nephrol.* 2012;177:30–37. doi:10.1159/000336933.

261. Cimino C, Burnett Y, Vyas N, Norris AH. Post-dialysis parenteral antimicrobial therapy in patients receiving intermittent high-flux hemodialysis. *Drugs.* 2021;81(5):555–574. doi:10.1007/s40265-021-01469-2.

262. Lewis SL, Nolin TD. New vancomycin dosing guidelines for hemodialysis patients: rationale, caveats, limitations. *Kidney360.* 2021;2(8):1313–1315. doi:10.34067/KID.0000192021.

263. Lavergne V, Ouellet G, Bouchard J, et al. Guidelines for reporting case studies on extracorporeal treatments in poisonings: methodology. *Semin Dial.* 2014;27(4):407–414. doi:10.1111/sdi.12251.

264. Ghannoun M, Hoffman RS, Gosselin S, Nolin TD, Lavergne V, Roberts DM. Use of extracorporeal treatments in the management of poisonings. *Kidney Int.* 2018;94(4):682–688. doi:10.1016/j.kint.2018.03.026.

265. King JD, Kern MH, Jaar BG. Extracorporeal removal of poisons and toxins. *Clin J Am Soc Nephrol.* 2019;14(9):1408–1415. doi:10.2215/CJN.02560319.

266. Decker BS, Goldfarb DS, Dargan PI, et al. Extracorporeal treatment for lithium poisoning: systematic review and recommendations from the EXTRIP Workgroup. *Clin J Am Soc Nephrol.* 2015;10(5):875–887. doi:10.2215/CJN.10021014.

267. Angioi A, Cabiddu G, Conti M, et al. Metformin associated lactic acidosis: a case series of 28 patients treated with sustained low-efficiency dialysis (SLED) and long-term follow-up. *BMC Nephrol.* 2018;19(1):77. doi:10.1186/s12882-018-0875-8.

268. Ahmed S, Kaplan A. Therapeutic plasma exchange using membrane plasma separation. *Clin J Am Soc Nephrol.* 2020;15(9):1364–1370. doi:10.2215/CJN.12501019.

269. Padmanabhan A, Connelly-Smith L, Aqui N, et al. Guidelines on the use of therapeutic apheresis in clinical practice—Evidence-based approach from the writing committee of the American Society for Apheresis: The Eighth Special Issue. *J Clin Apher.* 2019;34(3):171–354. doi:10.1002/jca.21705.

270. George JN, Nester CM. Syndromes of thrombotic microangiopathy. *N Engl J Med.* 2014;371(7):654–666. doi:10.1056/NEJMra1312353.

271. Walsh M, Merkel PA, Peh CA, et al. PEXIVAS Investigators: Plasma exchange and glucocorticoids in severe ANCA-associated vasculitis. *N Engl J Med.* 2020;382(7):622–631. doi:10.1056/NEJMoa1803537.

272. Keith PD, Wells AH, Hodges J, Fast SH, Adams A, Scott LK. The therapeutic efficacy of adjunct therapeutic plasma exchange for septic shock with multiple organ failure: a single-center experience. *Crit Care.* 2020;24(1):518. doi:10.1186/s13054-020-03241-6.

CHAPTER 13

Kidney Transplantation

Robert Stephen Brown ▦ Alexander Goldfarb-Rumyantzev ▦ Amtul Aala

Kidney transplantation represents a complex overlapping of immunology, nephrology, and surgery. We will initially describe the important role of tissue typing, tissue compatibility and histocompatibility testing in donor-recipient selection.

13.1 Tissue Typing and Compatibility

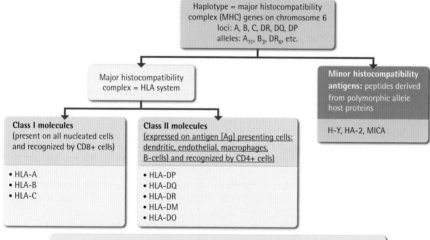

Histocompatibility Testing[1-3]

- Tissue typing
  - Serological (identifying Ag on cell membranes: reaction between cells of the subjects and antibodies to specific HLA antigens): microlymphocytotoxicity test
  - Molecular techniques (DNA typing): polymerase chain reaction (PCR) (DNA nomenclature: name has four digits, first two correlate with serologic name: A1, B3, etc.; last two indicate allelic name)
- HLA antibody (Ab) identification (panel reactive antibodies—PRA): cytotoxic test, ELISA, flow cytometry
- Crossmatching with T- and B-lymphocytes (to predict hyperacute rejection):
  - T cells do not constitutively express HLA class II so the result of a T-cell crossmatch generally reflects antibodies to HLA class I only
  - B cells on the other hand express both HLA class I and II so a positive B-cell crossmatch may be due to antibodies directed against HLA class I or II or both

- Microlymphocytotoxicity test with patient's serum and donor's lymphocytes (T & B)—screen for preformed Ab
- Flow cytometry (flow cytometric crossmatch [FCXM] method): more sensitive, allows the detection of antibodies against T-lymphocytes (anti-HLA class I antibodies) and B-lymphocytes (anti-HLA class I and/or HLA class II antibodies)
- Antiglobulin crossmatch

Lymphocytotoxicity test used in almost all of the above tests—complement-dependent cytotoxicity (CDC) assay:

Ag + Ab + complement $\rightarrow$ lysis of lymphocytes (may be used to look for a specific Ag or Ab)

13.2 Donor Selection and the Role of Tissue Matching

1. Blood type: while there are some transplant centers that transplant across ABO groups, typically it is required that donor and recipient would have the same blood type (though blood type O can be a universal donor). Also, multiple studies have demonstrated the safe and effective transplantation of blood group B kidney transplant recipients with kidneys from donors having the less immunogenic non-A1 subtype.

2. HLA match: higher degree of HLA match is associated with proportionally increased long-term graft survival.[4] Matching by the 6 alleles of HLA-A, -B, and −DR is considered matching compatibility for practical purposes.

3. Preformed donor antibodies: presence of preformed antibodies against donor-specific HLA antigens is a barrier to transplantation and an important cause of allograft loss, increasing the risk for early antibody mediated rejection.[5] Desensitization protocols can be used: plasmapheresis, IVIg, immunoabsorption (not presently in use in the USA), and rituximab.

13.3 Factors Affecting Transplant Graft Outcome[4,6,7]

Donor Characteristics:

- Live or deceased donor
- Age, BMI, race (worse outcome in Black or Hispanic donors), comorbidities, gender (better with kidneys from males), creatinine level[4]

Recipient Characteristics:

- Age, race (worse outcome in Black recipients), BMI, gender (better in males)
- First transplant (outcome of each consecutive transplant is generally worse)[4,8]
- RRT modality (PD or prior transplant are both better than HD)
- Timing of transplant—see charts below
- Duration of ESKD
- Cause of ESKD (e.g., SLE is associated with inferior outcome[9,10])
- Presence of CVD[11]
- Individual socioeconomic factors (education level, type of insurance, alcohol use)[12] and composite social adaptability index (higher index is associated with better outcome)[13]

Other Factors:

- HLA match of donor and recipient
- Cold ischemia time of kidney
- Procedure (worse outcome with kidney-pancreas, en-bloc transplant)[4]
- Higher transplant volume of transplant center
- State of the economy[14]
- Delayed graft function[15]

BMI, Body mass index; CVD, cardiovascular disease; ESKD, end-stage kidney disease; HLA, human leukocyte antigen; PD, peritoneal dialysis; RRT, renal replacement therapy; SLE, systemic lupus erythematosus.

13.4 Timing of Transplantation

First Transplant	Retransplantation
• Preemptive transplantation seems to be beneficial[4] • However, being on dialysis for up to 6 months is associated with the same outcome as preemptive transplantation[6]	• Unlike the first transplant, preemptive retransplantation might be associated with a higher risk of graft loss by 36%.[8] • However, among those on dialysis in between transplants, longer time on dialysis is associated with higher risk.

13.5 Preemptive Transplantation Versus Transplantation After Initial Period of Dialysis[6]

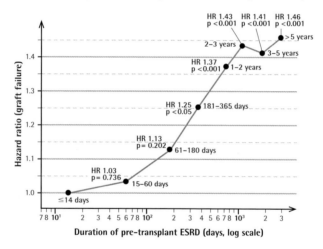

Preemptive transplantation vs. transplantation after initial period of dialysis[6]

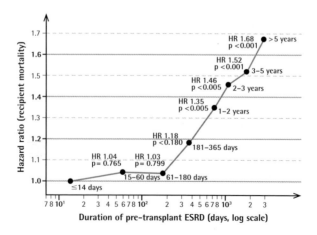

13.6 Immunosuppression

The following diagram is a schematic representation of the mechanism of action of the most commonly used immunosuppressive medications (see immunological pathways described at the end of this chapter).

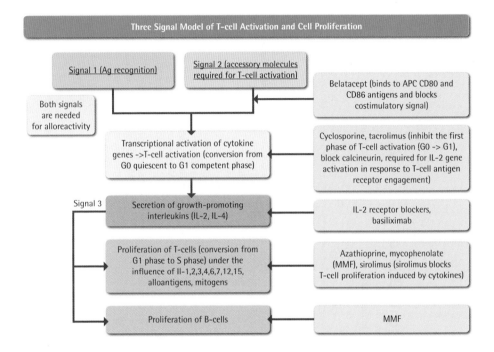

13.7 Action of Immunosuppressive Medications

The goal of immunosuppression therapy is to suppress the immune system to the point of avoiding rejection, but at the same time to minimize the potential side effects of excessive immune suppression.

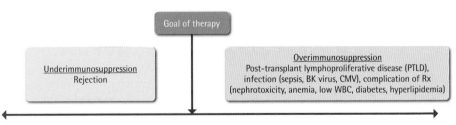

CMV, Cytomegalovirus; *WBC*, white blood cells.

This table represents a summary of the mechanisms of action, doses, and side effects of the most commonly used immunosuppressive medications.

Immunosuppressive Medications Commonly Utilized

	Mechanism	Initial Dose	Complications
Cyclosporine (Neoral, Sandimmune)	1. Binds with cyclophilin; this complex inhibits calcineurin ⟹ → expression of T-cell activation genes 2. Inhibits IL-2 driven proliferation of activated T-cells (inhibits IL-2 message); affects G0-G1 cell cycle 3. Enhances the expression of TGF-β	• PO: 8–15 mg/kg/day, change in 2-mg/kg increments according to level • IV daily dose = 1/3 PO daily dose • Levels may be influenced by drugs affecting p-450	• Nephrotoxicity (acute: reduction of renal blood flow b/o increased sympathetic tone and RA system; chronic: interstitial fibrosis after 6–12 months of treatment b/o chronic ischemia and toxicity and enhanced apoptosis) • HTN • Hyperlipidemia • Diabetes (less than tacrolimus) • Infections (CMV, BK virus, bacterial, etc.) • ↓T-cell proliferation • Tremors • Hirsutism • Hepatotoxicity • CNS toxicity • Gingival hypertrophy • Renal vascular damage • Malignancies • Drug–drug interaction reduces mycophenolate level[16]
Tacrolimus (FK506, Prograf)	1. Similar to cyclosporine; binds with FKBP12; blocks calcineurin 2. Inhibits IL-2 (inhibits IL-2 message), -3, -4, and TNF production 3. Affects G0-G1 cell cycle	• 0.15–0.3 mg/kg/day	Similar to cyclosporine: • Nephrotoxicity (same as for cyclosporine) • Neurotoxicity (tremor, low seizure threshold, headaches, nightmares) • HTN (less than cyclosporine) • Hyperlipidemia (less than cyclosporine and sirolimus) • GI: diarrhea, anorexia • Glucose intolerance/DM • Infections (CMV, BK virus, bacterial, etc.) • Hyperkalemia • Malignancies

Drug	Mechanism	Dosing	Side Effects
Sirolimus (Rapamycin)	1. Binds with FKBP12, interferes with TOR (target of rapamycin) and blocks T-cell activation; blocks IL-2 response 2. Affects G1-S cell cycle	• Start at 2 mg/day and follow levels	• Hypercholesterolemia, hypertriglyceridemia (treat with statins) • Stomatitis (dose reduction or transient discontinuation [DC]) • Myelosuppression: pancytopenia including thrombocytopenia (more common in combination with MMF, responds to dose reduction or transient DC) • HTN (treatment of choice: ACEI/ARB, but may worsen anemia) • Wound/incision complications, lymphocele (more common with high levels, in DM and obesity; responds to dose reduction or transient DC) • Pneumonitis (interstitial lung disease/BOOP/pulmonary fibrosis: increased risk with higher level, may respond to dose reduction or DC) • May potentiate nephrotoxic effect of cyclosporine, increases MMF level (but not tacrolimus level) • Infections (CMV, BK virus, bacterial, etc.) • Asthenia, headaches, epistaxis, diarrhea, arthralgia • Proteinuria
Azathioprine (Imuran)	1. Inhibits purine nucleotide synthesis ⇒ inhibits gene replication and T-cell activation, suppresses myelocytes 2. Effectiveness is not blood-level–dependent	• Start at 3–4 mg/kg/day, adjust the dose to WBC count • IV daily dose = 1/2 PO daily dose	• Bone marrow suppression/leukopenia • Hepatitis, cholestasis—occasionally • Avoid concomitant allopurinol- bone marrow toxicity; check for thiopurine methyltransferase (TPMT) mutation before initiation to avoid bone marrow toxicity
Mycophenolate mofetil (MMF) (CellCept)	1. Binds to protein MPA, affects IMPDH, inhibits IL-2 production (inhibits IL-2 message) and response 2. Inhibits de novo pathway of purine biosynthesis by blocking inosine monophosphate dehydrogenase activity 3. Blocks proliferation of T- and B-cells, Ab formation, generation of cytotoxic T-cells	• 1000 mg PO twice daily (1500 mg twice daily when greater immune suppression is desired with cyclosporine)	• GI: dyspepsia, diarrhea, hepatic injury, inflammatory colitis • Hematological: leukopenia, anemia • CMV (as all other immunosuppressives) • Infections (CMV, BK virus, bacterial, etc.) • Malignancies • Congenital malformations (avoid in pregnancy)

Continued on following page

	Mechanism	Initial Dose	Complications
Corticosteroids	1. Inhibit the expression of cytokine genes: IL-1, -2, -3, -6, TNF-alpha, gamma-interferon 2. Nonspecific immunosuppressive effect	• Taper to 5 mg/day, or stop early if on early steroid withdrawal protocol (center specific)	• Osteoporosis • Hyperlipidemia, glucose intolerance • Neuropsychological (anxiety) • Infections (opportunistic) • Impaired wound healing • Growth impairment in children
Nonlymphocyte-depleting antibodies; IL-2 inhibitors; daclizumab (Zenapax), basiliximab (Simulect)	1. Monoclonal Ab's against IL-2 receptors; used for induction therapy	• Zenapax 1 mg/kg on day of surgery, postop at 2-wk intervals up to 4 doses • Simulect: 20 mg on day of surgery, again on POD#4	• Zenapax: hyperlipidemia, diabetes, CMV • Simulect: anaphylaxis, infections
Lymphocyte-depleting antibodies (ATG, TMG, OKT3)	1. Ab's against CD3. For patients with high risk: retransplant, Blacks, sensitized (PRA >30%), as induction in pancreas transplant	• Dose may vary; e.g., for induction with ATG, 1.25 mg/kg IV every other day for 3 doses	• Malignancies, e.g., PTLD: greatest risk EBV donor positive to recipient negative • Anaphylaxis, serum sickness • Bone marrow suppression (leukopenia, thrombocytopenia) • Infections (CMV)
CTLA 4-Ig (Belatacept)	1. Costimulatory blocker, selectively blocks T-cell activation	• 5–10 mg/kg (monthly maintenance dosing)	• PTLD (black box warning EBV D+/R-) • PML • Infections

ACEi, Angiotensin-converting-enzyme inhibitor; *ARB*, angiotensin II receptor blocker; *b/o*, because of; *BOOP*, bronchiolitis obliterans organizing pneumonia; *CMV*, cytomegalovirus; *CNS*, central nervous system; *DC*, discontinuation; *DM*, diabetes mellitus; *GI*, gastrointestinal; *HTN*, hypertension; *IMPDH*, inosine-5′-monophosphate dehydrogenase; *IV*, intravenous; *MMF*, mycophenolate mofetil; *MPA*, mycophenolic acid; *OKT3*, muromonab-CD3; *PML*, progressive multifocal leukoencephalopathy; *PO*, by mouth; *POD*, postoperative day; *PTLD*, posttransplant lymphoproliferative disease; *RA*, renin angiotensin; *TMG*, thymoglobulin; *TNF*, tumor necrosis factor; *TPMT*, thiopurine methyltransferase; *WBC*, white blood cell.

Typical initial posttransplant medications:

Initial immunosuppressive regimen

Induction:
➢ ATG or Simulect
Maintenance:
➢ CNIs (tacrolimus or cyclosporine) or CTLA-4-Ig (Belatacept)
   and
➢ Antimetabolite (mycophenolate mofetil or azathioprine) or mTOR-I (sirolimus or everolimus) and
➢ Prednisone (sometimes rapidly withdrawn)

Prophylactic medications

• Antiviral: CMV/herpes (valganciclovir for moderate and high risk, acyclovir for low risk; dose based on serum creatinine) for 3–6 months
• Bacterial and PCP prophylaxis (Trimethoprim-sulfamethoxazole 1 single-strength tablet daily) for 12 months
• Fungal prophylaxis, e.g., oral candidiasis (fluconazole or nystatin) for 1 month
• Steroid ulcer prophylaxis (H2-blockers)

Other

• Antihypertensive medications
• Diabetic medications
• Iron, magnesium/phosphate supplements if needed
• Lipid-lowering medications

Advantages of CCBs in post-Tx patients for HTN

• Vasodilatory
• Stimulate natriuresis
• Protective effect on DGF
• Reduce hyperfiltration, renal hypertrophy, proximal tubular hypermetabolism, renal calcinosis
• Inhibition of cyclosporine-induced platelet aggregation and release of thromboxane
• IMPORTANT: Nondihydropyridine CCBs (e.g., verapamil, diltiazem) increase calcineurin inhibitor levels.

CCBs, Calcium channel blockers; *CMV,* cytomegalovirus; *CNIs,* calcineurin inhibitors; *DGF,* delayed graft function; *HTN, hypertension; PCP,* pneumocystis pneumonia.

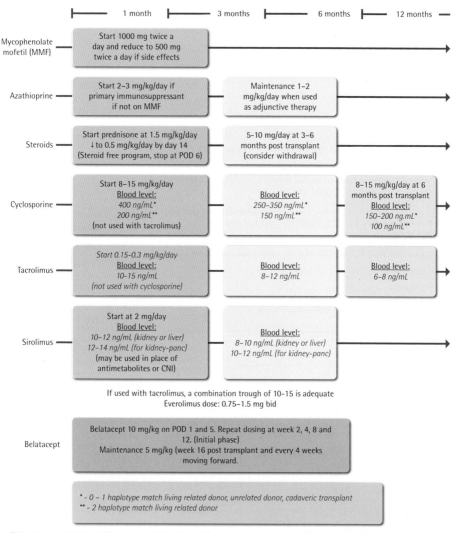

CNI, calcineurin inhibitors; DGF, delayed graft function; PCP, pneumocystis pneumonia; PO, by mouth; POD, post operative day.

13.8 Complications of Maintenance Immunosuppressive Medications

	Cyclosporine	Tacrolimus	MMF	Sirolimus
HTN	+++	++	–	–
Hyperlipidemia	++	+	–	+++
DM	+	+++	–	–
Nephrotoxicity	+++	+++	–	Associated with proteinuria and enhances toxicity of cyclosporine and tacrolimus

	Cyclosporine	Tacrolimus	MMF	Sirolimus
Diarrhea	+	++	+++	++ in combination with MMF
Anemia, leukopenia	–	–	++	++ especially in combination with MMF

MMF, Mycophenolate mofetil.

Why convert from CNI (tacrolimus/cyclosporine) to sirolimus or belatacept[17,18]:

Sirolimus:
- It inhibits growth factor mediated proliferation of cells involved in the chronic allograft nephropathy (CAN) pathogenesis
- It reduces the degree of intimal thickening
- It helps to avoid underimmunosuppression
- It is less nephrotoxic (creatinine preserved but can cause proteinuria)

Belatacept:
- Donor vascular disease or CNI nephrotoxicity
- Patients with non-compliance of CNI
- Non inferior to CNI in graft and patient survival
- Belatacept ineligible in EBV D+/R- transplant

Indications

- Nephrotoxicity of CNI (acute and chronic)
- Post-transplant diabetes
- Thrombotic microangiopathy (HUS)
- Poor initial graft function/extended criteria donor (old, HTN, DM)/DGF/ischemic damaged kidneys/anatomic or surgical damage
- Side effects of CNI (hirsutism, gingival hyperplasia, neurotoxicity)
- Renal dysfunction in non-renal transplant patients
- Others: polyoma, PTLD, etc.
- Kaposi's sarcoma—treatable with sirolimus

Conversion protocol

From CNI to Sirolimus
Abrupt conversion (in ATN, diabetes, HUS)
- Stop CNI, after 24 hr start sirolimus at loading dose 10 mg QD x2, then 5 mg QD
- Level after 3rd dose and weekly
- Can decrease MMF if leukopenia

CNI overlap (in chronic allograft nephropathy)
- Decrease CNI by ½, start sirolimus at 5 mg/day
- Level after 3rd dose and weekly
- Discontinue CNI when either sirolimus is therapeutic (8–12 ng/mL) or taper over 2–4 weeks

Wait 24 hrs before starting sirolimus for CsA levels >250 ng/mL or tacro level >14 ng/mL
For kidney-pancreas: Zenapax bridge (2 mg/kg) at day 0 and 14
May reduce MMF as levels are higher in combination with sirolimus

---

Conversion protocol

From CNI to belatacept
Abrupt conversion (in ATN, diabetes, HUS)
- Start bela at 10 mg/kg on Day 1 with no CNI dose change
- Continue bela 10 mg/kg on POD 5 with 50% CNI reduction
- Continue bela 10 mg/kg on POD 14 and discontinue CNI
- Continue bela 10 mg/kg on POD 28
- Reduce bela to 5 mg/kg on POD 42
- Continue bela 5 mg/kg every 4 weeks thereafter

Standard conversion (CNI overlap)
- Start bela at 5 mg/kg on Day 1 with no CNI dose change
- Continue bela 5 mg/kg on POD 15 with 40%–60% CNI reduction
- Continue bela 5 mg/kg on POD 28 with 20%–30% CNI reduction
- Continue bela 5 mg/kg on POD 42 and discontinue CNI
- Continue bela to 5 mg/kg on POD 57
- Continue bela 5 mg/kg every 4 weeks thereafter

ATN, Acute tubular necrosis; *CAN*, chronic allograft nephropathy; *CNI*, calcineurin inhibitor; *DGF*, delayed graft function; *DM*, diabetes mellitus; *EBV*, Epstein-Barr virus; *HTN*, hypertension; *HUS*, hemolytic uremic syndrome; *MMF*, mycophenolate mofetil; *POD*, post-operative day; *PTLD*, posttransplant lymphoproliferative disease.

Medications That ↑ CNI Level	Medications That ↓ CNI Level
• Calcium-channel blockers, nondihydropyridines (e.g., verapamil, diltiazem, nicardipine) • Antifungals (ketoconazole, fluconazole, itraconazole) • Antibiotics: erythromycin and other macrolides • Histamine blockers (cimetidine) • Proton pump inhibitors (omeprazole) • Hormones (corticosteroids, oral contraceptives) • Grapefruit or grapefruit juice	• Antituberculosis medications (rifampin, INH) • Anticonvulsants (barbiturates, phenytoin, carbamazepine) • Antibiotics (nafcillin, IV trimethoprim, IV sulfa, imipenem, cephalosporins)

13.9 Early Kidney Transplant Complications and Allograft Dysfunction

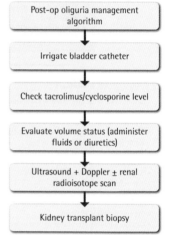

Early complications of transplantation

- Mechanical
  - Leak (bleeding, lymphocele, urine leak)
  - Ureteral obstruction
  - Vascular thrombosis of artery or vein
- Medical
  - Delayed graft function
  - Rejection (humoral or cellular)
  - Infection
  - Drug toxicity (cyclosporine/tacrolimus toxicity, associated thrombotic microangiopathy with HUS)
  - Volume depletion
  - De novo / recurrent renal disease
  - Other: ATN, prerenal failure, intrarenal conditions not specific for transplant kidney

Post-op oliguria management algorithm
↓
Irrigate bladder catheter
↓
Check tacrolimus/cyclosporine level
↓
Evaluate volume status (administer fluids or diuretics)
↓
Ultrasound + Doppler ± renal radioisotope scan
↓
Kidney transplant biopsy

ATN, Acute tubular necrosis; *HUS,* hemolytic uremic syndrome; *US,* ultrasound.

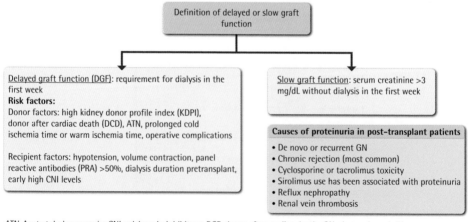

Definition of delayed or slow graft function

Delayed graft function (DGF): requirement for dialysis in the first week
Risk factors:
Donor factors: high kidney donor profile index (KDPI), donor after cardiac death (DCD), ATN, prolonged cold ischemia time or warm ischemia time, operative complications

Recipient factors: hypotension, volume contraction, panel reactive antibodies (PRA) >50%, dialysis duration pretransplant, early high CNI levels

Slow graft function: serum creatinine >3 mg/dL without dialysis in the first week

Causes of proteinuria in post-transplant patients
- De novo or recurrent GN
- Chronic rejection (most common)
- Cyclosporine or tacrolimus toxicity
- Sirolimus use has been associated with proteinuria
- Reflux nephropathy
- Renal vein thrombosis

ATN, Acute tubular necrosis; *CNI,* calcineurin inhibitors; *DCD,* donor after cardiac death; *GN,* glomerulonephritis; *KDPI,* High Kidney Donor Profile Index; *PRA,* panel reactive antibodies.

13.10 Acute Rejection

Acute rejection is one of the common early complications of renal transplant. Chronic rejection, while indicated in the following diagram for completeness, will be discussed in more detail below.

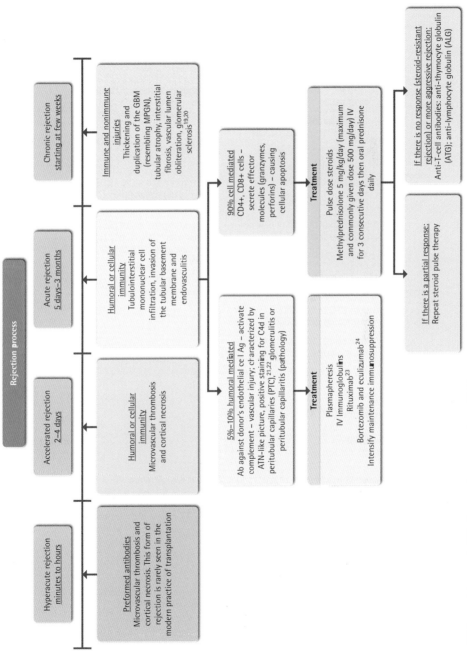

ATN, Acute tubular necrosis; GBM, glomerular basement membrane; MPGN, membranoproliferative glomerulonephritis; PTC, peritubular capillaries.

13.11 A 2018 Reference Guide to the Banff Classification of Renal Allograft Rejection[25]

Antibody-mediated rejection (ABMR):

	Morphological	Immunological	Serological
Acute ABMR	Microvascular inflammation (g > 0 and/or PTC > 0)	Linear C4d staining in PTCs	Donor specific antibodies (DSAs)
	Intimal or transmural arteritis (v > 0)	At least moderate microvascular inflammation ([g + PTC] ≥ 2)	
	Acute TMA in the absence of any other cause	Increased expression of gene transcripts in biopsy tissue indicative of endothelial injury	
	Acute tubular injury in the absence of any other apparent cause		
Chronic active ABMR	TG (cg > 0), if no evidence of chronic TMA	Linear C4d staining in PTCs	DSAs
	Severe PTC basement membrane multilayering	At least moderate microvascular inflammation ([g + PTC] ≥ 2)	
	Arterial intimal fibrosis of new on-set, excluding other causes	Increased expression of gene transcripts in the biopsy tissue indicative of endothelial injury	
Chronic ABMR	TG (cg > 0), if no evidence of chronic TMA	A prior documented diagnosis of active or chronic active ABMR	DSAs
	Severe PTC basement membrane multilayering		
	Arterial intimal fibrosis of new on-set, excluding other causes		

T cell-mediated rejection (TCMR):

	Description	Banff Scores
Acute TCMR		
Type IA	Moderate tubulitis and at least moderate interstitial inflammation	t2i2 or t2i3
Type IB	Severe tubulitis and at least moderate interstitial inflammation	t3i2 or t3i3
Type IIA	Mild to moderate intimal arteritis	v1
Type IIB	Severe intimal arteritis (>25% of the luminal area)	v2
Type III	"Transmural" arteritis and/or fibrinoid necrosis	v3
Chronic active TCMR		
Grade IA	Moderate tubulitis and at least moderate total cortical inflammation and at least moderate scarred cortical inflammation and other known causes ruled out	t2, ti ≥ 2, and i-IFTA ≥ 2

	Description	Banff Scores
Grade IB	Severe tubulitis and at least moderate total cortical inflammation and at least moderate scarred cortical inflammation and other known causes ruled out	t3, ti $\geq$ 2, and i-IFTA $\geq$ 2
Grade II	Arterial intimal fibrosis with mononuclear cell inflammation, formation of neointima	cv1, cv2, or cv3

cg, Chronic glomerulopathy (GBM double contours); *g*, glomerulitis; *I*, interstitial inflammation; *PTC*, peritubular capillaritis; *t*, tubulitis; *TG*, transplant glomerulopathy; *TMA*, thrombotic microangiopathy; *v*, vasculitis.

13.12 Complications of Renal Transplant

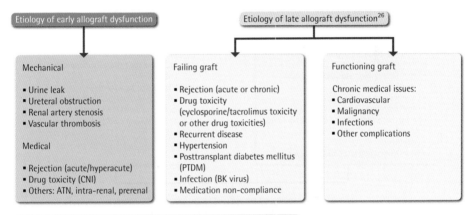

Etiology of early allograft dysfunction

Etiology of late allograft dysfunction[26]

Mechanical

- Urine leak
- Ureteral obstruction
- Renal artery stenosis
- Vascular thrombosis

Medical

- Rejection (acute/hyperacute)
- Drug toxicity (CNI)
- Others: ATN, intra-renal, prerenal

Failing graft

- Rejection (acute or chronic)
- Drug toxicity (cyclosporine/tacrolimus toxicity or other drug toxicities)
- Recurrent disease
- Hypertension
- Posttransplant diabetes mellitus (PTDM)
- Infection (BK virus)
- Medication non-compliance

Functioning graft

Chronic medical issues:
- Cardiovascular
- Malignancy
- Infections
- Other complications

Five entities that describe the status of an affected renal allograft[27]

- Rejection: graft injury secondary to T-cell mediated rejection (tubulitis, endothelialitis, interstitial infiltrates) or alloantibody-mediated rejection.
- Allograft nephropathy: tubular atrophy, interstitial fibrosis, fibrous intimal thickening of the arteries
- Transplant glomerulopathy
- Specific diseases (recurrent[28] or de novo renal disease, BK nephropathy,[29] HUS, calcineurin inhibitor toxicity as a primary disease,[30] diabetic nephropathy, hypertensive renal disease
- Accelerating processes: HTN causing acceleration of other diseases, calcineurin inhibitor causing acceleration of other diseases, diabetes, proteinuria, lipid abnormalities

ATN, Acute tubular necrosis; *CNI*, calcineurin inhibitors; *HTN*, hypertension; *HUS*, hemolytic uremic syndrome; *PTDM*, posttransplant diabetes mellitus.

13.13 Chronic Allograft Nephropathy

Chronic allograft nephropathy (CAN) is defined as a gradual progressive decline in renal function usually associated with proteinuria and HTN leading to graft failure. It is caused by immunological and nonimmunological factors.

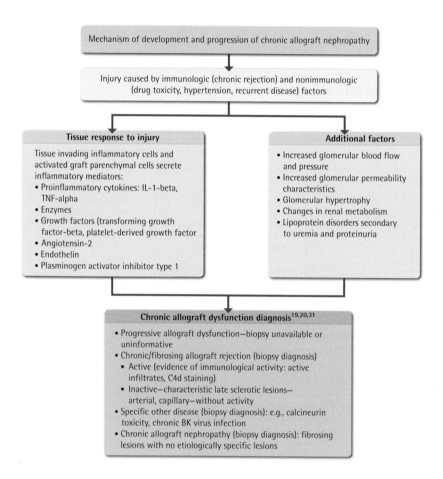

Mechanism of development and progression of chronic allograft nephropathy

Injury caused by immunologic (chronic rejection) and nonimmunologic (drug toxicity, hypertension, recurrent disease) factors

Tissue response to injury

Tissue invading inflammatory cells and activated graft parenchymal cells secrete inflammatory mediators:
• Proinflammatory cytokines: IL-1-beta, TNF-alpha
• Enzymes
• Growth factors (transforming growth factor-beta, platelet-derived growth factor
• Angiotensin-2
• Endothelin
• Plasminogen activator inhibitor type 1

Additional factors

• Increased glomerular blood flow and pressure
• Increased glomerular permeability characteristics
• Glomerular hypertrophy
• Changes in renal metabolism
• Lipoprotein disorders secondary to uremia and proteinuria

Chronic allograft dysfunction diagnosis[19,20,31]

• Progressive allograft dysfunction—biopsy unavailable or uninformative
• Chronic/fibrosing allograft rejection (biopsy diagnosis)
  ▪ Active (evidence of immunological activity: active infiltrates, C4d staining)
  ▪ Inactive—characteristic late sclerotic lesions—arterial, capillary—without activity
• Specific other disease (biopsy diagnosis): e.g., calcineurin toxicity, chronic BK virus infection
• Chronic allograft nephropathy (biopsy diagnosis): fibrosing lesions with no etiologically specific lesions

Chronic allograft nephropathy pathology
(typically tubular atrophy, interstitial fibrosis, intimal vascular thickening)

Light microscopy
• Glomerular lesions and sclerosis
  ▪ Wrinkling and collapse of the glomerular tuft
  ▪ Glomerular hypertrophy
  ▪ Mesangial matrix expansion
  ▪ Thickening of the GBM
  ▪ Focal glomerulosclerosis
  ▪ Chronic transplant glomerulopathy (may be a form of chronic rejection): double
    contours of the basement membrane, mesangiolysis, progressive sclerosing changes
• Tubulo-interstitial and vascular lesions
  ▪ Atherosclerosis/hyperplastic vasculopathy: concentric fibrous intimal thickening
    (migration of fibroblasts into the intima -> local proliferation and deposition of
    extracellular matrix proteins) often with vessel wall infiltration with macrophages,
    lymphocytes, foam cells; thickening of the internal elastic lamina
  ▪ Multilayering of peritubular capillaries
  ▪ Interstitial fibrosis and tubular atrophy and cell drop out

Immunofluorescence

Nondiagnostic pattern of Ig deposition (linear IgG deposition along GBM, granular
deposits of IgA, IgG in peripheral capillary loops)

Electron microscopy

Circumferential multilamination of the peritubular capillary basement membranes

Specific features of chronic rejection

Immune/inflammatory damage to the allograft; one of the causes of chronic allograft
nephropathy:
• Intimal proliferation/thickening, with intimal lymphocytes, and splintering
  and disruption of the elastic lamina with formation of neo-media and neointima
• Duplication of basement membrane (chronic allograft glomerulopathy)
• Duplication of capillary lamina densa in peritubular capillaries
• Peritubular capillary staining for C4d
• Overexpression of VCAM-1 on peritubular capillaries

GBM, Glomerular basement membrane.

13.14 Risk of Recurrent Disease in Transplanted Kidney[32]

Most diseases affecting the native kidney may recur in the kidney transplant with the notable
exception of a few, including polycystic kidney disease, hereditary nephritis, and Alport
syndrome.

	Risk of Recurrence	Graft Loss from Recurrence	Predictors of Recurrence	Treatment
Focal segmental glomerular sclerosis[32,33]	20%–50%	13%–20%	Younger age, rapid progression of original disease with development of end-stage renal failure within 3 years, mesangial hypercellularity of native kidney, Caucasian race, history of previous graft failure due to recurrence	Plasma exchange, steroids, ACEi, possibly rituximab, changing from sirolimus back to CNI; Preemptive perioperative plasma exchange in those with high risk
Membranous glomerulopathy[34]	10%–30%	10%–15%	Higher titers of anti-phospholipase A2 receptor (PLA2R) autoantibodies; initial concerns of the risk of recurrence with living related donors, presence of HLA-DR3 in the recipient, and the aggressiveness of native disease have not been substantiated	No role for additional immunosuppression, rituximab seems beneficial[35]
Membranoproliferative glomerulonephritis, type I	20%–30%	15% (in a second graft, 80%)	HLA-B8 DR3, living related donors and previous graft loss from recurrence	ASA, dipyridamole, possibly rituximab, eculizumab
Membranoproliferative glomerulonephritis, type II	80%–100%	15%–30%	Male gender, RPGN of original disease, nephrotic syndrome	Plasma exchange, possibly rituximab, eculizumab for C3 glomerulopathy
IgA nephropathy[32,36]	15%–60% (risk is increased 20%–100% in second transplant)	1%–10%	No single parameter including age, gender, race, HLA (although B35 and DR4 were suggested), typing, pretransplant course or biochemical characteristic of serum IgA can predict recurrence	In crescentic: plasma exchange, cytotoxics; otherwise, no effective therapy except for ACEi/ARB
Henoch-Schönlein purpura	30%–75%	20%–40%	Same as IgA nephropathy	Plasma exchange,[37] possibly steroids
ANCA-associated glomerulonephritis/vasculitis[36]	17%	6%–8%	Persistent ANCA positivity	It is advisable to defer kidney transplantation until the disease is inactive. Patients with renal relapses—cyclophosphamide. Patients with cellular crescents and high ANCA titer—cyclophosphamide + plasma exchange ± IV Ig

Disease				Treatment
Anti-GBM nephritis	Up to 50% if antibodies were still present; <5% if not	Rare	Recurrence is about 50% when circulating antibodies are still present before transplantation	Pulse steroids, plasma exchange, cyclophosphamide, Ab immunoadsorption
Hemolytic uremic syndrome	13%–25%	40%–50%	Precipitating environmental factors: infections including cytomegalovirus, influenza virus, parvovirus	Plasma exchange, eculizumab, possibly steroids
Lupus nephritis	Histological recurrence up to 30%, but clinically significant recurrent disease occurs in 2%–9%	2%–4%	African American non-Hispanic ancestry, female gender, and young age. Patients with antiphospholipid autoantibodies and kidneys from living donors	Postpone renal transplantation until the disease becomes quiescent for at least 6–9 months, MMF for recurrence
Granulomatosis with polyangiitis (formerly Wegener's granulomatosis)	Up to 70%		No clear risk factors	Cyclophosphamide + plasma exchange
Alport syndrome, hereditary nephritis	<10% de novo "anti-GBM" RPGN	100%	No clear risk factors	Same as anti-GBM nephritis
Diabetes mellitus[38]	Histological features recur in most if not all patients		Steroids, CNI, or mTORi immunosuppressives, obesity, infections (Hepatitis C, cytomegalovirus), hypomagnesemia. Increased age, male, African American and Hispanic ancestry, HLA mismatch, deceased donor	Diabetic nephropathy treatment

ACEi, Angiotensin-converting-enzyme inhibitors; ANCA, antineutrophilic cytoplasmic autoantibody; ARB, angiotensin II receptor blocker; CNI, calcineurin inhibitors; HLA, human leukocyte antigen; MMF, mycopherolate mofetil; mTORi, mammalian target of rapamycin inhibitor; RPGN, rapidly progressive glomerulonephritis.

13.15 Causes of Graft Failure During 10 Years of Follow-Up[39]

Chronic rejection/CAN	26%–40%
Death with graft functioning	30%–53%
Recurrent renal disease	3%–6%
Acute rejection	0.6%–7.5%
De novo renal disease	0.2%–1%
Noncompliance with immunosuppressives	2%–10%
Other	3%–10%

CAN, Chronic allograft nephropathy.

Transplant Outcomes (2019 OPTN/SRTR Data Shown in Table and Figure Below[40])

Survival in deceased donor transplant

	1 year	5 years
Graft survival	93%	78%
Patient survival	96%	85%

Survival in living donor transplant

	1 year	5 years
Graft survival	97%	88%
Patient survival	99%	92%

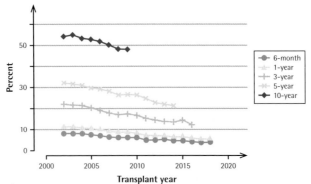

Transplant outcomes (2019 OPTN/SRTR data[40])

A Graft failure among adult deceased donor kidney transplant recipients

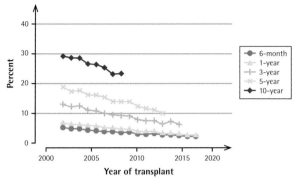

B Death-censored graft failure among adult deceased donor kidney transplant recipients

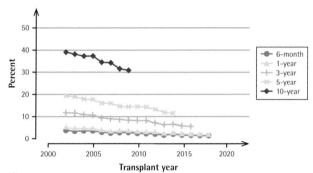

C Graft failure among adult living donor kidney transplant recipients

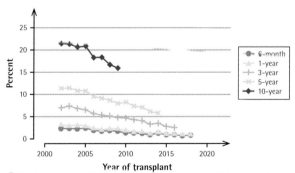

D Death-censored graft failure among adult living donor kidney transplant recipients

	Major causes of transplant recipient mortality[39]		
Cardiovascular disease	**Malignancy**	**Infection**	**Liver disease and hepatitis**
Identify and study newly symptomatic patients with angiography Noninvasive tests every 1– 2 years if necessary	<u>Most common:</u> squamous cell carcinomas of the skin; non-Hodgkin's lymphomas; in situ carcinomas of the uterine cervix, vulva, and perineum; renal carcinomas; other carcinomas: 1.5-fold increased risk of developing cancers seen in the general population (e.g., carcinomas of the lung and colon) Note: those who had cancer before Tx; are over age 55 years; have had intensive immunosuppressive therapy or many years of immunosuppressive therapy are at greater risk	High risk for post-transplant infections: diabetes mellitus; poor renal function; malnutrition; increased immunosuppressive therapy (ALG, ATGAM, or OKT3); leukopenia; splenectomy, and seronegativity for CMV	Viral: HBV, HCV, herpes simplex, EBV, and CMV Meds: azathioprine, cyclosporine, and tacrolimus can cause a picture of cholestatic jaundice; and azathioprine and CMV have been associated with veno-occlusive disease; ACEI, HMG-CoA reductase inhibitors, azole antifungals, isoniazid, high doses of acetaminophen, and alcohol

ACEi, Angiotensin-converting-enzyme inhibitors; *ALG*, Anti-lymphocyte globulin; *ATGAM*, Anti-thymocyte globulin (equine); *CMV*, cytomegalovirus; *EBV*, Epstein-Barr virus; *HBV*, hepatitis B virus; *HCV*, hepatitis C virus; *OKT3*, Muromonab-CD3; *Tx*, transplant.

Major Causes of Posttransplant Morbidity

- Hypertension
- Hyperlipidemia
- Posttransplant diabetes mellitus
- Neoplasms (e.g., skin cancers, PTLD, Kaposi's sarcoma—sirolimus is effective treatment)
- Electrolyte disturbances: hyperkalemia, hypomagnesemia, hypophosphatemia
- Musculoskeletal disorders
- Erythrocytosis (can usually be controlled with ACEi)
- GI problems
- Ocular disease
- Nonmalignant skin disease (basal cell epitheliomas very commonly)
- Psychiatric disease
- Allograft failure

ACEi, Angiotensin-converting-enzyme inhibitors; *GI*, gastrointestinal; *PTLD*, posttransplant lymphoproliferative disease.

13.16 Malignancies

By 20 years posttransplant[39]:

- Nearly 50% of recipients had ≥1 skin cancer
- Over 10% of recipients had a nonskin, non-PTLD malignancy
- Over 2% of recipients developed PTLD

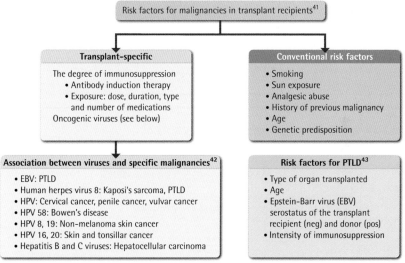

Risk factors for malignancies in transplant recipients[41]

Transplant-specific

The degree of immunosuppression
- Antibody induction therapy
- Exposure: dose, duration, type and number of medications
Oncogenic viruses (see below)

Conventional risk factors

- Smoking
- Sun exposure
- Analgesic abuse
- History of previous malignancy
- Age
- Genetic predisposition

Association between viruses and specific malignancies[42]

- EBV: PTLD
- Human herpes virus 8: Kaposi's sarcoma, PTLD
- HPV: Cervical cancer, penile cancer, vulvar cancer
- HPV 58: Bowen's disease
- HPV 8, 19: Non-melanoma skin cancer
- HPV 16, 20: Skin and tonsillar cancer
- Hepatitis B and C viruses: Hepatocellular carcinoma

Risk factors for PTLD[43]

- Type of organ transplanted
- Age
- Epstein-Barr virus (EBV) serostatus of the transplant recipient (neg) and donor (pos)
- Intensity of immunosuppression

PTLD, Posttransplant lymphoproliferative disease.

13.17 Posttransplant Infectious Complications and Prophylaxis

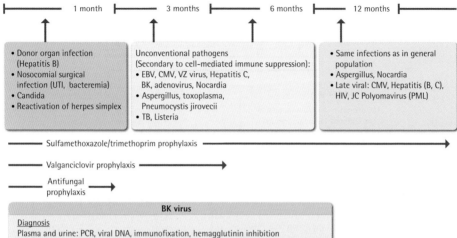

Post-transplant infectious complications and prophylaxis

| | 1 month | | 3 months | | 6 months | | 12 months | |

- Donor organ infection (Hepatitis B)
- Nosocomial surgical infection (UTI, bacteremia)
- Candida
- Reactivation of herpes simplex

Unconventional pathogens (Secondary to cell-mediated immune suppression):
- EBV, CMV, VZ virus, Hepatitis C, BK, adenovirus, Nocardia
- Aspergillus, toxoplasma, Pneumocystis jirovecii
- TB, Listeria

- Same infections as in general population
- Aspergillus, Nocardia
- Late viral: CMV, Hepatitis (B, C), HIV, JC Polyomavirus (PML)

— Sulfamethoxazole/trimethoprim prophylaxis →

— Valganciclovir prophylaxis →

— Antifungal prophylaxis →

BK virus

Diagnosis
Plasma and urine: PCR, viral DNA, immunofixation, hemagglutinin inhibition
Transplant Biopsy: signs of tubular injury, presence of intranuclear viral inclusions, immunohistochemistry to demonstrate infected tubular epithelial cells

Rx
1) Reduce or stop immunosuppression: decrease MMF dose by 50%
2) Follow PCR titers
3) Other medical therapies with no clear benefit: fluoroquinolones, leflunomide, cidofovir
4) IVIG has shown possible benefit

COVID-19

Novel coronavirus disease 2019 caused by SARS-CoV-2 was first identified in Wuhan, China in Dec 2019. It has since become a global pandemic.

Diagnosis
PCR test for SARS-CoV-2 nasopharyngeal swab
Antigen tests (rapid point-of-care tests are less sensitive)

Rx
Prophylactic and Treatments as shown
Prophylaxis for immune compromised before exposure:
Tixagevimab–cilgavimab (intramuscular Evusheld)

Treatments, approved to date: Remdesivir, nirmatrelvir/ritonavir, molnupiravir, baricitinib, or monoclonal antibodies (sotrovimab, bebtelovimab, bamlanivimab and etesevimab, casirivimab and imdevimab)

Supportive care in solid organ transplant recipients anti-inflammatory therapy with dexamethasone with or without remdesivir, tocilizumab or baricitinib in severe cases
Reduction in immunosuppression

CMV, cytomegalovirus; EBV, Epstein Barr virus; MMF, mycophenolate mofetil; PCR, polymerase chain reaction; PML, progressive multifocal leukoencephalopathy; UTI, urinary tract infection.

13.18 Immunosuppression Withdrawal After Graft Failure

As it has been demonstrated that it is of potential benefit to go on dialysis in between transplants for those with repeat transplants,[8] one of the potential mechanisms involves the withdrawal of immunosuppressive therapy. However, there are risks associated with immunosuppression withdrawal.

Complications of Immunosuppression Withdrawal
- Acute rejection, possibly requiring transplant nephrectomy (even after allograft failure)
- Secondary adrenal insufficiency after withdrawing prednisone
- Loss of residual renal function supported by allograft
- Sensitization in those who are candidates for another transplantation, transplant nephrectomy might limit sensitization

Strategies for Immunosuppression Withdrawal
- Early allograft failure (i.e., less than 1 year after surgery): immediate withdrawal of immunosuppression combined with preemptive nephrectomy may be advisable.
- Later allograft failure: immediately withdraw cyclosporine or tacrolimus and azathioprine or mycophenolate mofetil; subsequently taper prednisone by 1 mg/month until the prednisone is discontinued, carefully watching for symptoms of adrenal insufficiency.
- Those who develop symptoms of allograft rejection with withdrawal can be treated as for acute rejection (3 days of pulse doses of Solu-Medrol), then transplant nephrectomy may be advisable.

13.19 Pancreas Transplantation

Indications for Pancreas Transplant
- Diabetes requiring insulin (c-peptide <0.2 nmol/L, type I DM)
- Frequent hypoglycemic episodes
- Early development of secondary diabetic complications
- Brittle DM: inability to manage with insulin regimens

Types of Pancreas Transplant
- Simultaneous pancreas and kidney transplant (SPK)
- Pancreas transplantation after kidney transplantation (PAK)
- Pancreas transplant alone (PTA)

Benefits of Pancreas Transplant
- Improved quality of life
- Freedom from exogenous insulin
- Normalization of HbA1c
- Lack of frequent monitoring, lack of dietary restrictions
- Stabilization or improvement in secondary complications

13.20 General Transplant Patient Management

- Maintenance of well-being: exercise, nutrition, appetite, weight, etc.
- Monitor kidney allograft function
- Immunosuppression: regimen, drug levels, side effects (e.g., tremor, osteoporosis, diabetes, taper prednisone, etc.)

- Infection prophylaxis: symptoms of infection, adjustment of immunosuppressive medications, discontinuation of antimicrobial prophylaxis
- Blood pressure control
- Treatment of other primary diseases (e.g., diabetes, coronary artery disease)
- Anemia or posttransplant erythrocytosis management
- Monitor cholesterol levels and treat if indicated
- Chronic kidney disease (CKD) management, if transplant is failing
- Primary care: bone disease, vaccinations (pneumococcus, 2–3 years; flu,1 year, COVID-19), stool for occult blood (yearly)
- Cancer screening and prophylaxis: particularly with long-term or intense immunosuppression
  - Sunscreen and skin exam (yearly)
  - Mammography (yearly)
  - Pap smears (every 2–3 years)
  - Colonoscopy (every 5 years)
  - PSA and chest xray (uncertain data)

13.21 Elements of Hematopoiesis: Types and Origin of Cells Participating in Immune Response

Elements of hematopoiesis: types and origin of cells participating in immune response

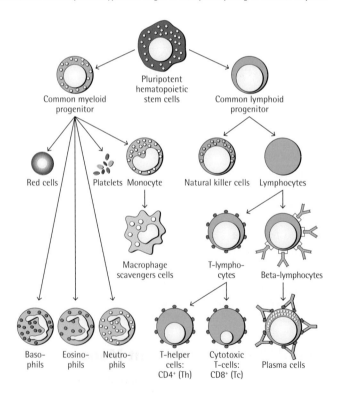

Pluripotent hematopoietic stem cells

Common myeloid progenitor

Common lymphoid progenitor

Red cells   Platelets Monocyte   Natural killer cells   Lymphocytes

Macrophage scavengers cells

T-lympho-cytes

Beta-lymphocytes

Baso-phils   Eosino-phils   Neutro-phils   T-helper cells: CD4+ (Th)   Cytotoxic T-cells: CD8+ (Tc)   Plasma cells

13.22 Lymphocytes and Their Role in Immune Response[19,44]

	Function	Receptors Expressed
Natural killer cells	Lysis of virally infected cells and tumor cells	CD16, CD56, but not CD3
Helper T cells (Th)	Release cytokines and growth factors that regulate other immune cells	TCR alpha-beta, CD3, and CD4
Cytotoxic T cells (Tc)	Lysis of virally infected cells, tumor cells and allografts	TCR alpha-beta, CD3, and CD8
Gamma-delta T cells	Immunoregulation and cytotoxicity	TCR gamma-delta and CD3
B cells	Secretion of antibodies	MHC class II, CD19, and CD21

13.23 The Role of Th Cells[45]

T-helper (Th) lymphocytes consist of Th1 and Th2 subsets. Th1 cells are effectors of cell-mediated immunity and secrete interferon-gamma (IFN-gamma) along with multiple other cytokines. IFN-gamma in combination with IL-12 recruits new Th1 cells in cooperation with interleukin-12 produced by monocytes. IFN-gamma also inhibits differentiation of Th cells into Th2. Th2 cells, on the other hand, act more as suppressors of immune response; they produce IL-4 and IL-10 along with other cytokines, which inhibit IFN-gamma secretion and cell immunity. In addition to Th1 and Th2, there are other Th cell types: Th3, Th17 (produce IL-17, important in autoimmune disease), and ThFH.

After the Th cell has been activated by the antigen presenting cell (APC), cells that are derived from monocytes, macrophages, B lymphocytes or activated endothelial cells or may be dendritic cells, the Th cell undergoes the process of differentiation into one of the Th subtypes and secretes multiple cytokines, involved in a complex process of regulation of the immune response, as depicted on the picture below.

The Role of Th Cells in Regulating Immune Response

Role of Cytokines in Developing Tolerance

In addition to the immunological reaction that leads to rejection of allogenic tissue, there are mechanisms of developing immunological tolerance that prevent an allograft from being rejected. This process is also regulated by cytokines.
- IL-2—essential for T-cell apoptosis
- IFN-gamma—down-regulates the proliferation of activated T-cells
- IL-4 + IL-13—converts T-cells into suppressor cells (Th1 → Th2 deviation)

13.24 Th-cell Activation

As indicated earlier, activated Th cells undergo the process of differentiation and secrete regulatory cytokines. The process of activating the Th cell is a function of the antigen-presenting cell (APC) in which two signals are necessary to activate the Th cell, as indicated on the diagram below.

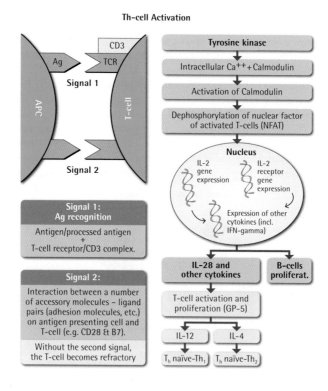

Th–cell Activation

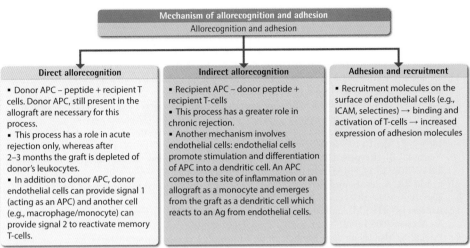

APC, antigen presenting cell; ICAM, intracellular adhesion molecule.

References

1. Delgado JC, Eckels DD. Positive B-cell only flow cytometric crossmatch: implications for renal transplantation. *Exp Mol Pathol*. 2008;85(1):59–63. doi:10.1016/j.yexmp.2008.03.009.
2. Sheldon S, Poulton K. HLA typing and its influence on organ transplantation. *Methods Mol Biol*. 2006;333:157–174. doi:10.1385/1-59745-049-9:157.
3. Takemoto SK. HLA matching in the new millennium. *Clin Transpl*. 2003;387–403.
4. Goldfarb-Rumyantzev AS, Scandling JD, Pappas L, Smout RJ, Horn S. Prediction of 3-yr cadaveric graft survival based on pre-transplant variables in a large national dataset. *Clin Transplant*. 2003;17(6): 485 497. doi:10.1046/j.0902-0063.2003.00051.x.
5. Everly MJ. Donor-specific anti-HLA antibody monitoring and removal in solid organ transplant recipients. *Clin Transpl*. 2011;319–325.
6. Goldfarb-Rumyantzev A, Hurdle JF, Scandling J, et al. Duration of end-stage renal disease and kidney transplant outcome. *Nephrol Dial Transplant*. 2005;20(1):167–175. doi:10.1093/ndt/gfh541.
7. Goldfarb-Rumyantzev AS, Hurdle JF, Scandling JD, Baird BC, Cheung AK. The role of pretransplantation renal replacement therapy modality in kidney allograft and recipient survival. *Am J Kidney Dis*. 2005;46(3):537–549. doi:10.1053/j.ajkd.2005.05.013.
8. Goldfarb-Rumyantzev AS, Hurdle JF, Baird BC, et al. The role of pre-emptive re-transplant in graft and recipient outcome. *Nephrol Dial Transplant*. 2006;21(5):1355–1364. doi:10.1093/ndt/gfk061.
9. Tang H, Chelamcharla M, Baird BC, Shihab FS, Koford JK, Goldfarb-Rumyantzev AS. Factors affecting kidney-transplant outcome in recipients with lupus nephritis. *Clin Transplant* 2008;22(3): 263–272. doi:10.1111/j.1399-0012.2007.00781.x.
10. Chelamcharla M, Javaid B, Baird BC, Goldfarb-Rumyantzev AS. The outcome of renal transplantation among systemic lupus erythematosus patients. *Nephrol Dial Transplant*. 2007;22(12):3623–3630. doi:10.1093/ndt/gfm459.
11. Petersen E, Baird BC, Shihab F, et al. The impact of recipient history of cardiovascular disease on kidney transplant outcome. 2007;53(5):601–608. doi:10.1097/MAT.0b013e318145bb4a.
12. Goldfarb-Rumyantzev AS, Koford JK, Baird BC, et al. Role of socioeconomic status in kidney transplant outcome. *Clin J Am Soc Nephrol*. 2006;1(2):313–322. doi:10.2215/CJN.00630805.
13. Garg J, Karim M, Tang H, et al. Social adaptability index predicts kidney transplant outcome: a single-center retrospective analysis. *Nephrol Dial Transplant*. 2012;27(3):1239–1245. doi:10.1093/ndt/gfr445.
14. Gueye AS, Baird BC, Shihab F, et al. The role of the economic environment in kidney transplant outcomes. *Clin Transplant*. 2009;23(5):643–652. doi:10.1111/j.1399-0012.2009.01024.x.

15. Lebranchu Y, Halimi JM, Bock A, et al. Delayed graft function: risk factors, consequences and parameters affecting outcome-results from MOST, a Multinational Observational Study. *Transplant Proc.* 2005;37(1):345–347. doi:10.1016/j.transproceed.2004.12.297.

16. Van Gelder T. How cyclosporin reduces mycophenolic acid exposure by 40% while other calcineurin inhibitors do not. *Kidney Int.* 2021;100(6):1185–1189. doi:10.1016/j.kint.2021.06.036.

17. Saunders RN, Metcalfe MS, Nicholson ML. Rapamycin in transplantation: a review of the evidence. *Kidney Int.* 2001;59(1):3–16. doi:10.1046/j.1523-1755.2001.00460.x.

18. Martin ST, Tichy EM, Gabardi S. Belatacept: a novel biologic for maintenance immunosuppression after renal transplantation. *Pharmacotherapy.* 2011;31(4):394–407. doi:10.1592/phco.31.4.394.

19. Fletcher JT, Nankivell BJ, Alexander SI. Chronic allograft nephropathy. *Pediatr Nephrol.* 2009;24(8): 1465–1471. doi:10.1007/s00467-008-0869-z.

20. Nankivell BJ, Kuypers DR. Diagnosis and prevention of chronic kidney allograft loss. *Lancet.* 2011;378(9800):1428–1437. doi:10.1016/S0140-6736(11)60699-5.

21. Colvin RB. Antibody-mediated renal allograft rejection: diagnosis and pathogenesis. *J Am Soc Nephrol.* 2007;18(4):1046–1056. doi:10.1681/ASN.2007010073.

22. Racusen LC, Haas M. Antibody-mediated rejection in renal allografts: lessons from pathology. *Clin J Am Soc Nephrol.* 2006;1(3):415–420. doi:10.2215/CJN.01881105.

23. Parajuli S, Mandelbrot DA, Muth B, et al. Rituximab and monitoring strategies for late antibody-mediated rejection after kidney transplantation. *Transplant Direct.* 2017;3(12):e227. doi:10.1097/TXD.0000000000000746.

24. Kaneku H. Annual literature review of donor-specific HLA antibodies after organ transplantation. *Clin Transpl.* 2011;311–318.

25. Roufosse C, Simmonds N, Clahsen-van Groningen M, et al. A 2018 reference guide to the Banff classification of renal allograft pathology. *Transplantation.* 2018;102(11):1795–1814. doi:10.1097/TP.0000000000002366.

26. Halloran PF, Melk A, Barth C. Rethinking chronic allograft nephropathy: the concept of accelerated senescence. *J Am Soc Nephrol.* 1999;10(1):167–181. doi:10.1681/ASN.V101167.

27. Halloran PF. Call for revolution: a new approach to describing allograft deterioration. *Am J Transplant.* 2002;2(3):195–200. doi:10.1034/j.1600-6143.2002.20301.x.

28. Golgert WA, Appel GB, Hariharan S. Recurrent glomerulonephritis after renal transplantation: an unsolved problem. *Clin J Am Soc Nephrol.* 2008;3(3):800–807. doi:10.2215/CJN.04050907.

29. Dall A, Hariharan S. BK virus nephritis after renal transplantation. *Clin J Am Soc Nephrol.* 2008;3 Suppl 2(Suppl 2):S68–S75. doi:10.2215/CJN.02770707.

30. Gaston RS. Chronic calcineurin inhibitor nephrotoxicity: reflections on an evolving paradigm. *Clin J Am Soc Nephrol.* 2009;4(12):2029–2034. doi:10.2215/CJN.03820609.

31. Racusen LC, Solez K, Colvin R. Fibrosis and atrophy in the renal allograft: interim report and new directions. *Am J Transplant.* 2002;2(3):203–206. doi:10.1034/j.1600-6143.2002.20303.x.

32. Lim WH, Shingde M, Wong G. Recurrent and de novo glomerulonephritis after kidney transplantation. *Front Immunol.* 2019;10:1944. doi:10.3389/fimmu.2019.01944.

33. Hickson LJ, Gera M, Amer H, et al. Kidney transplantation for primary focal segmental glomerulosclerosis: outcomes and response to therapy for recurrence. *Transplantation.* 2009;87(8):1232–1239. doi:10.1097/TP.0b013e31819f12be.

34. Passerini P, Malvica S, Tripodi F, Cerutti R, Messa P. Membranous nephropathy (MN) recurrence after renal transplantation. *Front Immunol.* 2019;10:1326. doi:10.3389/fimmu.2019.01326.

35. Dahan K, Debiec H, Plaisier E, et al. Rituximab for severe membranous nephropathy: a 6-month trial with extended follow-up. *J Am Soc Nephrol.* 2017;28(1):348–358. doi:10.1681/ASN.2016040449.

36. Choy BY, Chan TM, Lai KN. Recurrent glomerulonephritis after kidney transplantation. *Am J Transplant.* 2006;6(11):2535–2542. doi:10.1111/j.1600-6143.2006.01502.x.

37. Lee J, Clayton F, Shihab F, Goldfarb-Rumyantzev A. Successful treatment of recurrent Henoch-Schonlein purpura in a renal allograft with plasmapheresis. *Am J Transplant.* 2008;8(1):228–231. doi:10.1111/j.1600-6143.2007.02022.x.

38. Thomas MC, Mathew TH, Russ GR. Glycaemic control and graft loss following renal transplantation. *Nephrol Dial Transplant.* 2001;16(10):1978–1982. doi:10.1093/ndt/16.10.1978.

39. Matas AJ, Gillingham KJ, Humar A, et al. 2202 kidney transplant recipients with 10 years of graft function: what happens next? *Am J Transplant.* 2008;8(11):2410–2419. doi:10.1111/j.1600-6143.2008.02414.x.

40. OPTN/SRTR 2019 Annual Data Report: Kidney. *Health Resources and Services Administration Scientific Registry of Transplant Recipients.* https://srtr.transplant.hrsa.gov/annual_reports/2019/Kidney.aspx#KI_tx_adult_egfr_12M_ld_b64. Accessed August 31, 2021.

41. Dantal J, Pohanka E. Malignancies in renal transplantation: an unmet medical need. *Nephrol Dial Transplant.* 2007;22(suppl 1):i4–i10. doi:10.1093/ndt/gfm085.

42. Morath C, Mueller M, Goldschmidt H, Schwenger V, Opelz G, Zeier M. Malignancy in renal transplantation. *J Am Soc Nephrol.* 2004;15(6):1582–1588. doi:10.1097/01.asn.0000126194.77004.9b.

43. Quinlan SC, Pfeiffer RM, Morton LM, Engels EA. Risk factors for early-onset and late-onset post-transplant lymphoproliferative disorder in kidney recipients in the United States. *Am J Hematol.* 2011;86(2):206–209. doi:10.1002/ajh.21911.

44. Berrington JE, Barge D, Fenton AC, Cant AJ, Spickett GP. Lymphocyte subsets in term and significantly preterm UK infants in the first year of life analysed by single platform flow cytometry. *Clin Exp Immunol.* 2005;140(2):289–292. doi:10.1111/j.1365-2249.2005.02767.x.

45. Chinen J, Buckley RH. Transplantation immunology: solid organ and bone marrow. *J Allergy Clin Immunol.* 2010;125(2 suppl 2):S324–S335. doi:10.1016/j.jaci.2009.11.014.

CHAPTER 14

Hypertension

Robert Stephen Brown ▪ Alexander Goldfarb-Rumyantzev ▪ Min Zhuo

14.1 Staging of Hypertension (HTN) According to ACC/AHA[1]

BP Value	Stage	Treatment
<120/80	Normal	
120–129/<80	Elevated blood pressure	Does not require drugs, but early interventions of lifestyle modifications[2] (weight loss, low salt, and/or DASH diet, increased physical activity, and limiting alcohol) could reduce BP
130–139/80–89	HTN stage 1	Pharmacological therapy is indicated if ≥135/85 or ≥130/80 + at least one risk factor (established cardiovascular disease or at high risk, type 2 diabetes, CKD, age ≥65)
≥140/≥90	HTN stage 2	May start with two drugs if baseline SBP is ≥15 mmHg above goal

BP, Blood pressure; *CKD*, chronic kidney disease; *SBP*, systolic blood pressure.

14.2 Resistant, Refractory, and Accelerated HTN and HTN in Pregnancy

Classification	Definition	Treatment
Resistant HTN	BP above goal despite three agents of different classes, including a diuretic[3]	Evaluate for causes and adherence to therapy (see below) and lifestyle modifications as listed above; consider ambulatory BP monitoring
Refractory HTN	BP uncontrolled despite ≥5 agents, including chlorthalidone and a mineralocorticoid receptor antagonist[4]	Refer to a specialized HTN clinic; same as resistant HTN plus sympatholytic Rx may be effective in this group; renal sympathetic denervation and carotid sinus stimulation are investigational treatments
HTN urgency	Asymptomatic BP ≥180/120	MAP reduction ≤25%–30% over first 2–4 hours BP control to 140/90 or 130/80 over several days

Classification	Definition	Treatment
HTN emergency (accelerated or malignant HTN)	Symptomatic with retinal hemorrhages, papilledema, neurological symptoms, encephalopathy, and/or malignant nephrosclerosis; BP ≥180/120 (usually but not required)	Hospitalization, target BP <180/120 for the first hour and <160/110 for the first day (MAP reduction 10%–20% for the first hour and 5%–15% for the first day); overly aggressive reduction in BP may cause coronary, cerebral, or renal ischemia; evaluate for secondary causes of HTN
HTN in pregnancy	BP ≥140/≥90 but must differentiate: • Chronic essential HTN (presenting at <20 weeks) • Preeclampsia (new onset >20 weeks but may be superimposed on chronic HTN) • Transient (gestational) HTN near term	Treatment is indicated if BP ≥160/110, but others suggest treatment if BP ≥140/90,[5,6] end organ damage, or preeclampsia (see Rx below and Chapter 10)

BP, Blood pressure; *HTN*, hypertension; *MAP*, mean arterial pressure.

14.3 Which Blood Pressure Reading Should Be Followed?

- Systolic blood pressure (BP) has a better association with cardiovascular disease (CVD) events than diastolic BP in older adults; in younger patients (age <60 years), diastolic BP is significantly associated with CVD risk.[7]
- Twenty-four-hour BP monitoring is the gold standard; otherwise, office-based BP measurement may be used. Home BP could be used to complement office measurement.
- If there is a discrepancy between office and home BP, 24-hour BP monitoring should be obtained (to rule out white coat or masked HTN).
- Consider ambulatory BP monitoring to evaluate the circadian rhythm of BP readings (e.g., higher values while awake and lower values at nighttime = BP "dipping"); control of nighttime rather than daytime BP seems most associated with better outcomes.
- Goal BP in patients with established CVD is 125 to 130/80 (office measurement) or 120 to 125/80 (other measurements).

14.4 Causes of Resistant or Refractory Hypertension to Consider

- Secondary HTN (see below)
- Improper BP measurements (e.g., inappropriate cuff size) or "white coat" HTN
- Calcification or sclerosis of brachial arteries (falsely high by arm sphygmomanometer)
- Nonadherence to anti-HTN medications
- Use of other drugs (over-the-counter meds, such as nonsteroidal antiinflammatory drugs [NSAIDs] and decongestants)
- Dietary indiscretion of salt or alcohol

- Volume overload with inadequate diuretic therapy
- Comorbidities (e.g., obesity, obstructive sleep apnea)

14.5 Evaluation of Secondary Causes of Hypertension (Especially in Young Onset, Resistant, or Accelerated HTN)

- **Patient studies:**
  - History—HTN related to drugs: hormonal contraceptives, NSAIDs, cocaine, amphetamines, sympathomimetics, corticosteroids, licorice, epoetin, excessive alcohol
  - Endocrinopathies—hyperthyroidism, Cushing syndrome, pheochromocytoma
  - Sleep study if obstructive sleep apnea is considered
  - Ambulatory 24-hour BP monitoring ("white coat" labile HTN, nighttime dipping)
- **Laboratory tests:**
  - All patients:
    - Creatinine (renal function)
    - Urinalysis (detect proteinuria, kidney disease)
    - Electrolytes/glucose (hypokalemia, metabolic alkalosis, or diabetes may suggest hypermineralocorticoid state)
  - Specific studies (based on findings):
    - Aldosterone, renin levels (primary hyperaldosteronism or secondary hyperreninemic state; for example, renal artery stenosis, kidney tumor)
    - Thyroid stimulating hormone (TSH; hyperthyroidism)
    - Cortisol (Cushing syndrome)
    - Plasma or urine catecholamines (pheochromocytoma)
    - Drug screening (e.g., cocaine)
- **Radiological imaging:**
  - Renal ultrasound (US) with Doppler (cystic/anatomic diseases, obstructive uropathy, signs of renal artery stenosis)
  - CT or MR angiogram (detect/confirm renal artery stenosis, fibromuscular dysplasia, coarctation of the aorta)
  - Radiocontrast angiography (confirm main or segmental renal artery stenosis)
  - Adrenal vein aldosterone and cortisol levels for laterality of adrenal adenomas

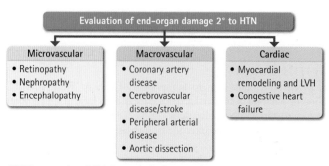

HTN, Hypertension; LVH, left ventricular hypertrophy.

14.6 Selection of Initial Therapy in Patients With No Specific Indications[3]

STAGE 1

Thiazide diuretic, or angiotensin converting enzyme inhibitor (ACEi), or angiotensin receptor blocker (ARB), or calcium channel blocker (CCB)

STAGE 2

Long-acting CCB and ACEi or ARB[8]
ACEi/ARB and a thiazide diuretic (chlorthalidone preferred)
Selection of initial therapy based on demographics:
- In Blacks, ACEi may be less effective in lowering BP than either a thiazide-type diuretic or a CCB.
- Blacks and Asians have greater rates of angioedema and cough as side effects with ACEi.[9]
- In older adults, HTN and isolated systolic HTN should be treated; lower initial doses should be used; could start initial therapy with a long-acting CCB and adding an ACEi/ARB if needed; in the absence of a specific indication (e.g., heart failure), beta blockers should not be used as the primary therapy for HTN; avoid orthostatic hypotension; alpha blockers should generally be avoided unless indicated for symptoms of prostatic hypertrophy.

14.7 Treatment Based on Specific Indications or Comorbid Conditions

14.7.1 PATIENTS WITH KIDNEY DISEASE[10]

- Target SBP: < 120[11]
- In patients with proteinuric renal disease: ACEi or ARB slows progression of chronic kidney disease (CKD); ACEi or ARB should be administered using the highest approved dose that is tolerated.
- Combination therapy with an ACEi and an ARB is associated with an increased risk of adverse events among patients with diabetic nephropathy.[12] Aliskiren has been shown to decrease proteinuria, but the long-term effect on CKD needs elucidation.[13]
- Thiazide diuretics become less effective when the glomerular filtration rate (GFR) is less than 30 mL/min/1.73m^2. In such patients, loop diuretics are preferred as initial therapy to achieve BP control by relieving hypervolemia.
- A mineralocorticoid receptor antagonist (spironolactone or eplerenone) is an effective agent for the treatment of resistant HTN in patients with CKD.
- In CKD patients: ≥3 drugs including a diuretic are commonly needed to achieve a goal SBP ≤120.

14.7.2 PATIENTS WITH DIABETES MELLITUS

- With proteinuria: ACEi or ARB first to slow progression of CKD.
- Sodium-glucose co-transporter-2 inhibitors (SGLT-2i), such as canagliflozin, empagliflozin, and dapagliflozin, have been shown to decrease proteinuria, slow the progression of CKD, and lower the risk of end-stage kidney disease (ESKD) and death from renal causes in patients with or without type 2 diabetes.

- In patients with CKD and type 2 diabetes, treatment with finerenone (a nonsteroidal selective mineralocorticoid receptor antagonist) resulted in lower risks of CKD progression and cardiovascular events though systolic blood pressures decreased by only about 2-3 mm Hg.[14,15]
- Thiazide diuretics may be needed but may worsen glucose tolerance: potassium depletion may impair pancreatic islet beta-cell insulin release and thiazides may increase insulin resistance of target tissues (avoid hypokalemia by potassium repletion and use low-dose diuretic with co-administration of ACEi or ARB).
- If beta blockers are indicated, they may have deleterious metabolic consequences: increased severity and duration of hypoglycemic episodes in type 1 diabetes mellitus (DM) by impairing the hepatic glycogenolytic response to adrenal epinephrine release in hypoglycemia (decrease this effect by using cardioselective beta blockers at low doses). Beta blockers may elevate plasma triglycerides (though beta blockers with intrinsic sympathomimetic [partial agonist] activity [e.g., pindolol or acebutolol] are less likely to cause this effect).

14.7.3 PATIENTS WITH RESISTANT OR REFRACTORY HTN

- Low-sodium diet should be stressed (test for 24-hour urinary Na excretion).
- Diuretics (counter the volume expansion caused by other anti-HTN agents and potentiate their effect). Start with thiazides, use loop diuretics in those with low GFR, and consider adding aldosterone blockade with spironolactone or eplerenone or potassium-sparing collecting-duct sodium channel blockade with amiloride or triamterene.
- Combine effects of different anti-HTN medication classes: renin-angiotensin-aldosterone antagonism with ACEi, ARB, or beta blocker (e.g., labetalol or carvedilol); long-acting CCB; CNS acting agent (e.g., clonidine); or direct vasodilator (e.g., hydralazine or minoxidil).
- Consider investigational use of endovascular radiofrequency renal sympathetic denervation[16] or electrical stimulation of carotid sinus baroreceptors in severe cases. Neither is approved for treatment of HTN in the United States.

14.7.4 PATIENTS WITH HTN EMERGENCY (ACCELERATED OR MALIGNANT HTN)

- Start with parenteral IV administration: commonly a direct vasodilator (nitroprusside), an alpha and beta sympatholytic (labetalol), a CCB with vasodilator activity (nicardipine or clevidipine), or a postsynaptic dopamine receptor agonist (fenoldopam).
- Other IV medications that can be used include esmolol, enalaprilat, hydralazine, and urapidil.
- Use a loop diuretic for volume overload.
- Follow with oral agents as for resistant HTN, combining effects of different classes (e.g., labetalol, amiloride, clonidine, prazosin, hydralazine).

14.7.5 PATIENTS WITH HEART FAILURE

- In heart failure with a reduced ejection fraction (HFrEF), HTN should be treated with a renin-angiotensin system inhibitor (e.g., neprilysin inhibitor [sacubitril], ACEi, or ARB), a beta blocker (e.g., carvedilol), and a mineralocorticoid receptor antagonist (spironolactone or eplerenone).
- The combination of hydralazine and isosorbide dinitrate might be effective in Black patients on standard therapies.[17]
- Use diuretics for peripheral or pulmonary edema.

- Use a long acting CCB (e.g., amlodipine, felodipine) if needed.
- In heart failure with a preserved ejection fraction (HFpEF), optimal therapy of HTN is uncertain but usually includes diuretics and a mineralocorticoid receptor antagonist.

14.7.6 PATIENTS WITH SLEEP APNEA

- Nasal continuous positive airway pressure may be effective treatment of HTN.
- Prescribe weight reduction for obesity.
- Otherwise, conventional antihypertensive treatment should be undertaken.

14.7.7 PATIENTS WITH OBSTRUCTIVE AIRWAYS DISEASE (COPD OR ASTHMA)

- Beta-adrenergic antagonists can increase airway reactivity and should be considered second-line therapy unless there is another indication (e.g., coronary artery disease), in which case a selective beta-1-blocker should be preferred.

14.7.8 PATIENTS WITH DYSLIPIDEMIA

- Thiazides may increase serum cholesterol levels, especially LDL, however the effect is generally dose dependent; co-administration of an ACEi blunts or abolishes thiazide-induced metabolic abnormalities.
- Beta blockers cause an elevation in serum triglyceride levels (beta blockers with intrinsic sympathomimetic [partial agonist] activity [e.g., pindolol or acebutolol] are less likely to cause this effect).
- ACEi and calcium channel antagonists have little effect on lipids.
- Alpha-1-antagonists may elevate HDL.

14.7.9 PREGNANT PATIENTS

- BP $\geq$160/110 should be pharmacologically treated with consideration when BP is $\geq$140/90.
- Methyldopa: centrally alpha agonist, may cause sedation
- Hydralazine: long-term safety data
- Long-acting CCB: for example, amlodipine or extended-release nifedipine
- Labetalol: combined alpha and beta blocker, can cause bronchoconstriction
- Diuretics controversial; okay for volume overload
- Acute treatment: parenteral labetalol, hydralazine, or nicardipine
- ACEi, nitroprusside: contraindicated in pregnancy

14.7.10 PATIENTS WITH PHEOCHROMOCYTOMA

- Preoperative management: alpha-adrenergic blockade (e.g., oral phenoxybenzamine for control of BP and tachyarrhythmias)
- If alpha-blockade alone does not normalize BP and HR, beta blockers may be added (e.g., propranolol, nadolol). Beta-blockade may be used only after effective alpha-blockade is in place to prevent unopposed alpha-adrenergic mediated vasoconstriction by elevated circulating catecholamines.
- Preoperative management should include intravascular volume expansion. Some patients with pheochromocytoma are volume contracted; encourage high-sodium diet.
- CCB could be used when BP is still uncontrolled.

14.7.11 PATIENTS WITH OTHER CONDITIONS

- Atrial fibrillation: beta blockers help control heart rate.
- Essential tremor: beta blockers have beneficial effect on tremor.
- Prostatic hypertrophy: alpha blockers help with voiding hesitancy.
- Obese patients: weight reduction is a primary goal of Rx.
- Scleroderma (progressive systemic sclerosis): ACEi is preferred therapy, with captopril used most commonly, or an ARB if ACEi isn't tolerated; CCB or a direct vasodilator added if necessary; beta blockers may aggravate Raynaud phenomenon so should be avoided.

14.7.12 RENAL ARTERY STENOSIS (RAS): CAUSES, EVALUATION, AND TREATMENT

14.7.12.1 Causes of RAS

- Atherosclerosis (most common: 90% of cases)
- Fibromuscular dysplasia
- Other: vasculitis, neurofibromatosis, congenital bands, extrinsic compression, and radiation

14.7.12.2 Evaluation of Patient for RAS

- Renal US with Doppler: detects RAS with ~80% sensitivity
- US-resistive indices helpful to predict outcome of intervention (better when <0.8; poorer when >0.8)
- Radiocontrast CT angiography
- MR angiography
- Radiocontrast aortography and selective renal arteriography to confirm RAS, particularly for segmental or fibromuscular arterial disease
- Renal vein renin levels to assess lateralization when findings are indecisive (false positives and negatives have decreased this test's usefulness)
- Radionuclide renography to assess differential renal blood flow and function (as a percentage of overall renal function)

14.7.12.3 Treatment of RAS

Medical Therapy
- ACEi or ARB is effective in >85% of patients but has risk of a hemodynamic decrease in renal function, particularly with bilateral RAS
- Often need to combine Rx with a diuretic
- Should urge smoking cessation, lipid-lowering Rx, and aspirin or antiplatelet agents, if indicated
- Concerns: progression of disease, long-term ischemic damage

Interventional Therapy. Revascularization is not indicated in all patients since overall results are similar to medical Rx; should be considered in those with hemodynamically significant RAS with worsening renal function, HTN that is difficult to control, intolerance to optimal medical therapy, unexplained flash pulmonary edema, or refractory heart failure.
- Percutaneous intervention: balloon angioplasty, with or without stenting; stent placement for atherosclerotic RAS for a higher initial primary success rate and higher patency rate at 6 months[18]
- Renal artery stenting did not confer a significant benefit with respect to the prevention of major renal and cardiovascular events when added to medical therapy in people with atherosclerotic RAS and HTN or CKD[19–21]

- Surgical therapy might be equally or more effective than percutaneous intervention in the treatment of atherosclerotic disease[22]
- Surgical revascularization may be indicated for certain cases not amenable to percutaneous angioplasty: unilateral aortorenal bypass surgery and extraanatomical bypass (bypass originates from the celiac or mesenteric branches)

14.7.13 HYPERTENSIVE NEPHROPATHY (HYPERTENSIVE NEPHROSCLEROSIS)

Hypertensive nephropathy is thought to be the second most common cause of ESKD after diabetic nephropathy.[23] If HTN is poorly controlled, renal insufficiency may progress slowly over years with benign nephrosclerosis, the nephropathy associated with benign hypertension, whereas with malignant hypertension, malignant nephrosclerosis is a rapidly progressive renal disease with ESKD that may occur in weeks.

14.7.14 PREDICTORS OF KIDNEY INJURY

- Severity of HTN
- Presence of comorbid conditions (e.g., diabetes)
- Male gender
- Black race (a coexisting condition of genetic focal segmental glomerular sclerosis may be a contributing cause of progressive nephropathy; see Chapter 8)

14.7.15 MECHANISM OF KIDNEY INJURY

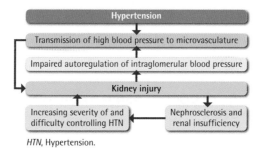

HTN, Hypertension.

14.7.16 CLINICAL FEATURES OF HYPERTENSIVE NEPHROPATHY/ NEPHROSCLEROSIS

- Proteinuria
- Renal insufficiency
- Hematuria (usually with malignant HTN)
- Possible association with other hypertensive end-organ damage (hypertensive retinopathy, left ventricular hypertrophy, and congestive heart failure)

14.7.17 PATHOLOGY OF NEPHROSCLEROSIS

- Vascular wall medial thickening, arteriolar hyaline deposits, intimal fibrosis
- Focal glomerular ischemic changes with variable thickening and wrinkling of the basement membranes

- Segmental or global sclerosis, subtotal podocyte foot process effacement
- Tubular atrophy and interstitial fibrosis

GOALS OF THERAPY TO DELAY PROGRESSION OF RENAL FAILURE

- Control BP (achieving target BP is more important for protection of renal function than the selection of particular class of antihypertensive used)
- Reduce albuminuria (when present, ACEi or ARB;[24] the use of aliskiren or aldosterone antagonists remains uncertain)
- Low-sodium and possibly "Mediterranean" vegetarian diet

14.7.18 MEDICATIONS AFFECTING ADRENERGIC RECEPTORS

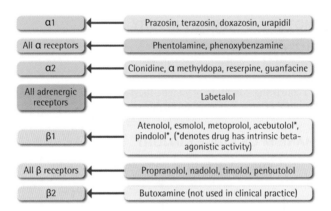

14.7.19 MEDICATIONS BLOCKING RENIN-ANGIOTENSIN-ALDOSTERONE SYSTEM

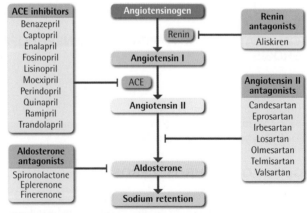

ACE, Angiotensin-converting-enzyme.

14.7.20 CLASSES OF CALCIUM CHANNEL BLOCKERS

Class	Agents	
Nondihydropyridines	Verapamil, diltiazem	Negative chronotropic actions: affects sinoatrial and AV nodes to slow conduction and ↓ heart rate. Avoid in angina and impaired ventricular function.
Dihydropyridines	Nifedipine, nicardipine, isradipine, nimodipine, nisoldipine, nitrendipine, felodipine, amlodipine besylate	Negative inotropic actions, vasodilators. In systolic dysfunction, avoid nifedipine, but amlodipine and felodipine are acceptable.

14.7.21 COMBINATIONS OF CALCIUM CHANNEL BLOCKERS WITH BETA BLOCKERS

When combining a CCB with a beta blocker, a dihydropyridine CCB is desirable as the compensatory tachycardia of the dihydropyridine CCB is opposed by β-blockade whereas verapamil or diltiazem added to a beta blocker is undesirable due to the common side effect of negative chronotropy.

14.7.22 DIURETICS

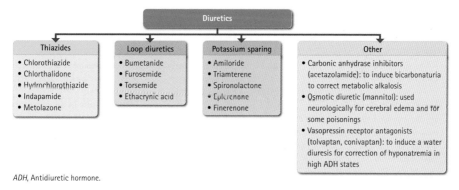

ADH, Antidiuretic hormone.

References

1. Whelton PK, Carey RM, Aronow WS, et al. 2017 ACC/AHA/AAPA/ABC/ACPM/AGS/APhA/ASH/ASPC/NMA/PCNA Guideline for the Prevention, Detection, Evaluation, and Management of High Blood Pressure in Adults: a report of the American College of Cardiology/American Heart Association Task Force on Clinical Practice Guidelines. *Hypertension*. 2018;71(6):e13–e115. doi:10.1161/HYP.0000000000000065.
2. Elmer PJ, Obarzanek E, Vollmer WM, et al. Effects of comprehensive lifestyle modification on diet, weight, physical fitness, and blood pressure control: 18-month results of a randomized trial. *Ann Intern Med*. 2006;144(7):485–495. doi:10.7326/0003-4819-144-7-200604040-00007.
3. Reboussin DM, Allen NB, Griswold ME, et al. Systematic review for the 2017 ACC/AHA/AAPA/ABC/ACPM/AGS/APhA/ASH/ASPC/NMA/PCNA Guideline for the Prevention, Detection, Evaluation, and Management of High Blood Pressure in Adults: a report of the American College of Cardiology/American Heart Association Task Force on Clinical Practice Guidelines. *Circulation*. 2018;138(17):e595–e616. doi:10.1161/CIR.0000000000000601.

4. Dudenbostel T, Siddiqui M, Oparil S, Calhoun DA. Refractory hypertension: a novel phenotype of antihypertensive treatment failure. *Hypertens (Dallas, Tex 1979)*. 2016;67(6):1085–1092. doi:10.1161/HYPERTENSIONAHA.116.06587.

5. Reddy S, Jim B. Hypertension and pregnancy: management and future risks. *Adv Chronic Kidney Dis*. 2019;26(2):137–145. doi:10.1053/j.ackd.2019.03.017.

6. Magee LA, von Dadelszen P. State-of-the-art diagnosis and treatment of hypertension in pregnancy. *Mayo Clin Proc*. 2018;93(11):1664–1677. doi:10.1016/j.mayocp.2018.04.033.

7. Li F-R, He Y, Yang H-L, et al. Isolated systolic and diastolic hypertension by the 2017 American College of Cardiology/American Heart Association guidelines and risk of cardiovascular disease: a large prospective cohort study. *J Hypertens*. 2021;39(8):1594–1601. doi:10.1097/HJH.0000000000002805.

8. Jamerson K, Weber MA, Bakris GL, et al. Benazepril plus amlodipine or hydrochlorothiazide for hypertension in high-risk patients. *N Engl J Med*. 2008;359(23):2417–2428. doi:10.1056/NEJMoa0806182.

9. Wright JTJ, Dunn JK, Cutler JA, et al. Outcomes in hypertensive black and nonblack patients treated with chlorthalidone, amlodipine, and lisinopril. *JAMA*. 2005;293(13):1595–1608. doi:10.1001/jama.293.13.1595.

10. Kidney Disease: Improving Global Outcomes (KDIGO) Blood Pressure Work Group. KDIGO 2021 Clinical Practice Guideline for the Management of Blood Pressure in Chronic Kidney Disease. *Kidney Int*. 2021;99(3S):S1–S87. doi:10.1016/j.kint.2020.11.003.

11. Zhuo M, Yang D, Goldfarb-Rumyantzev A, Brown RS. The association of SBP with mortality in patients with stage 1-4 chronic kidney disease. *J Hypertens*. 2021;39(11):2250–2257. doi:10.1097/HJH.0000000000002927.

12. Fried LF, Emanuele N, Zhang JH, et al. Combined angiotensin inhibition for the treatment of diabetic nephropathy. *N Engl J Med*. 2013;369(20):1892–1903. doi:10.1056/nejmoa1303154.

13. Woo K-T, Choong H-L, Wong K-S, et al. Aliskiren and losartan trial in non-diabetic chronic kidney disease. *J Renin Angiotensin Aldosterone Syst*. 2014;15(4):515–522. doi:10.1177/1470320313510584.

14. Bakris GL, Agarwal R, Anker SD, et al. Effect of finerenone on chronic kidney disease outcomes in type 2 diabetes. *N Engl J Med*. 2020;383(23):2219–2229. doi:10.1056/NEJMoa2025845.

15. Ruilope LM, Agarwal R, Anker SD, et al; FIDELIO-DKD Investigators. Blood Pressure and Cardiorenal Outcomes With Finerenone in Chronic Kidney Disease in Type 2 Diabetes. *Hypertension*. 2022;79(12):2685–2695. doi: 10.1161/HYPERTENSIONAHA.122.19744.

16. Kandzari DE, Böhm M, Mahfoud F, et al. Effect of renal denervation on blood pressure in the presence of antihypertensive drugs: 6-month efficacy and safety results from the SPYRAL HTN-ON MED proof-of-concept randomised trial. *Lancet*. 2018;391(10137):2346–2355. doi:10.1016/S0140-6736(18)30951-6.

17. Taylor AL, Ziesche S, Yancy C, et al. Combination of isosorbide dinitrate and hydralazine in blacks with heart failure. *N Engl J Med*. 2004;351(20):2049–2057. doi:10.1056/NEJMoa042934.

18. van de Ven PJ, Kaatee R, Beutler JJ, et al. Arterial stenting and balloon angioplasty in ostial atherosclerotic renovascular disease: a randomised trial. *Lancet*. 1999;353(9149):282–286. doi:10.1016/S0140-6736(98)04432-8.

19. Cooper CJ, Murphy TP, Cutlip DE, et al. Stenting and medical therapy for atherosclerotic renal-artery stenosis. *N Engl J Med*. 2014;370(1):13–22. doi:10.1056/NEJMoa1310753.

20. Wheatley K, Ives N, Gray R, et al. Revascularization versus medical therapy for renal-artery stenosis. *N Engl J Med*. 2009;361(20):1953–1962. doi:10.1056/NEJMoa0905368.

21. Zeller T, Krankenberg H, Erglis A, et al. A randomized, multi-center, prospective study comparing best medical treatment versus best medical treatment plus renal artery stenting in patients with hemodynamically relevant atherosclerotic renal artery stenosis (RADAR)—one-year results of a pre-ma. *Trials*. 2017;18(1):380. doi:10.1186/s13063-017-2126-x.

22. Lawrie GM, Morris GCJ, Glaeser DH, DeBakey ME. Renovascular reconstruction: factors affecting long-term prognosis in 919 patients followed up to 31 years. *Am J Cardiol*. 1989;63(15):1085–1092. doi:10.1016/0002-9149(89)90083-0.

23. United States Renal Data System. *2020 USRDS Annual Data Report: Epidemiology of Kidney Disease in the United States*. National Institutes of Health. Bethesda, MD; 2020. https://adr.usrds.org/2020.

24. Agodoa LY, Appel L, Bakris GL, et al. Effect of ramipril vs amlodipine on renal outcomes in hypertensive nephrosclerosis: a randomized controlled trial. *JAMA*. 2001;285(21):2719–2728. doi:10.1001/jama.285.21.2719.

CHAPTER 15

Nephrolithiasis and Nephrocalcinosis

Robert Stephen Brown ■ Alexander Goldfarb-Rumyantzev

15.1 Kidney Stones[1-3]

Kidney stone disease is common, with a risk of 10% to 15% occurring more commonly in men, but with an increasing incidence in women. Stone formation is recurrent in 50% of those with one stone.[4,5] In addition to causing the pain of renal colic, kidney stone disease also may lead to complicated interventions to remove stones, urosepsis, or an increased incidence of chronic kidney disease.

Types[6-13] and predisposing causes[14-21] of kidney stones.

Kidney stone composition Urinary crystal photomicrographs	Percentage of stones (approx.)	Predisposing causes
Calcium Oxalate (or May be Mixed With Calcium Phosphate)		
	70% (more common in men)	• Hypercalciuria • Hyperuricosuria • Hyperoxaluria • Hypocitraturia • Hypercalcemic states (primary hyperparathyroidism, vitamin D/calcium overdose) • Anatomic kidney abnormalities (e.g., medullary sponge kidney) • Low fluid intake and certain diets (increased animal protein or high vitamin C intake)
Calcium Phosphate		
	10%	• Hypercalciuria • Type 1 "distal" RTA • Hypercalcemic states (primary hyperparathyroidism, vitamin D/calcium overdose) • Anatomic kidney abnormalities (e.g., medullary sponge kidney)

Continued on following page

Kidney stone composition Urinary crystal photomicrographs	Percentage of stones (approx.)	Predisposing causes
Uric Acid		
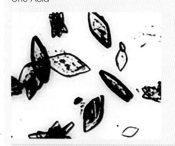	10% in United States Up to 40% in hot "stone belt" areas	• Hyperuricosuria • Chronic diarrheal conditions (uric acid excreted in a decreased volume of highly concentrated acidic urine to compensate for stool losses of $NaHCO_3$)
Struvite or "infection stone" ("triple phosphate"; i.e., magnesium ammonium phosphate and calcium carbonate-apatite crystal)		
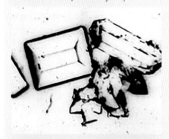 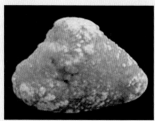	<5% (more common in women)	• Chronic UTI with a urea-splitting organism (e.g., *Proteus* or *Klebsiella*)
Cystine		
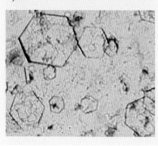	<1% (more common in children)	Cystinuria

Kidney stone composition Urinary crystal photomicrographs	Percentage of stones (approx.)	Predisposing causes
Drugs		
	<1%	• Acyclovir high-dose Rx (urinary crystal shown with light and polarized microscopy) • Amoxicillin • Atazanavir • Indinavir • Methotrexate • Sulfadiazine • Triamterene

RTA, Renal tubular acidosis; *UTI*, urinary tract infection.

*Urine photomicrographs of calcium oxalate, uric acid, and triple phosphate crystals courtesy of late H. Richard Nesson, MD.

15.1.1 PRESENTING SYMPTOMS AND SIGNS OF KIDNEY STONES

- Flank pain, severe and colicky in nature
- Pain often accompanied by restlessness, nausea and vomiting
- Hematuria, gross or microscopic
- Stone passage: occurrence may/may not be recognized, so best to strain urine to catch stone

15.1.2 DETECTION OF KIDNEY STONES[22,23]

Noncontrast CT is best, preferably using a reduced radiation dose[24] (virtually all stones are radiopaque by CT and can usually evaluate obstruction without radiocontrast). Ultrasound (US) is less sensitive but can evaluate obstruction, avoids radiation, and can be used in pregnancy. Abdominal X-ray (KUB) can only detect larger radioopaque calcium-containing and some cystine stones so is no longer an imaging of choice. Intravenous pyelography (IVP) is less sensitive than CT, uses radiation, and requires radiocontrast.

15.1.3 INITIAL WORKUP OF KIDNEY STONES[4,25]

- History and exam for predisposing risk factors
- Serum electrolytes (HCO_3), calcium, phosphate, creatinine (r/o RTA, hypercalcemia, evaluate renal function)
- Urinalysis to look for pH, hematuria, infection, and crystals
- Stone analysis if stone is available

- Radiology: see Detection of Kidney Stones, but if medullary sponge kidney is to be detected because there are multiple small stones or nephrocalcinosis, either CT or IVP with radiocontrast will be needed
- Assess daily urine output (UO) volume (UO of less than 1 L/day is common, and often the only Rx for first stone is to increase to 2 L/day)
- Metabolic workup to include 24-hour urine studies: often undertaken after recurrent stone formation or severe first presentation of stone episode

15.1.4 GENERAL PRINCIPLES OF THERAPY FOR STONE DISEASE

15.1.4.1 Acute Therapy[5]

- Pain relief: nonsteroidal antiinflammatory drugs (NSAIDs), narcotic analgesics
- Intravenous fluid in dehydrated patients, also increases urine flow
- 80% of stones 7 mm or less will pass without intervention
- Medications that increase successful stone passage: alpha blockers (tamsulosin) and calcium channel blockers (CCBs; nifedipine most commonly) are most useful with stones measuring 5 to 10 mm[26,27]

15.1.4.2 Indications for Hospitalization/Interventional Procedure

- Intractable pain and vomiting
- Severe urinary tract infection (UTI) or sepsis
- Complete ureteral obstruction for >3 days
- Partial obstruction of a solitary kidney
- Obstruction or infection may indicate need for temporary ureteral stent placement or nephrostomy

15.1.4.3 Urological Interventions[28–32]

- Extracorporeal shock wave lithotripsy (ESWL) has better success with smaller stones
- Ureteroscopic lithotripsy (useful for ureteral stones)
- Percutaneous nephrolithotomy (successful for larger stones but with increased complication rate than lithotripsy, equal success to open surgical procedures)
- Laparoscopic or open surgical stone removal

15.1.4.4 General Stone Management

- Specific stone therapy as noted below when stone composition is known
- Fluid intake to increase urine output to >2 L/day
- Dietary considerations:
  - Reduce fructose and sugar-containing beverage consumption which may increase calcium stone occurrence;
  - Replace sweet and dairy fluids with coffee, tea, and water;
  - Reduce high intake of vitamin D and calcium supplementation but maintain normal calcium diet; and
  - Reduce intake of animal protein.

15.1.4.5 Follow-Up

- Reassess effects of specific therapy when indicated with urinary and plasma chemistries in 2 months and yearly.
- Consider radiological assessment for new stone formation at 1 year.
- Whenever recurrent stone disease is uncomplicated by infection, obstruction, or underlying disorders, the major risks for patients are the occurrence of painful episodes and the possibility

of requiring urological interventions for stone passage. In general, renal function has been thought to be well preserved, but recent data suggest that those with one or more kidney stones have about double the risk of developing chronic kidney disease (CKD) or end-stage kidney disease (ESKD), with the added hazard appearing to be greater in women than in men.[33,34]

15.1.5 PREDISPOSING CAUSES OF STONE FORMATION

15.1.5.1 Hypercalciuria or Idiopathic Hypercalciuria[15,35]

15.1.5.1.1 Defining the Defect
- Urinary calcium:
    - In men: >300 mg/day,
    - In women: >250 mg/day, or
    - >4 mg/kg/day in all.

15.1.5.1.2 Mechanisms Involved
- Absorptive: increased gastrointestinal (GI) absorption of calcium—can be assessed by urinary calcium to creatinine ratio of >0.2 mg/mg after an oral calcium load
- Resorptive: increased bone resorption—may have elevated parathyroid hormone (PTH) without hypercalcemia
- Renal "leak": decrease in renal tubular calcium reabsorption—can be assessed by fasting urinary calcium >0.11 mg/100 mL/min of creatinine clearance (CrCl)
- Hypophosphatemia: renal phosphate wasting may stimulate increased 1,25-dihydroxy-vitamin D, enhancing GI absorption of calcium

15.1.5.1.3 Treatment of Specific Causes of Recurrent Stones
Bone density studies of hypercalciuric patients have generally shown decreased bone density in all of the four mechanistic categories listed above, making evaluation of mechanism clinically unnecessary, with treatment as follows:
- Reduce dietary Na to <2 g/day to increase renal tubular reabsorption of calcium.
- Maintain a normal, rather than a low, calcium diet to bind dietary oxalates and avoid osteopenia since decreased bone mineral density and increased bone fractures have been shown[36], but avoid added calcium and vitamin D products.
- Thiazide diuretics (e.g., hydrochlorothiazide, 25–50 mg twice daily) decrease urinary calcium excretion by up to 50% with a demonstrated reduction in stone incidence.[37,38]
- Avoid hypokalemia, which reduces urinary citrate. Potassium citrate may be used to prevent thiazide-induced hypocitraturia.
- Amiloride can be used with a thiazide instead of potassium citrate to reduce urinary excretion of both potassium and calcium.
- An alternative therapy, neutral sodium phosphate (500 mg four times daily) corrects the low serum phosphate in the hypophosphatemic form of hypercalciuria, which may decrease calcium excretion.[39] It also increases urinary pyrophosphate excretion to solubilize calcium, but has not been shown to decrease stone occurrence.

15.1.5.2 Hypocitraturia[40,41]

15.1.5.2.1 Defining the Defect
- Urinary citrate <320 mEq/day

15.1.5.2.2 Mechanisms Involved
- Idiopathic or associated with renal tubular acidosis (RTA), cystic fibrosis, chronic metabolic acidosis (diarrhea, carbonic anhydrase inhibitors)

15.1.5.2.3 Treatment of Specific Causes of Recurrent Stones

- Potassium citrate has been demonstrated to decrease stone occurrence (10–20 mEq three times daily for urinary citrate <320 mEq/day, 20 mEq 3–4 times daily for urinary citrate <150 mEq/day).[42]

15.1.5.3 Hyperuricosuria (May Be Associated With Either Uric Acid or Calcium Oxalate Stones)[10,43,44]

15.1.5.3.1 Defining the Defect

- Urinary uric acid >750 to 800 mg/day

Note: Uric acid stones can occur with normal excretion of uric acid due to low urine pH in chronic diarrheal states.

15.1.5.3.2 Mechanisms Involved

- Overproduction of uric acid may occur with or without gout, certain enzyme defects, high purine intake, myeloproliferative and hemolytic disorders, cytotoxic drugs, and alcoholism.

15.1.5.3.3 Treatment of Specific Causes of Recurrent Stones

- For hyperuricosuria, allopurinol has been shown to decrease both uric acid stone and hyperuricosuric calcium oxalate stone occurrence.
- For uric acid stones with normal uric acid excretion or with intolerance to allopurinol or febuxostat, alkalinize the urine to pH >6.5 to increase urate solubility ($NaHCO_3$ or sodium or potassium citrate, 1–3 mEq/kg/day, usually given in 4 doses).
- Avoid purine-rich foods.

15.1.5.4 Cystinuria[11,12,45]

15.1.5.4.1 Defining the Defect

- Urinary cystine >400 mg/day or cystine crystals in urinary sediment
- Cystine stone formation

15.1.5.4.2 Mechanisms Involved

- Several genetic defects in cystine and dibasic amino acid transport decreasing renal tubular cystine reabsorption

15.1.5.4.3 Treatment of Specific Causes of Recurrent Stones

- Dietary protein and sodium restriction decreases urinary cystine
- Alkalinization of urine to pH >7.0 to 7.5 with potassium citrate
- Bedtime dose of acetazolamide or potassium citrate to maintain alkaline urine at night
- Fluid intake to very high urine output >3 to 4 L/day

If those measures fail:

- Thiol drug treatment with tiopronin (preferable), penicillamine, or perhaps captopril to decrease cystine by forming cysteine-drug disulfide bonds has been shown to decrease cystine stone occurrence.

15.1.5.5 Hyperoxaluria[40,46–50]

15.1.5.5.1 Defining the Defect

Urinary oxalate >45 mg/day

15.1.5.5.2 Mechanisms Involved

- Primary hyperoxaluria (three types of genetic defects: rare, but overproduction may be as much as >>100 mg/day)

- May be associated with idiopathic hypercalciuria
- Secondary: intestinal hyperabsorption in malabsorption syndromes, postbypass surgery, inflammatory bowel disease, pancreatic insufficiency, and cystic fibrosis
- High-dose vitamin C intake increases endogenous oxalate production

15.1.5.5.3 Treatment of Specific Causes of Recurrent Stones
- Low-oxalate diet (restrict dietary intake of spinach and other leafy vegetables, cranberries, tea, cocoa, and nuts)
- Avoid high-dose vitamin C intake

To decrease intestinal absorption of oxalate:
- Low-fat diet helps reduce free oxalate in the intestine
- Calcium carbonate or citrate, 1 to 4 g/day with meals, binds oxalate in the intestine with a greater proportional decrease in urinary oxalate than increase in urinary calcium
- Cholestyramine, an oxalate-binding resin, at a dose of 8 to 16 g/day may help
- Restoration of small bowel continuity, if possible (if prior bypass surgery)

For primary hyperoxaluria:
- Pyridoxine at high dose (100–800 mg/day) for hereditary deficiency type 1
- Neutral sodium phosphate and potassium citrate as above may help decrease urinary supersaturation of calcium oxalate
- Segmental liver transplant, to correct the enzyme defect, combined with a kidney transplant for renal failure, has been successfully utilized in patients with hereditary hyperoxaluria
- A new treatment for primary hyperoxaluria type 1 (PH1) with an RNA interference agent that targets glycolate oxidase, lumasiran injected subcutaneously, has been shown to reduce hepatic oxalate overproduction, decreasing plasma and urinary oxalate.[51]

15.1.5.6 Struvite Stone Crystalluria (Magnesium Ammonium Phosphate "Triple Phosphate")[52,53]

15.1.5.6.1 Defining the Defect
- Chronic urinary infection with a urea-splitting organism, urine pH > 7.0, struvite stone, or staghorn

15.1.5.6.2 Mechanisms Involved
- Urease-producing bacteria break down urea to ammonia, leading to alkaline urine and struvite crystallization with ammonium, magnesium, calcium carbonate, and phosphate

15.1.5.6.3 Treatment of Specific Causes of Recurrent Stones
- Eradication of infection, if possible, with long-term antimicrobial therapy
- Urease inhibitor therapy (acetohydroxamic acid decreases stone formation but often causes side effects)
- Removal of stones with lithotripsy, percutaneous nephrolithotomy, or open surgery
- Evaluate for an underlying additional stone-forming disorder (e.g., hypercalciuria)

15.1.6 NEPHROCALCINOSIS

Nephrocalcinosis is the deposition of calcium phosphate and/or calcium oxalate (the latter often described as oxalosis) in the kidney parenchyma, usually in the renal medulla and less commonly in the renal cortex. Nephrocalcinosis may be associated with hypercalcemia, hypercalciuria, hyperphosphatemia, hyphosphaturia, or hyperoxaluria. When severe, nephrocalcinosis can result in ESKD.

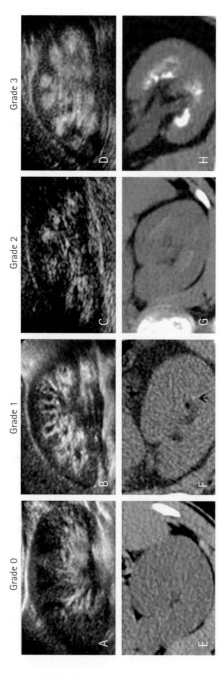

Representative images for nephrocalcinosis grading system. Panels A–D are US images corresponding to grades 0, 1, 2, and 3, respectively. Panels E–H are CT images corresponding to grades 0, 1, 2, and 3 respectively. The arrow in panel F points to a single punctate calcification in the medullary pyramids typical of grade 1 nephrocalcinosis. (Courtesy of Boyce AM, et al.[54])

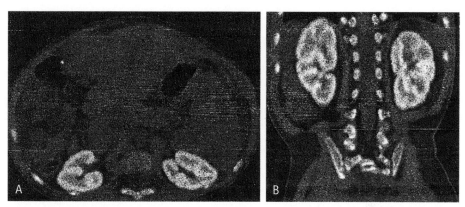

Severe nephrocalcinosis. (A, B): Axial section and coronal reformat of precontrast CT abdomen shows bilateral extensive nephrocalcinosis. (Courtesy of Ethiraj D, et al.[55])

15.1.6.1 Diagnosis of Nephrocalcinosis

The diagnosis of nephrocalcinosis is made by radiological imaging most commonly, but at times by kidney biopsy. US is quite sensitive to mild or moderate nephrocalcinosis, but CT scan is usually the gold standard for radiographic confirmation.[54,55] Characteristic images of kidneys with nephrocalcinosis as detected by either US or CT scan are depicted in the two figures above.

15.1.6.2 Causes of Nephrocalcinosis[56,57]

Primarily medullary calcification:
- Hypercalcemia associated with hyperparathyroidism, sarcoidosis,[58] milk alkali syndrome, high-dose vitamin D, or congenital hypothyroidism
- Hypercalciuria associated with Type 1 "distal" renal tubular acidosis[59]; medullary sponge kidney; long-term, high-dose loop diuretics (neonatal more commonly than adults)[60]; inherited tubular diseases (e.g., familial hypomagnesemia[61] or Bartter syndrome[62]); chronic hypokalemia[63]; or beta thalassemia[64]
- Hyperphosphatemia associated with oral sodium phosphate laxatives or tumor lysis syndrome
- Hyperphosphaturia associated with X-linked or autosomal dominant or recessive hypophosphatemic rickets[65] or various inherited tubular diseases
- Primary or secondary hyperoxaluria (e.g., following gastric bypass); also may cause cortical oxalosis with ESKD[66]

Secondary cortical nephrocalcinosis:
- Superimposed upon renal cortical necrosis, infection, infarction, and other tissue injuries[67]

15.1.6.3 Treatment of Nephrocalcinosis[56,68,69]

Treatment relies upon correcting the underlying disorder. For example:
- High fluid intake (urine output >2 L/day
- Decrease hypercalcemia, hypercalciuria, hyperphosphatemia, hypophosphaturia, or hyperoxaluria
- Potassium citrate for Type 1 "distal" RTA
- Corticosteroid treatment of sarcoidosis
- Avoid sodium phosphate bowel preparations and vitamin D overdoses

References

1. Song L, Maalouf NM, Feingold KR, et al. Nephrolithiasis. *Endotext* [Internet]. South Dartmouth (MA): MDText.com, Inc.; 2000.
2. Cavanaugh C, Perazella MA. Urine sediment examination in the diagnosis and management of kidney disease: core curriculum 2019. *Am J Kidney Dis*. 2019;73(2):258–272. doi:10.1053/j.ajkd. 2018.07.012.
3. Sakhaee K, Maalouf NM, Sinnott B. Clinical review: kidney stones 2012: pathogenesis, diagnosis, and management. *J Clin Endocrinol Metab*. 2012;97(6):1847–1860. doi:10.1210/JC.2011-3492.
4. Johri N, Cooper B, Robertson W, Choong S, Rickards D, Unwin R. An update and practical guide to renal stone management. *Nephron Clin Pract*. 2010;116(3):c159–c171. doi:10.1159/000317196.
5. Wilcox CR, Whitehurst LA, Somani BK, Cook P. Kidney stone disease: an update on its management in primary care. *Br J Gen Pract*. 2020;70(693):205–206. doi:10.3399/BJGP20X709277.
6. Pozdzik A, Maalouf N, Letavernier E, et al. Meeting report of the "Symposium on kidney stones and mineral metabolism: calcium kidney stones in 2017." *J Nephrol*. 2019;32(5):681–698. doi:10.1007/ S40620-019-00587-1.
7. Beara-Lasic L, Goldfarb DS. Recurrent calcium kidney stones. *Clin J Am Soc Nephrol*. 2019;14(9): 1388–1390. doi:10.2215/CJN.02550319.
8. Worcester EM, Coe FL. Clinical practice. Calcium kidney stones. *N Engl J Med*. 2010;363(10): 954–963. doi:10.1056/NEJMCP1001011.
9. Abou-Elela A. Epidemiology, pathophysiology, and management of uric acid urolithiasis: a narrative review. *J Adv Res*. 2017;8(5):513–527. doi:10.1016/j.jare.2017.04.005.
10. Moe OW, Xu LHR. Hyperuricosuric calcium urolithiasis. *J Nephrol*. 2018;31(2):189–196. doi:10.1007/ S40620-018-0469-3.
11. Eisner BH, Goldfarb DS, Baum MA, et al. Evaluation and medical management of patients with cystine nephrolithiasis: a consensus statement. *J Endourol*. 2020;34(11):1103–1110. doi:10.1089/END.2019.0703.
12. Moore SL, Cook P, de Coninck V, et al. Outcomes and long-term follow-up of patients with cystine stones: a systematic review. *Curr Urol Rep*. 2019;20(6):27. doi:10.1007/S11934-019-0891-7.
13. Daudon M, Frochot V, Bazin D, Jungers P. Drug-induced kidney stones and crystalline nephropathy: pathophysiology, prevention and treatment. *Drugs*. 2018;78(2):163–201. doi:10.1007/S40265-017-0853-7.
14. Wang Z, Zhang Y, Zhang J, Deng Q, Liang H. Recent advances on the mechanisms of kidney stone formation (review). *Int J Mol Med*. 2021;48(2):149. doi:10.3892/IJMM.2021.4982.
15. Howles SA, Thakker RV. Genetics of kidney stone disease. *Nat Rev Urol*. 2020;17(7):407–421. doi:10.1038/S41585-020-0332-X.
16. Daudon M, Frochot V. Crystalluria. *Clin Chem Lab Med*. 2015;53(suppl 2):S1479–S1487. doi:10.1515/ CCLM-2015-0860.
17. Ferraro PM, Curhan GC. More good news: coffee prevents kidney stones. *Am J Kidney Dis*. 2022;79(1):3–4. doi:10.1053/J.AJKD.2021.07.002.
18. Yuan S, Larsson SC. Coffee and caffeine consumption and risk of kidney stones: a Mendelian randomization study. 2022;79(1):9–14.e1. doi:10.1053/j.ajkd.2021.04.018.
19. Singh P, Harris PC, Sas DJ, Lieske JC. The genetics of kidney stone disease and nephrocalcinosis. *Nat Rev Nephrol*. 2022;18(4):224–240. doi:10.1038/s41581-021-00513-4.
20. Santoriello D, Al-Nabulsi M, Reddy A, Salamera J, D'Agati VD, Markowitz GS. Atazanavir-associated crystalline nephropathy. *Am J Kidney Dis*. 2017;70(4):576–580. doi:10.1053/J.AJKD.2017.02.376.
21. Huynh LM, Dianatnejad S, Tofani S, et al. Metabolic diagnoses of recurrent stone formers: temporal, geographic and gender differences. *Scand J Urol*. 2020;54(6):456–462. doi:10.1080/21681805.2020.18 40430.
22. Mandeville JA, Gnessin E, Lingeman JE. Imaging evaluation in the patient with renal stone disease. *Semin Nephrol*. 2011;31(3):254–258. doi:10.1016/J.SEMNEPHROL.2011.05.006.
23. Moore CL, Carpenter CR, Heilbrun ME, et al. Imaging in suspected renal colic: systematic review of the literature and multispecialty consensus. *Ann Emerg Med*. 2019;74(3):391–399. doi:10.1016/J. ANNEMERGMED.2019.04.021.
24. Moore CL, Bhargavan-Chatfield M, Shaw MM, Weisenthal K, Kalra MK. Radiation dose reduction in kidney stone CT: a randomized, facility-based intervention. *J Am Coll Radiol*. 2021;18(10): 1394–1404. doi:10.1016/J.JACR.2021.05.004.

25. Ferraro PM, Unwin R, Bonny O, Gambaro G. Practice patterns of kidney stone management across European and non-European centers: an in-depth investigation from the European Renal Stone Network (ERSN). *J Nephrol.* 2021;34(4):1337–1346. doi:10.1007/S40620-020-00854-6.

26. Wang RC, Smith-Bindman R, Whitaker E, et al. Effect of tamsulosin on stone passage for ureteral stones: a systematic review and meta-analysis. *Ann Emerg Med.* 2017;69(3):353–361.e3. doi:10.1016/J. ANNEMERGMED.2016.06.044.

27. Velázquez N, Zapata D, Wang HHS, Wiener JS, Lipkin ME, Routh JC. Medical expulsive therapy for pediatric urolithiasis: systematic review and meta-analysis. *J Pediatr Urol.* 2015;11(6):321–327. doi:10.1016/J.JPUROL.2015.04.036.

28. Kim CH, Chung DY, Rha KH, Lee JY, Lee SH. Effectiveness of percutaneous nephrolithotomy, retrograde intrarenal surgery, and extracorporeal shock wave lithotripsy for treatment of renal stones: a systematic review and meta-analysis. *Medicina (Kaunas).* 2020;57(1):1–23. doi:10.3390/MEDICINA57010026.

29. Tsai SH, Chung HJ, Tseng PT, et al. Comparison of the efficacy and safety of shockwave lithotripsy, retrograde intrarenal surgery, percutaneous nephrolithotomy, and minimally invasive percutaneous nephrolithotomy for lower-pole renal stones: a systematic review and network meta-analysis. *Medicine (Baltimore).* 2020;99(10):e19403. doi:10.1097/MD.0000000000019403.

30. Veser J, Jahrreiss V, Seitz C. Innovations in urolithiasis management. *Curr Opin Urol.* 2021;31(2): 130–134. doi:10.1097/MOU.0000000000000850.

31. Rassweiler J, Rassweiler MC, Klein J. New technology in ureteroscopy and percutaneous nephrolithotomy. *Curr Opin Urol.* 2016;26(1):95–106. doi:10.1097/MOU.0000000000000240.

32. Miernik A, Hein S, Adams F, Halbritter J, Schoenthaler M. [Stone treatment tomorrow and the day after]. *Urologe A.* 2016;55(10):1309–1316. doi:10.1007/S00120-016-0227-X.

33. Uribarri J. Chronic kidney disease and kidney stones. *Curr Opin Nephrol Hypertens.* 2020;29(2):237–242. doi:10.1097/MNH.0000000000000582.

34. El-Zoghby ZM, Lieske JC, Foley RN, et al. Urolithiasis and the risk of ESRD. *Clin J Am Soc Nephrol.* 2012;7(9):1409–1415. doi:10.2215/CJN.03210312.

35. Alexander RT, Fuster DG, Dimke H. Mechanisms underlying calcium nephrolithiasis. *Annu Rev Physiol.* 2022;84:559–583. doi:10.1146/ANNUREV-PHYSIOL-052521-121822.

36. Denburg MR, Leonard MB, Haynes K, et al. Risk of fracture in urolithiasis: a population-based cohort study using the health improvement network. *Clin J Am Soc Nephrol.* 2014;9(12):2133–2140. doi:10.2215/ CJN.04340514.

37. Reilly RF, Peixoto AJ, Desir V G. The evidence-based use of thiazide diuretics in hypertension and nephrolithiasis. *Clin J Am Soc Nephrol.* 2010;5(10):1893–1903. doi:10.2215/CJN.04670510.

38. Dhayat NA, Faller N, Bonny O, et al. Efficacy of standard and low dose hydrochlorothiazide in the recurrence prevention of calcium nephrolithiasis (NOSTONE trial): protocol for a randomized double-blind placebo-controlled trial. *BMC Nephrol.* 2018;19(1):349. doi:10.1186/s12882-018-1144-6.

39. Irzyniec T, Boryń M, Kasztalska J, Nowak-Kapusta Z, Maciejewska-Paszek I, Grochowska-Niedworok E. The effect of an oral sodium phosphate load on parathyroid hormone and fibroblast growth factor 23 secretion in normo- and hypercalciuric stone-forming patients. *Clin Nutr.* 2020;39(12):3804–3812. doi:10.1016/J.CLNU.2020.04.020.

40. Youssef RF, Martin JW, Sakhaee K, et al. Rising occurrence of hypocitraturia and hyperoxaluria associated with increasing prevalence of stone disease in calcium kidney stone formers. *Scand J Urol.* 2020;54(5):426–430. doi:10.1080/21681805.2020.1794955.

41. Wiegand A, Fischer G, Seeger H, et al. Impact of potassium citrate on urinary risk profile, glucose and lipid metabolism of kidney stone formers in Switzerland. *Clin Kidney J.* 2019;13(6):1037–1048. doi:10.1093/CKJ/SFZ098.

42. Fink HA, Wilt TJ, Eidman KE, Garimella PS, et al. Medical management to prevent recurrent nephrolithiasis in adults: a systematic review for an American College of Physicians Clinical Guideline. *Ann Intern Med.* 2013;158(7):535–543. doi: 10.7326/0003-4819-158-7-201304020-00005.

43. Wiederkehr MR, Moe OW. Uric acid nephrolithiasis: a systemic metabolic disorder. *Clin Rev Bone Miner Metab.* 2011;9(3–4):207–217. doi:10.1007/S12018-011-9106-6.

44. Adomako E, Moe OW. Uric acid and urate in urolithiasis: the innocent bystander, instigator, and perpetrator. *Semin Nephrol.* 2020;40(6):564–573. doi:10.1016/j.semnephrol.2020.12.003.

45. Servais A, Thomas K, Dello Strologo L, et al. Cystinuria: clinical practice recommendation. *Kidney Int.* 2021;99(1):48–58. doi:10.1016/J.KINT.2020.06.035.

46. Spradling K, Vernez SL, Khoyliar C, et al. Prevalence of hyperoxaluria in urinary stone formers: chronological and geographical trends and a literature review. *J Endourol.* 2016;30(4):469–475. doi:10.1089/end.2015.0676.

47. Abu-Ghanem Y, Kleinmann N, Erlich T, Winkler HZ, Zilberman DE. The impact of dietary modifications and medical management on 24-hour urinary metabolic profiles and the status of renal stone disease in recurrent stone formers. *Isr Med Assoc J.* 2021;23(1):12–16.

48. Witting C, Langman CB, Assimos D, et al. Pathophysiology and treatment of enteric hyperoxaluria. *Clin J Am Soc Nephrol.* 2021;16(3):487–495. doi:10.2215/CJN.08000520.

49. Shee K, Stoller ML. Perspectives in primary hyperoxaluria—historical, current and future clinical interventions. *Nat Rev Urol.* 2022;19(3):137–146. doi:10.1038/S41585-021-00543-4.

50. Burns Z, Knight J, Fargue S, Holmes R, Assimos D, Wood K. Future treatments for hyperoxaluria. *Curr Opin Urol.* 2020;30(2):171. doi:10.1097/MOU.0000000000000709.

51. Garrelfs SF, Frishberg Y, Hulton SA, et al. Lumasiran, an RNAi therapeutic for primary hyperoxaluria type 1. *N Engl J Med.* 2021;384(13):1216–1226. doi:10.1056/NEJMOA2021712.

52. Cohen TD, Preminger GM. Struvite calculi. *Semin Nephrol.* 1996;16(5):425–434. doi:10.1148/radiology.193.3.702.

53. Iqbal MW, Shin RH, Youssef RF, et al. Should metabolic evaluation be performed in patients with struvite stones? *Urolithiasis.* 2017;45(2):185–192. doi:10.1007/S00240-016-0893-6.

54. Boyce AM, Shawker TH, Hill SC, et al. Ultrasound is superior to computed tomography for assessment of medullary nephrocalcinosis in hypoparathyroidism. *J Clin Endocrinol Metab.* 2013;98(3):989. doi:10.1210/JC.2012-2747.

55. Ethiraj D, Indiran V. Images in clinical urology primary hyperoxaluria-imaging of renal oxalosis. *Urology.* 2019;134:e3–e4. doi:10.1016/j.urology.2019.09.020.

56. Vaidya SR, Yarrarapu SNS, Aeddula NR. Nephrocalcinosis. [Updated Aug 13, 2021]. In: *StatPearls* [Internet]. Treasure Island (FL): StatPearls Publishing; 2022. https://www.ncbi.nlm.nih.gov/books/NBK537205.

57. Kumbar L, Yee J. Nephrocalcinosis: a diagnostic conundrum. *Am J Kidney Dis.* 2018;71(4):A12–A14. doi:10.1053/J.AJKD.2017.11.025.

58. Bergner R, Löffler C. Renal sarcoidosis: approach to diagnosis and management. *Curr Opin Pulm Med.* 2018;24(5):513–520. doi:10.1097/MCP.0000000000000504.

59. Soares SBM, de Menezes Silva LAW, de Carvalho Mrad FC, Simões e Silva AC. Distal renal tubular acidosis: genetic causes and management. *World J Pediatr.* 2019;15(5):422–431. doi:10.1007/S12519-019-00260-4.

60. Kim YG, Kim B, Kim MK, et al. Medullary nephrocalcinosis associated with long-term furosemide abuse in adults. *Nephrol Dial Transplant.* 2001;16(12):2303–2309. doi:10.1093/NDT/16.12.2303.

61. Vall-Palomar M, Madariaga L, Ariceta G. Familial hypomagnesemia with hypercalciuria and nephrocalcinosis. *Pediatr Nephrol.* 2021;36(10):3045–3055. doi:10.1007/S00467-021-04968-2.

62. Li Cavoli G, Mulè G, Rotolo U. Renal involvement in psychological eating disorders. *Nephron Clin Pract.* 2011;119(4):c338–c341; discussion c341. doi:10.1159/000333798.

63. Nuñez-Gonzalez L, Carrera N, Garcia-Gonzalez MA. Molecular basis, diagnostic challenges and therapeutic approaches of Bartter and Gitelman syndromes: a primer for clinicians. *Int J Mol Sci.* 2021;22(21):11414. doi:10.3390/ijms222111414.

64. Piccoli GB, De Pascale A, Randone O, et al. Revisiting nephrocalcinosis: a single-centre perspective. A northern Italian experience. *Nephrology (Carlton).* 2016;21(2):97–107. doi:10.1111/NEP.12535.

65. Bitzan M, Goodyer PR. Hypophosphatemic rickets. *Pediatr Clin North Am.* 2019;66(1):179–207. doi:10.1016/J.PCL.2018.09.004.

66. Buysschaert B, Aydin S, Morelle J, Gillion V, Jadoul M, Demoulin N. Etiologies, clinical features, and outcome of oxalate nephropathy. *Kidney Int Rep.* 2020;5(9):1503–1509. doi:10.1016/J.EKIR.2020.06.021.

67. Malakar S, Negi B, Singh G, Sharma T. Nephrocalcinosis in a patient with extrapulmonary tuberculosis—a rare entity. *J Fam Med Prim Care.* 2019;8(1):296–298. doi:10.4103/jfmpc.jfmpc_385_18.

68. Weigert A, Hoppe B. Nephrolithiasis and nephrocalcinosis in childhood-risk factor-related current and future treatment options. *Front Pediatr.* 2018;6:98. doi:10.3389/FPED.2018.00098.

69. Dickson FJ, Sayer JA. Nephrocalcinosis: a review of monogenic causes and insights they provide into this heterogeneous condition. *Int J Mol Sci.* 2020;21(1):369. doi:10.3390/IJMS21010369.

CHAPTER 16

Laboratory Values for Nephrology

Robert Stephen Brown ■ Alexander Goldfarb-Rumyantzev

It should be recognized that normal laboratory values may vary among different clinical laboratories, measurement techniques, and of importance, the state of the subject when the sample is collected (e.g., fasting or postprandial, supine or standing, high-salt or low-salt intake, hydrated or not). So the reference ranges below may vary, but offer a guide to distinguish values that fall outside the range listed and investigate a probable abnormality.

16.1 Adrenocorticotropic Hormone (ACTH)

Adrenocorticotropic Hormone (ACTH), Plasma

Reference Range

9 to <120 pg/mL [SI units: 2 to <26 pmol/L]

Description

ACTH is a polypeptide hormone of the anterior lobe of the pituitary gland (hypophysis) that stimulates growth of the adrenal cortex or secretion of its hormones. Indicator used in the differential diagnosis of hypercortisolism and adrenocortical insufficiency.
- **Increased:** central Cushing syndrome—pituitary ACTH secreting adenoma (usually microadenomas), hypothalamic hyperfunction (increased corticotropin-releasing hormone), ACTH therapy, Addison's disease, ectopic ACTH syndrome
- **Decreased:** adrenal Cushing syndrome (adrenal adenoma, adrenal hyperplasia, adrenal carcinoma), iatrogenic hypercortisolism (long-term glucocorticoid therapy)

16.2 Albumin

Albumin, Serum

Reference Range

3.5–5.0 g/dL [SI units: 35–50 g/L]

Description

Albumin is a transport protein for small molecules, including bilirubin, calcium, magnesium, progesterone, and various medications. Its oncotic pressure serves to keep the fluid in the blood and avoid it leaking out into the tissues. The test helps assess protein absorption or malnutrition of the body and determine whether the patient has liver or kidney disease.
- **Increased:** dehydration, shock
- **Decreased:** cystic fibrosis, proteinuric glomerular kidney disease, cirrhosis, Hodgkin's disease, malnutrition, nephrotic syndrome, multiple myeloma, inflammatory bowel disease, leukemia, collagen-vascular diseases

16.3 Albumin/Creatinine Ratio

Albumin/Creatinine Ratio, Urine

Reference Range

	On Spot (random sample) Urine	24-Hour Urine Collection
• Normal:	<30 mg/g • <17 mg/g (men) • <25 mg/g (women)	• <30 mg/24 hr
• Microalbuminuria:	30–300 mg/g (either sex) • 17–300 mg/g (men) • 25–300 mg/g (women)	• 30–300 mg/24 hr
• Macroalbuminuria:	>300 mg/g	• >300 mg/24 hr

Description

It is used to measure albuminuria as a sign of kidney disease, or in diabetes and hypertension as a marker which may lead to kidney disease and/or cardiovascular risk.

Microalbuminuria: chronic kidney disease, diabetes mellitus, congestive cardiac failure, acute or chronic obstructive airways disease, hypertension, malignancy

16.4 Aldosterone

Aldosterone, Plasma and Urine

Reference Range

• Plasma: supine 2–9 ng/dL [SI units: 55–250 pmol/L]
  Standing: 7–20 ng/dL [SI units: 195–555 pmol/L]
• Urine: 5–19 mcg/day [SI units: 14–53 nmol/day]

Description

Adrenal glands release the hormone aldosterone which maintains blood volume and pressure. Blood pressure increases when aldosterone increases the tubular reabsorption of sodium by the kidneys. It also causes renal excretion of potassium. Renin levels should usually be measured simultaneously to assess whether a high aldosterone is primary (with low renin) or secondary (with high renin).

• **Increased:** primary hyperaldosteronism, secondary hyperaldosteronism, very low-sodium diet
• **Decreased:** Addison's disease, very high-sodium diet, hyporeninemic hypoaldosteronism

16.5 Alkaline Phosphatase

Alkaline Phosphatase, Serum

Reference Range

30–140 U/L [SI units: 0.5–2.5 μkat/L] (for adults)

Description

This is a group of enzymes that hydrolyze many orthophosphoric monoesters and are present ubiquitously (liver, kidney, bones, intestine, and placenta).

• **Increased:** physiological—during growth, last trimester of pregnancy, rickets, osteomalacia, ulcerative colitis, bowel perforation, fatty liver, hepatitis, hyperparathyroidism, bone resorption, hyperthyroidism
• **Decreased:** vitamin D intoxication, pernicious anemia, hypothyroidism, celiac sprue, malnutrition, fibrate therapy

16.6 Amylase

Reference Range

* 30–110 U/L [SI units: 0.4–1.4 μkat/L]

Description

Enzyme amylase is generated in the pancreas and salivary glands. It is released into the blood on injury to the pancreas (diseased or inflamed), or less commonly, the parotid gland. It helps in assimilation of carbohydrates.
* **Increased:** acute pancreatitis, pancreatic duct obstruction, alcohol ingestion, mumps, parotitis, renal disease, cholecystitis, peptic ulcers, intestinal obstruction, mesenteric thrombosis, postoperative abdominal surgery
* **Decreased:** liver damage, pancreatic destruction (pancreatitis, cystic fibrosis)

16.7 Angiotensin-Converting Enzyme (ACE)

Angiotensin-Converting Enzyme (ACE), Serum

Reference Range

<40 U/L [SI units: <670 nkat/L]

Description

This is an important enzyme in the renin-angiotensin-aldosterone system and the kallikrein-kinin system. ACE's effects are based on the direct vasoconstrictive effect of angiotensin II conversion from angiotensin I as well as increased catabolism of the vasodilatory bradykinins. ACE is found in the endothelial cells of the vascular system, particularly in the lungs and kidneys. It is an indicator in the diagnosis and course of sarcoidosis.

Increased: sarcoidosis (Besnier-Boeck-Schaumann disease), silicosis, asbestosis, tuberculosis, alcoholic liver disease, Gaucher disease, kidney diseases, hyperparathyroidism, hyperthyroidism, diabetes mellitus

16.8 Anion Gap

Reference Range

* 8–12 mEq/L [SI units: 8–12mmol/L]

Description

The anion gap is the difference between the major positive and negative ions in serum, plasma, and urine.
Calculate: Anion gap = $(Na^+) - (HCO_3^- + Cl^-)$
* **Increased:** lactic acidosis, high anion gap metabolic acidosis (e.g., DR. MAPLES mnemonic: Diabetic ketoacidosis, Renal failure, Methanol, Aspirin, Paraldehyde/Propylene glycol/Pyroglutamic acid, Lactic acid, Ethylene glycol/Ethanol ketoacidosis, Starvation ketoacidosis)
* **Decreased:** hypoalbuminemia, multiple myeloma, increased potassium, calcium or magnesium, lithium or bromide toxicity

16.9 Antinuclear Antibody (ANA)

Reference Range

Negative ≤1:40

Description

The ANA detects antibodies to all nuclear antigens present in serum by an indirect immunofluorescence assay. Since the test is nonspecific, it may be positive in many autoimmune conditions and at low titers (1:40–1:80) in up to 20%–25% of normal persons. When positive at higher titers, autoimmune or connective tissue diseases are more likely, but more specific antibody testing is needed for better differentiation (shown below).

- **Positive:** connective tissue disease—systemic lupus erythematosus (anti-dsDNA; anti-Sm), drug-induced lupus (anti-histone), Sjögren's syndrome (anti-Ro/La), rheumatoid arthritis (rheumatoid factor; anti-CCP), scleroderma or systemic sclerosis (anti-Scl-70; anti-centromere), mixed connective tissue disease (anti-RNP), polymyositis or dermatomyositis (anti-PM-1; anti-Jo-1). Other conditions: autoimmune hepatitis, primary biliary cirrhosis (antimitochondrial), chronic hepatitis C, ulcerative colitis, Crohn's disease, subacute bacterial endocarditis
- **Negative:** negative predictive value for lupus

16.10 Antineutrophil Cytoplasmic Antibody (ANCA)

Reference Range

Positive: confirm with anti-PR3 and anti-MPO titers

Description

ANCA tests for autoantibodies to antigens in neutrophil cytoplasm; c-ANCA staining diffusely in the cytoplasm and p-ANCA in a perinuclear pattern.

- **Positive:** c-ANCA, usually anti-proteinase 3 (PR3)—granulomatosis with polyangiitis (formerly Wegener's), pauci-immune glomerulonephritis, Churg-Strauss syndrome; p-ANCA, usually anti-myeloperoxidase (MPO)—microscopic polyangiitis, pauci-immune necrotizing "renal-limited vasculitis" glomerulonephritis (may be positive in anti-GBM nephritis also), Churg-Strauss syndrome, drug-induced vasculitis, other connective tissue diseases, ulcerative colitis, Crohn's disease, autoimmune hepatitis, sclerosing cholangitis

16.11 Bilirubin

Reference Range

- Total: 0.3–1.2 mg/dL [SI units: 5–20 μmol/L]
- Direct: 0–0.3 mg/dL [SI units: 0–5.1 μmol/L]
- Indirect: 0.2–0.6 mg/dL [SI units: 3.4–10.2 μmol/L]

Description

Bile is produced by the liver and contains yellowish pigment bilirubin.

- **Increased total:** hepatic damage (hepatitis, toxins, cirrhosis), biliary obstruction, hemolysis, fasting, Gilbert's syndrome, hemolytic anemia
- **Increased direct (conjugated):** biliary obstruction/cholestasis, drug-induced cholestasis

16.12 Bicarbonate (HCO$_3^-$)

HCO$_3^-$, Serum (also called total CO$_2$)

Reference Range

- Arterial: 22–27 mEq/L [SI units: 22–27 mmol/L]
- Venous: 23–29 mEq/L [SI units: 23–29 mmol/L]

Description

Bicarbonate is a buffer that maintains the pH of the blood from getting too acidic or too alkaline (basic).
- **Increased:** severe vomiting, pulmonary insufficiency, Cushing syndrome, hyperaldosteronism, metabolic alkalosis, respiratory acidosis (compensatory)
- **Decreased:** Addison's disease, chronic diarrhea, diabetic ketoacidosis, kidney failure, salicylate toxicity, ethylene glycol or methanol poisoning, metabolic acidosis, respiratory alkalosis (compensatory)

16.13 Blood Urea Nitrogen (BUN)

Reference Range

- 7–20 mg/dL [SI units: 2.5–7.14 mmol/L]

Description

The test evaluates the amount of urea nitrogen in the blood to evaluate kidney function. Urea is a by-product of protein breakdown produced by the liver.
- **Increased:** acute kidney injury, renal failure, prerenal azotemia (hypotension, septic shock, volume depletion), postrenal (obstruction), gastrointestinal (GI) bleeding, catabolic states, drugs (corticosteroids, amino acid infusions), high protein intake
- **Decreased:** starvation, liver failure, pregnancy, infancy, overhydration

16.14 BUN:Creatinine Ratio

Reference Range

- Between 10:1 and 20:1

Description

- **Increased:** prerenal failure, GI bleeding, catabolic states, postrenal obstruction, steroids, tetracycline
- **Decreased:** hepatic insufficiency, rhabdomyolysis (creatinine rises more than BUN), malnutrition

16.15 Calcium

Calcium, Serum

Reference Range

Calcium, total serum
- 8.5–10.2 mg/dL [SI units: 2.0–2.6 mmol/L]
Calcium, ionized serum
- 4.8–5.3 mg/dL [SI units: 1.2–1.4 mmol/L]

Continued on following page

Description

Calcium is essential for the proper contraction of the muscles and blood vessels and for the efficient conduction of impulses through the nervous system and in the secretion of hormones by the endocrine system. Bones and teeth act as the chief stores of calcium in the body along with blood and other tissues of the body. Serum calcium is approximately 50% ionic and 50% bound to albumin and anions.

- **Increased:** malignancies—non-Hodgkin's lymphoma, multiple myeloma, breast and other cancers, primary hyperparathyroidism, tertiary hyperparathyroidism, hyperthyroidism, adrenal insufficiency, Paget's disease, 1, 25 dihydroxy vitamin D overproduction (tuberculosis, sarcoidosis, fungal diseases, berylliosis); drugs–hypervitaminosis of A or D, calcitriol, lithium, thiazides, theophylline toxicity, tamoxifen, milk-alkali syndrome
- **Decreased:** hypoparathyroidism, insufficient vitamin D, hypomagnesemia, renal tubular acidosis, hypoalbuminemia, chronic renal failure (phosphate retention), acute pancreatitis, alcoholism

16.16 Calcitonin

Reference Range

- Males <19 pg/mL [SI units: <19 ng/L]
- Females <14 pg/mL [SI units: <14 ng/L]

Description

Calcitonin is a hormone produced in the C cells of the thyroid gland that downregulates blood calcium, opposing the action of parathyroid hormone (PTH) and vitamin D.

- **Increased:** malignant diseases—medullary thyroid cancer, lung cancer, insulinomas, VIPomas; non-malignant diseases—newborns, pregnancy, renal failure, Zollinger-Ellison syndrome (associated with men), pernicious anemia

16.17 Chloride

Chloride, Serum

Reference Range

- 95–105 mEq/L [SI units: 95–105 mmol/L]

Description

Chloride is the major anion maintaining the electrical and acid-base balance of the body and regulating the renal tubular reabsorption and maintenance of sodium and fluids in the body.

- **Increased:** metabolic acidosis (nonanion gap), respiratory alkalosis (compensated), renal tubular acidosis
- **Decreased:** Addison's disease, burns, congestive heart failure, dehydration, excessive sweating, metabolic alkalosis, respiratory acidosis (compensated), syndrome of inappropriate antidiuretic hormone (SIADH) secretion and other hyponatremic states

Chloride, Urine

Reference Range

- 110–250 mEq/day [SI units: 110–250 mmol/day]
- Varies with diet
- <20 mEq/L suggests vomiting, gastric suction, excessive sweating with chloride depletion

Description

Same as above for chloride.
- **Increased:** metabolic alkalosis, potassium depletion, Addison's disease, increased salt intake, Gitelman or Bartter syndrome
- **Decreased:** vomiting, volume depletion, Cushing syndrome, Conn syndrome, congestive heart failure, malabsorption syndrome, diarrhea, decreased salt intake

16.18 Complement (C3, C4)

Serum Complement (C3, C4)

Reference Range

C3: 90–180 mg/dL [SI units: 0.9–1.8 g/L]
C4: 10–40 mg/dL [SI units: 0.1–0.4 g/L]

Description

The complement system is part of the body's immune and inflammatory response and testing is used to evaluate immune and autoimmune disorders. While normal increases occur in infectious illnesses, complement is most often measured to detect autoimmune conditions that lower serum complement levels by binding and/or consumption of complement components.
- **Increased:** acute response to infection or injury
- **Decreased:** lupus, Sjögren's syndrome, cryoglobulinemia, immune complex and membranoproliferative glomerulonephritis, serum sickness, hemolysis, and inherited complement disorders

16.19 Creatinine Excretion and Clearance

Reference Range

Normal creatinine production and excretion:
- Males: 15–20 mg/kg/24 hr
- Females: 10–15 mg/kg/24 hr
Normal creatinine clearance:
- Males: 97–137 mL/min [SI units: 1.6–2.2 mL/s] decreasing with age
- Females: 88–128 mL/min [SI units: 1.4–2.1 mL/s] decreasing with age

Description

The creatinine clearance (CrCl) test helps detect and diagnose kidney dysfunction and disorders of renal perfusion. It is a measure of the efficiency of the filtration process of the kidneys, evaluated by comparing the level of creatinine excreted in the urine to the creatinine levels in the blood.
Creatinine clearance = UCr (in mg/dL) × UVol (in mL/min)/SCr (in mg/dL)
- **Increased:** high protein intake, early diabetes mellitus, burns, CO poisoning, hypothyroidism, pregnancy
- **Decreased:** acute and chronic kidney injury or renal failure, congestive heart failure, volume depletion

16.20 Creatinine

Creatinine, Serum

Reference Range

- Males: 0.7–1.2 mg/dL [SI units: 61.8–106 µmol/L]
- Females: 0.6–1.1 mg/dL [SI units: 53–97 µmol/L]

Description

Creatinine is a breakdown product of muscle metabolism that is filtered out of the blood by the kidneys. The test is used to measure the functioning of the kidneys. If kidney function is reduced creatinine levels rise in the blood.

- **Increased:** acute or chronic renal failure, urinary tract obstruction, drugs that decrease kidney function or tubular creatinine secretion (e.g., trimethoprim), body-building or creatine intake
- **Decreased:** muscle atrophy, protein starvation, liver disease, pregnancy

16.21 Cystatin C

Cystatin C, Serum

Reference Range

- Males: 0.56–0.98 mg/L
- Females: 0.52–0.90 mg/L

Description

Cystatin C is a 120-amino acid basic protein secreted by all nucleated cells and removed by glomerular filtration. It can be used to estimate glomerular filtration rate (GFR; see Chapter 11) with less effect of age, race, and muscle mass than creatinine, but it is affected by body composition, cancer, and various other conditions.

- **Increased:** acute or chronic renal failure, HIV, increased body mass index (BMI), high C-reactive protein, hyperthyroidism, corticosteroid use, and other disorders
- **Decreased:** atherosclerotic vascular disease, cyclosporine

16.22 Fractional Excretion of Sodium (FENa %)

Reference Range

- <1% normally

Description

FENa is the quantity (percentage) of sodium excreted in the urine compared to the amount filtered by the kidney and is used as a test to distinguish prerenal from renal causes of kidney injury/failure.

FeNa = Na^+ excreted/Na^+ filtered = $(UNa \times SCr \times 100)/(SNa \times UCr)$

- **Increased:** acute tubular necrosis (>1%, often >3%)
- **Decreased:** prerenal azotemia (<1%) normal physiology (low sodium diet, volume depletion)

16.23 Ferritin

Ferritin, Serum

Reference Range

15–200 ng/mL [SI units: 33–450 pmol/L]

Description

Ferritin is a protein that stores iron. The amount of ferritin gives an indication of the amount of iron stored in the blood.
- **Increased:** hemochromatosis and iron overload, inflammation, liver disease, chronic infection, autoimmune disorders, hemolytic anemia, sideroblastic anemia
- **Decreased:** iron deficiency

16.24 Glomerular Filtration Rate (GFR)

Reference Range

Measured GFR in young adults (decreasing with age):
- Males: 115–145 mL/min/1.73 m^2
- Females: 105–140 mL/min/m^2
Estimated GFR: >60 mL/min/1.73 m^2

Description

The GFR test measures functioning of the kidneys and progression of chronic kidney disease. Glomerular filtration is the process by which the kidneys filter the blood, removing excess wastes and fluids. GFR can be measured directly, as with inulin or iothalamate, or estimated from serum creatinine and/or cystatin C using a calculator at http://www.kidney.org/professionals/kdoqi/gfr.cfm.
- **Increased:** pregnancy, early diabetes
- **Decreased:** acute or chronic kidney disease, volume depletion, hypotension, congestive heart failure (CHF)

16.25 Glucose

Glucose, Blood

Reference Range

- Fasting blood glucose: 65–100 mg/dL [SI units: 3.6–5.5 mmol/L]
- Random blood glucose: <125 mg/dL [SI units: <6.88 mmol/L]
- Impaired fasting glucose: 100–125 mg/dL [SI units: 5.5–6.88 mmol/L]

Description

Measuring glucose levels in the blood gives an indication of carbohydrate metabolism and balance of glycogen breakdown, gluconeogenesis, and glucose uptake mediated largely by insulin.
- **Increased:** acromegaly, acute stress (e.g., response to trauma, heart attack, and stroke), chronic kidney failure, Cushing syndrome, diabetes mellitus, excessive food intake, hyperthyroidism, pancreatic cancer, pancreatitis
- **Decreased:** adrenal insufficiency, excessive alcohol, severe liver disease, hypopituitarism, hypothyroidism, insulin overdose, insulinomas, starvation

Glucose, Urine

Reference Range

- Negative

Description

The glucose test is used to measure the glucose levels in urine. Urinary excretion of glucose is called glycosuria or glucosuria.
- **Increased:** diabetes mellitus, gestational diabetes, acromegaly, estrogens, chloral hydrate, corticosteroids, inherited renal glycosuria, sodium-glucose co-transporter 2 (SGLT2) inhibitors.

16.26 Hemoglobin (Hb)

Reference Range

- Males: 13.8–17.2 g/dL [SI units: 138–172 g/L]
- Females: 12.1–15.1 g/dL [SI units: 121–151 g/L]

Description

Hemoglobin is the oxygen-carrying pigment and major protein in erythrocytes. Hemoglobin forms an unstable, reversible bond with oxygen. Oxyhemoglobin (oxygenated state) transports oxygen from the lungs to the tissues where it releases its oxygen and converts to deoxyhemoglobin (deoxygenated state).
- **Increased:** polycythemia, volume depletion, hypoxia, high-altitude living
- **Decreased:** anemia (hemorrhagic, hemolytic, or failure of red blood cell [RBC] production)

16.27 Hematocrit

Hematocrit, Whole Blood

Reference Range

- Males: 40%–52%
- Females: 36%–48%

Description

Hematocrit (Hct) indicates packed cell volume (PCV), or the proportion of the blood by volume that consists of RBCs, expressed as a percentage.
- **Increased:** polycythemia, volume depletion, hypoxia, high-altitude living
- **Decreased:** anemia (hemorrhagic, hemolytic, or failure of RBC production)

16.28 Iron

Iron, Serum

Reference Range

- Males: 65–175 mcg/dL [11.6–31.3 µmol/L]
- Females: 50–170 mcg/dL [9.0–30.4 µmol/L]

Description

The total iron content of the body is approximately 38 mg/kg in women and 50 mg/kg in men. The iron stores in the body are erythrocytes (approx. 3000 mg); myoglobin (approx. 120 mg); cytochromes (approx. 3–8 mg); and liver/spleen (approx. 300–800 mg). Daily turnover through synthesis and conversion of hemoglobin is 25 mg. Uptake occurs mainly through uptake of bivalent iron in the small intestine. Considerable iron loss is possible through menstruation, hemodialysis, and pregnancy.
- **Increased:** hemochromatosis, hemolytic anemia, sideroblastic anemia, lead poisoning, liver disease
- **Decreased:** iron deficiency, chronic illness, poor diet, intestinal disease (problems with GI absorption), hemodialysis, parasitic diseases

16.29 Ketones

Ketones, Urine

Reference Range

- Negative
- When ketones are present in the urine, the results are usually listed as small, moderate, or large with these approximate corresponding values:
  - Small: <20 mg/dL
  - Moderate: 30–40 mg/dL
  - Large: >80 mg/dL

Description

Ketones are made in excess when fat is metabolized preferentially more than carbohydrates to supply energy.

- **Increased:** anorexia, fasting, diabetic ketoacidosis, high-fat or low-carbohydrate diets, starvation, vomiting over a long period of time, alcoholism, acute or severe illness, burns, fever

16.30 Lactate

Lactate, Plasma or Serum

Reference Range

5.0–18 mg/dL [SI units: 0.6–2.0 mmol/L]

Description

Lactic acid is produced from the metabolism of glucose when pyruvic acid is converted to lactic acid. Since the H^+ ion will be picked up by the body's buffers, excess lactate will reduce the serum bicarbonate, causing an anion gap metabolic acidosis. Note that lactate measurement only detects L-lactate, not D-lactic acidosis from bacterial metabolism in short bowel syndromes or GI bacterial overgrowth.

- **Increased** (>4.0 mmol/L): tissue ischemia (shock, sepsis), drugs (metformin, zidovudine, stavudine, didanosine), alcoholism, malignancy

16.31 Magnesium

Magnesium, Serum

Reference Range

1.5–2.6 mEq/L [SI units: 0.62–1.07 mmol/L]

Description

Distribution of magnesium within the body has some similarity to potassium, with approximately 1% (mainly in ionized form, 30% protein bound) in the serum, approximately 40% in the skeletal muscles, and approximately 60% in the bones. Magnesium is important for many enzymes, including the activation of Na^+ K^+ ATPase (significant for cardiac dysrhythmias), adenylate cyclase, pyruate dehydrogenase, calcium ATPase, and others.

- **Increased:** renal insufficiency, uncontrolled diabetes mellitus, Addison's disease, hypothyroidism, drugs (magnesium-containing antacids or enema salts)
- **Decreased:** malabsorption syndromes, alcoholism, chronic inflammatory bowel diseases, sprue, chronic renal disease, diabetic acidosis, proton pump inhibitors, diuretics, nephrotoxic drugs, Gitelman syndrome

16.32 Osmolality

Osmolality, Plasma (P_{Osm})

Reference Range

- 275–295 mOsm/kg [SI units: 275–295 mmol/kg]

Description

The test is used for measuring blood osmolality, primarily proportional to sodium and its accompanying anion, glucose, and urea.
- **Increased:** dehydration, hyperglycemia, hypernatremia, kidney failure with azotemia, mannitol therapy, alcohol, ethylene glycol or methanol toxicity
- **Decreased:** excess hydration, hyponatremia, inappropriate antidiuretic hormone (ADH) secretion

Osmolality, Urine (U_{Osm})

Reference Range

- 50–1200 mOsm/kg [SI units: 50–1200 mmol/kg]

Description

The testing of urine osmolality is important in the diagnosis of conditions that cause an increased urinary volume. Urine osmolarity should be tested in renal concentration defects, diabetes insipidus, osmotic diuresis, and water diuresis. The human ADH is arginine-vasopressin (AVP) whose release is regulated by an increase in plasma osmolality or by a reduction in the intravascular volume (extracellular volume). AVP causes a reduction (antidiuresis) of water excretion. When plasma osmolality is <280 mOsmol/kg H_2O, AVP release should be low; when osmolality increases to >300 mOsmol/kg H_2O, AVP release is increased with concentrated urine to conserve water.
- **Increased:** congestive heart failure, hypernatremia, inappropriate ADH secretion, liver damage, shock
- **Decreased:** central diabetes insipidus, excess fluid intake, hypercalcemia, hypokalemia, kidney tubular damage

16.33 Parathyroid Hormone (PTH)

Reference Range

- 10–65 pg/mL [SI units: 10–65 ng/L]

Description

PTH is a peptide hormone formed in the parathyroid glands whose function is to raise serum calcium by causing bone resorption, intestinal calcium absorption, and calcium reabsorption by the renal tubules and to lower serum phosphate by inhibiting phosphate reabsorption by the renal tubules.
- **Increased:** osteitis fibrosa, extraskeletal calcification, calciphylaxis, chronic kidney disease, hypersecretion or adenoma of the parathyroid glands
- **Decreased:** osteomalacia, adynamic/aplastic bone lesions, low levels of magnesium in the blood, radiation to the parathyroid glands, sarcoidosis, vitamin D intoxication

16.34 pH

Reference Range

- Arterial: 7.36–7.44
- Venous: 7.33–7.43

Description

Blood gas analysis is done to determine the pH. Most commonly, analysis is done on arterial blood gas (ABG) to categorically determine the level of oxygenation and to assess whether disturbances in the pH and buffering system of arterial blood are due to respiratory or metabolic causes. Ideally, the pH of the blood should be maintained at 7.4 which is kept constant by buffers dissolved in the blood and respiration.

- **Increased:** metabolic alkalosis (e.g., vomiting, diuretics), respiratory alkalosis
- **Decreased:** metabolic acidosis, nonanion gap (DR. DOOFUS: Diarrhea; RTA; Drugs such as acetazolamide, topiramate, ifosfamide, or tenofovir; Obstructive uropathy; Other as recovery from hyperventilation; Fistulous ileal bladder; Uremia; Sniffing glue), or high anion gap (DR. MAPLES: Diabetic ketoacidosis; Renal failure; Methanol; Aspirin; Pyroglutamic acid, paraldehyde, or propylene glycol; Lactic acid; Ethylene glycol or ethanol ketoacidosis; Starvation ketoacidosis), respiratory acidosis

16.35 pO$_2$

Reference Range

- Arterial: 80–100 mmHg [SI units: 10.6–13.3 kPa]
- Venous: 37–47 mmHg [SI units: 5–6.3 kPa]

Description

pO$_2$ measures the partial pressures of oxygen in the blood. An ABG analysis evaluates how effectively the lungs are delivering oxygen to the blood.

- **Increased:** oxygen inhalation by O$_2$ mask or nasal cannula
- **Decreased:** chronic obstructive pulmonary disease (COPD), pneumonia, hypoventilation or increased alveolar-arterial gradient

16.36 pCO$_2$

Reference Range

- Arterial: 35–45 mmHg [SI units: 4.7–5.9 kPa]
- Venous: 36–48 mmHg [SI units: 4.7–6.4 kPa]

Description

pCO$_2$ measures the partial pressures of carbon dioxide in the blood. An ABG analysis evaluates how effectively the lungs are eliminating carbon dioxide.

- **Increased:** respiratory acidosis, hypoventilation, metabolic alkalosis (compensation)
- **Decreased:** respiratory alkalosis, hyperventilation, sepsis, liver disease, pregnancy, salicylate toxicity, metabolic acidosis (compensation)

16.37 Phosphorus

Phosphorus, Serum

Reference Range

- 2.7–4.5 mg/dL [SI units: 0.87–1.45mmol/L]

Description

85% of phosphate is contained in the bones and teeth, 14% in body cells, and 1% in the extracellular space. Energy-rich phosphates (ATPs) supply energy for metabolic reactions.
- **Increased:** acute and chronic renal failure, acidosis (lactic acidosis, diabetic ketoacidosis), phosphate administration, phosphate-containing laxatives, tumor lysis syndrome, osteolytic metastases, vitamin D overdose, hypoparathyroidism, pseudohypoparathyroidism, hyperthyroidism
- **Decreased:** primary hyperparathyroidism, renal tubular defects, postrenal transplantation, extracellular fluid (ECF) volume expansion, hyperaldosteronism, hypokalemia, hypercalcemia, hypomagnesemia, Cushing syndrome, mesenchymoma or neurofibroma (if FGF 23 secreting tumors), vomiting, diarrhea, malabsorption, drugs (steroid therapy, oral phosphate binders, oral contraceptives, estrogens, diuretics)

16.38 Potassium

Potassium, Serum

Reference Range

- 3.5–5.1 mEq/L [SI units: 3.5–5.1 mmol/L]

Description

Potassium is closely regulated between the intracellular and extracellular fluid compartments; most of the body stores are in muscle and bone. The potassium electrical potential across cardiac cell membranes is important to heart function. As such, severe hyperkalemia or hypokalemia needs immediate attention and treatment.
- **Decreased:** diarrhea, vomiting, severe sweating, Cushing syndrome, hyperaldosteronism, Bartter or Gitelman syndrome, Fanconi syndrome, diuretics, antibiotics (amphotericin, high-dose penicillin, gentamicin), magnesium deficiency
- **Increased:** Addison's disease, acute or chronic kidney failure, angiotensin-converting-enzyme inhibitors (ACEi), angiotensin II receptor blockers (ARBs), beta blockers, K-sparing diuretics (spironolactone, eplerenone, finerenone, amiloride, triamterene), trimethoprim

16.39 Protein/Creatinine Ratio

Protein/Creatinine Ratio, Urine

Reference Range

- Normal: <0.2
- Moderate proteinuria: 0.3–2.9
- Nephrotic range proteinuria: >3.0

Description

Protein/creatinine ratio measures all urinary proteins, not just albumin, so immune globulins and polypeptides are included. The test is helpful to assess the severity of proteinuria without collecting a 24-hour urine and to follow proteinuric kidney diseases.
- **Positive:** proteinuric glomerular diseases, renal tubular proteinuria, multiple myeloma and other dysglobulinemias

16.40 SaO$_2$

Oxygen Saturation (Hemoglobin)

Reference Range

- Arterial: >95%
- Venous: 60%–85%

Description

Oxygen saturation measures how much of the hemoglobin in the RBCs is carrying oxygen.
- **Increased:** oxygen inhalation by O$_2$ mask or nasal cannula
- **Decreased:** COPD, pneumonia, hypoventilation or increased alveolar-arterial gradient

16.41 Sodium

Sodium, Serum

Reference Range

- 135–145 mEq/L [SI units: 135–145 mmol/L]

Description

Sodium constitutes 90% to 95% of all cations in the blood plasma and interstitial fluid, and thus determines most of the osmolality and volume of the ECF.
- **Decreased:** Addison's disease, glucocorticoid deficiency, severe heart failure, cirrhosis, diarrhea, diuretics, burns, pancreatitis, acute hyperglycemia, salt-losing conditions, SIADH secretion, severe lipemia or hyperglobulinemia (may cause pseudohyponatremia)
- **Increased:** dehydration, Cushing syndrome, diabetes insipidus, hyperaldosteronism, osmotic diuresis, prolonged glucosuria

Sodium, Urine

Reference Range

- 40–220 mEq/day (varies with dietary intake)

Description

This test measures the amount of sodium excreted in urine during 24 hours, and in balance, sodium intake in the diet. Sodium maintains the water volume and electrolyte balance of the body.
- **Decreased:** volume depletion, congestive heart failure, liver disease, nephrotic syndrome, low salt intake
- **Increased:** diuretic use, Addison's disease, high salt intake

16.42 Specific Gravity

Specific Gravity, Urine

Reference Range

- 1.003–1.030 by dipstick

Description

This test measures the density of urine and is usually proportional to the osmolality or concentration of the urine. However, dense substances, such as radiocontrast or glucose, increase density and specific gravity much more than osmolality.
- **Increased:** dehydration, diarrhea, glucosuria, heart failure, renal arterial stenosis, shock, SIADH, heavy proteinuria, radiocontrast
- **Decreased:** excessive fluid intake, diabetes insipidus, hypercalcemia, hypokalemia, kidney tubular damage causing a urinary concentration defect

16.43 Total Iron Binding Capacity (TIBC)

Reference Range

• 250–425 mcg/dL [SI units: 44.8–76.1 μmol/L]

Description

TIBC is most frequently used to evaluate iron deficiency or iron overload. It is used along with a serum iron test to calculate transferrin saturation to determine how much iron is being carried in the blood.
• **Increased:** iron deficiency anemia, pregnancy, use of oral contraceptives
• **Decreased:** cirrhosis, hemolytic anemia, hypoproteinemia, inflammation, liver disease, malnutrition, pernicious anemia, sickle cell anemia, nephrotic syndrome

16.44 Transferrin Saturation

Reference Range

• Males: 15%–50%
• Females: 12%–45%

Description

Transferrin is capable of associating reversibly with iron and acting as an iron transporting protein. Transferrin saturation (%) = 100 × serum iron (mcg/dL) / TIBC (mcg/dL) is only diagnostically relevant in conjunction with iron and ferritin levels.
• **Increased:** iron overload or poisoning, hemochromatosis, hemolytic anemia, sideroblastic anemia, starvation, nephrotic syndrome, cirrhosis
• **Decreased:** iron deficiency anemia, chronic infection, chronic inflammation, uremia, third trimester of pregnancy

16.45 Uric Acid

Uric Acid, Serum

Reference Range

• Males: 3.4–7.5 mg/dL [SI units: 202–446 μmol/L]
• Females: 2.4–6.0 mg/dL [SI units: 143–357 μmol/L]

Description

Uric acid is produced from the breakdown of purines, requiring the enzyme xanthine oxidase, mainly located in the liver and small intestine. Uric acid elimination occurs about 80% in the kidney and about 20% in the intestines. Complications of hyperuricemia are acute gouty arthritis, chronic soft tissue and/or bone tophi, nephrolithiasis, and acute uric acid nephropathy.
• **Increased:** gout, multiple myeloma, metastatic cancer, leukemia, diet high in purines, diuretics, kidney insufficiency, chemotherapy treatment of hematological malignancies
• **Decreased:** allopurinol, pregnancy, probenecid, febuxostat

"Page numbers followed by "f" indicate figures and "t" indicate tables."

A

Abdominal X-ray (KUB), of kidney stones, 273
ABMR. *See* Antibody-mediated rejection
Accelerated hypertension, 264
  in pregnancy, 260–261t, 260–261
ACE. *See* Angiotensin-converting enzyme
ACEi. *See* Angiotensin-converting-enzyme
  inhibitors
Acid-base balance, in peritoneal dialysis, 211, 211t,
  212f
Acid-base disorders, 49–59
  complex (double or triple), 57
  diagnostic algorithm of, 49–51, 50f, 50t
  metabolic acidosis as, 51–55
  metabolic alkalosis as, 55–57
  potassium and, 57, 57t
Acid-base regulation, 19, 19f
Acidemia, 50f
Acidosis, 12–13t
  hyperkalemia and, 57f
  lactic
    in peritoneal dialysis, 211t
    treatment of, 55
    types of, 54–55, 54t
  metabolic, 50f, 51–55, 52f
    alkalinizing therapy for, 55
    causes of, 51
    compensation for, 50t
    non-anion gap, 52, 52f
    serum osmolar gap for, 51–52
  renal tubular
    GI losses *versus*, 52
    types of, 53–54, 53t, 54f
  respiratory, 50f, 50t
ACR. *See* Albumin to creatinine ratio
ACTH. *See* Adrenocorticotropic hormone
Acute complicated urinary tract infection (UTI),
  113t
Acute dialysis, indications for, 152–153
Acute glomerulonephritis, causing AKI, 85t
Acute interstitial nephritis (AIN), 86, 106–107
  causes of, 86, 106
  clinical presentation of, 107
  diagnosis of, 86, 107
  treatment of, 86, 107
Acute kidney injury (AKI), 73–91
  acute interstitial nephritis in, 86
  acute tubular necrosis in, 81–83
  associated with COVID-19, 87–88
  cause of, diagnostic steps to establish, 75–76, 75t
  chronic kidney disease *versus*, 75, 75t
  contrast-associated/induced, 81–83
    diagnosis of, 82, 82t
    incidence of, 81–82, 82t

Acute kidney injury *(Continued)*
    management of, 82–83
    pathophysiology of, 82
    risk factors for, 82
  definition of, 73
  diagnostic algorithm for, 76, 76f
  dialysis for, 152
    adequacy of conventional hemodialysis in, 156
    appropriateness of, 154
    continuous renal replacement therapy for,
      156–158
    modalities, 153–164
    peritoneal, 164
    potential negative effect of, 88
    recovery from, 156
    timing of initiation in, 154–156, 155t
  due to glomerular disease, 85–86, 85t
  epidemiology of, 73–74, 73f
  heme pigment-induced, 83, 83t
  indications for RRT in, 88
  induced by cancer/chemotherapy, 85, 85f
  induced by medications, 84, 84f
  initial diagnostic approach to, 76, 76f
  KDIGO stage-based clinical practice guideline
    for, 74–75, 74t
  nutritional considerations in patients with, 88–89
  postrenal, 87, 87t
  prerenal, 78–80
  red flags in, 78, 78t
  staging of, 74, 74t
  treatment of, 88–89
  urinary indices in, 77–78, 77t
    BUN/Cr, 78, 78t
    FENa, 77, 77t
Acute rejection, of kidney transplantation, 241, 241f
Acute renal failure (ARF)
  kidney biopsy for, 71
  in pregnancy, 126
  risk factors for, 121, 121t
Acute tubular necrosis (ATN), 81–83
  biomarkers of, 89, 89t
  causes of, 81t
  in HIV patients, 121
  ischemia/sepsis-associated, 81, 81t
Adrenal insufficiency (Addison's disease), 10t,
  12–13t
Adrenocorticotropic hormone (ACTH), 283, 283t
ADTKD. *See* Autosomal dominant
  tubulointerstitial kidney disease
Advanced sclerotic lupus nephritis, 122–123t
Aging kidney, with chronic kidney disease,
  136–137, 136f
AIN. *See* Acute interstitial nephritis
AKI. *See* Acute kidney injury

AKIKI. *See* Artificial Kidney Initiation in Kidney Injury
Albumin, 283, 283t
Albumin to creatinine ratio (ACR), 62–63, 63t, 284, 284t
Albuminuria, 63t
Aldosterone, 284, 284t
Alkalemia, 50f
Alkaline phosphatase, 284, 284t
Alkalinizing therapy, for metabolic acidosis, 55
Alkalosis
    hypokalemia and, 57f
    metabolic, 50f, 55–57, 56f
        causes of, 55–56
        compensation for, 50t
        diagnostic workup for, 56, 56f
        treatment of, 57
    respiratory, 50f, 50t
Allograft dysfunction, kidney transplantation, 240, 240f
Allopurinol, for urate-lowering therapy, 193
Alpha glutathione S-transferase (GST), urine, 89t
Alpha-blockers, in hemodialysis, 177–178t
Alport syndrome, 127–128t, 246t
Aluminum hydroxide, for hyperphosphatemia, 186t
Ambulatory BP monitoring, 261
Amiloride, for hypercalciuria, 275
Amylase, 285, 285t
Amyloidosis, 119
ANA. *See* Antinuclear antibody
ANCA. *See* Antineutrophil cytoplasmic antibody
ANCA-associated glomerulonephritis/vasculitis, 246t
Anemia
    in chronic kidney disease, 138–142
        causes of, 138–139, 139f
        differential diagnosis of causes of, 139, 139t
        treatment of, 140, 140f
        workup of, 138
    management of, dialysis and, 181, 181t
    shortness of breath and, 11–12t
Angiotensin II receptor blockers (ARBs), in hemodialysis, 177–178t
Angiotensin-converting enzyme (ACE), 285, 285t
Angiotensin-converting-enzyme inhibitors (ACEi), in hemodialysis, 177–178t
Anion gap, 285, 285t
Antibody-mediated rejection (ABMR), 242, 242t
Anticoagulation, in hemodialysis, 173–174, 173t
    assessing bleeding risk during, 173t
    sites of action of, 174f
Anti-GBM (glomerular basement membrane), 102t, 103t
Anti-GBM nephritis, 246t
Anti-HIV medications, drug-induced kidney disorders and, 121
Antineutrophil cytoplasmic antibody (ANCA), 286, 286t
Antinuclear antibody (ANA), 286, 286t
Antiplatelet agents, 9t

Apixaban, pharmacokinetic and pharmacodynamic properties of, 175t
ARBs. *See* Angiotensin II receptor blockers
Arcuate artery, 14f
Arcuate vein, 14f
ARF. *See* Acute renal failure
Arrhythmias, hemodialysis and, 176
Arteriolopathy, calcific uremic, 185–187, 187t
Arteriovenous fistula (AVF), for hemodialysis, 166–167, 168f
Arteriovenous graft (AVG), for hemodialysis, 166–167, 168f
Artificial Kidney Initiation in Kidney Injury (AKIKI), 154, 155t
Aspirin, 9t
Asthma, 11–12t
Atherosclerosis, end-stage kidney disease and, 176
ATN. *See* Acute tubular necrosis
Atrial fibrillation, 266
Autoimmune disease, 10t
Autosomal dominant tubulointerstitial kidney disease (ADTKD), 111, 111t, 127–128t
AVF. *See* Arteriovenous fistula
AVG. *See* Arteriovenous graft
Azathioprine (Imuran), 235–236t

B
B cells, 255t
Bacteria, in urine, 66t
Basiliximab (Simulect), 235–236t
Beckwith-Wiedemann syndrome, 127–128t
Behcet's disease, 86
Beta-blockers, in hemodialysis, 177–178t
Bicarbonate, 287, 287t
    therapy
        administration guidelines of, 55
        for chronic kidney disease, 148
        for lactic acidosis, 55
        potential complications of, 55
Bilirubin, 286, 286t
Biopsy, kidney, 71
    absolute contraindications for, 71
    complications of, 71
    indications for, 71
    relative contraindications for, 71
Bisphosphonates, for secondary hyperparathyroidism, 145
Bladder cancer, 9t, 12t
Bladder catheterization, for postrenal AKI, 87
Bleeding, during hemodialysis anticoagulation, 173t
Blood, in dipstick test, 61–62t
Blood buffering system, 49
Blood pressure, hypertension, 261
Blood type, of donor, 231
Blood urea nitrogen (BUN), 287, 287t
Bone, cellular components of, 142
Bone and mineral disorders, dialysis and, 184–187
Broad casts, in urine, 66t
Bronchospasm, 11–12t
BUN. *See* Blood urea nitrogen

BUN:creatinine ratio, 78, 78t, 287, 287t
Buprenorphine, for chronic kidney disease, 197t

C

C3 glomerulonephritis (C3GN), 100–101
C3 glomerulopathy, 100–101
C3GN. *See* C3 glomerulonephritis
CA-AKI. *See* Contrast-associated acute kidney injury
Calcific uremic arteriolopathy, 185–187, 187t
Calcimimetics, for secondary hyperparathyroidism, 145, 184
Calcineurin inhibitors, for FSGS, 99t
Calciphylaxis, 185–187, 187t
Calcitonin, 288, 288t
Calcium
    laboratory values of, 287–288t, 287–288
    renal handling of, 22–23, 23f
Calcium acetate, for hyperphosphatemia, 186t
Calcium and phosphate balance,
    regulation of, 36, 36f
Calcium channel blockers (CCBs)
    with beta blockers, 269, 269f
    classes of, 268–269, 269t
    in hemodialysis, 177–178t
Calcium oxalate
    in kidney stones, 271–273t
    in urine, 66t
Calcium phosphate
    in kidney stones, 271–273t
    in urine, 66t
Calcium-phosphate metabolism,
    in chronic kidney disease, 143, 143f
CAN. *See* Chronic allograft nephropathy
Cancer, AKI induced by, 85, 85f
Cancer screening, in end-stage kidney disease, 194, 194f
CAPD. *See* Continuous ambulatory peritoneal dialysis
Capsule, 14f
Carboplatin, 10t
Cardiomyopathy, 6t
Cardiorenal syndrome, 80, 80f, 80t
    diagnosis of, 80, 80t
    management of, 80
Catheter-related bloodstream infections (CRBSIs), 171, 171t
Catheters
    for dialysis, 169–170
        duration of, 169t
        infections of, 171, 171t
    for hemodialysis, complications of, 170t
    peritoneal dialysis
        in abdomen, 210f
        initiation of, 202f
        removal of, 209, 209t
CAVH. *See* Continuous arterio-venous hemofiltration
CCBs. *See* Calcium channel blockers
CCPD. *See* Continuous cycling peritoneal dialysis
CellCept. *See* Mycophenolate mofetil

Central diabetes insipidus, 8t
Central venous catheter (CVC)
    for hemodialysis, 166–167, 168f
    infection
        algorithm for, 172f
        prophylaxis for, 171, 171t
        malfunction, approach to, 170f
CERA. *See* Continuous erythropoiesis receptor activator
Charcoal hemoperfusion, 215
Chemotherapy, AKI induced by, 85, 85f
Chloride, 288–289t, 288–289
Chronic allograft nephropathy (CAN), 244–245, 244f, 245f
Chronic dialysis, indications for, 152–153
Chronic fluid overload, dialysis and, 178–179
Chronic interstitial nephritis (CIN), 107–108
Chronic kidney disease (CKD), 5t, 7–8t, 8t, 10t, 11–12t, 13t, 132–151
    aging kidney and, 136–137, 136f
    AKI *versus*, 75, 75t
    anemia in, 138–142
    calcium-phosphate metabolism in, 143, 143f
    estimated glomerular filtration rate and
        based on serum creatinine, 133, 134, 133–134
        based on serum cystatin C, 134
        comparison of methods to, 135
        controversies about, 135–136
        problems with, 134–135
    KDIGO stages of, 132–133, 132f, 133f
    management of patients with, 137–138
    mineral and bone disease in, 142–146
    nutrition in, 147–148
    osteoporosis management in, 146
    uremic coagulopathy and, 147
Chronic Kidney Disease Epidemiology
    Collaboration (CKD-EPI), 64, 134
Churg-Strauss syndrome, 86
CI-AKI. *See* Contrast-induced acute kidney injury
CIN. *See* Chronic interstitial nephritis
Cinacalcet, for secondary hyperparathyroidism, 184
Cirrhosis, 7t
Cisplatin, 10t
Citrate anticoagulation
    of continuous renal replacement therapy, 160, 160f
    pharmacokinetic properties of, 173t
CKD. *See* Chronic kidney disease
CKD-EPI. *See* Chronic Kidney Disease
    Epidemiology Collaboration
Clarithromycin, 10t
CLIA. *See* Clinical Laboratory Improvement Amendments
Clinical Laboratory Improvement Amendments (CLIA), 60
Coagulopathy, uremic, 147, 147t
Cockcroft-Gault equation, 134, 64, 133
Colchicine, for acute gout flares, 193
Complement (C3, C4), 289, 289t
Computed tomography (CT)
    of nephrocalcinosis, 278f, 279
    noncontrast, of kidney stones, 273

Congestive heart failure (CHF), 6t, 11–12t
Conn's syndrome. *See* Primary hyperaldosteronism
Continuous ambulatory peritoneal dialysis
    (CAPD), 203
Continuous arterio-venous hemofiltration
    (CAVH), 157, 157t
Continuous cycling peritoneal dialysis (CCPD),
    203
Continuous erythropoiesis receptor activator
    (CERA), for anemia in ESKD, 182t
Continuous hemodiafiltration (CVVHD), 157, 157t
Continuous renal replacement therapy (CRRT)
    for acute kidney injury, 156–158
    anticoagulation in, 160, 161f
    antimicrobials with no dosage adjustment in,
        160, 160t
    citrate anticoagulation of, 160f
    complications of, 162t
    guidelines of, 153
    indication for, 157, 157t
    options, 157, 157t
    in poisoning, 216t
    substitution fluid and dialysate solutions for,
        158, 158t
    transmembrane pressure in, 158, 159f
Continuous veno-venous hemofiltration (CVVH),
    157, 157t
Contrast-associated acute kidney injury
    (CA-AKI), 81–83
    diagnosis of, 82, 82t
    incidence of, 81–82, 82t
    management of, 82–83
    pathophysiology of, 82
    risk factors for, 82
Contrast-induced acute kidney injury (CI-AKI),
    81–83
    diagnosis of, 82, 82t
    incidence of, 81–82, 82t
    management of, 82–83
    pathophysiology of, 82
COPD exacerbation, 11–12t
Cortex, 14f
Corticosteroids
    for kidney transplantation, 235–236t
    for primary FSGS, 99t
COVID-19
    AKI associated with, 87–88
    end-stage kidney disease and, 194–196, 195t
CRBSIs. *See* Catheter-related bloodstream
    infections
CrCl. *See* Creatinine clearance
Creatinine, 290, 290t
    serum
        in AKI, 74, 74t
        equations to calculate eGFR based on,
            133, 134, 133–134
Creatinine clearance (CrCl), 63, 135t, 289, 289t
Crescentic glomerulonephritis, 95–96t, 102–103,
    102t
    treatment of, 103
CRRT. *See* Continuous renal replacement therapy

Cryoglobulinemia, 120t
    type 1, 119
Cryptococcus neoformans infection, 121
CTLA 4-Ig (Belatacept), 235–236t
Cushing syndrome, 6t, 7–8t
CVC. *See* Central venous catheter
CVVH. *See* Continuous veno-venous hemofiltration
CVVHD. *See* Continuous hemodiafiltration
Cyclosporine (Neoral, Sandimmune)
    for kidney transplantation, 235–236t
    for membranous nephropathy, 98f
    for primary FSGS, 99t
Cystatin C, 290, 290t
    serum, 89t, 134, 135t
Cystic kidney diseases, 109–111
Cystine crystals
    kidney stones and, 271–273t
    in urine, 66t
Cystinuria, 276
Cystitis, 113t
Cystoscopy, for postrenal AKI, 87
Cytotoxic T cells (Tc), 255t
Cytotoxic therapy, for membranous nephropathy, 98f

D
DAAs. *See* Direct-acting antivirals
Dabigatran, pharmacokinetic and
    pharmacodynamic properties of, 175t
Daclizumab (Zenapax), 235–236t
Darbepoetin, for anemia in ESKD, 182t
Dark field, 66
DDD. *See* Dense deposit disease
Delta/Delta calculation, 57
Dense deposit disease (DDD), 100–101
Depression, 10t
    end-stage kidney disease and, 198
Dextrose, 201–202, 202t
Diabetes mellitus, 8t, 263–264
    end-stage kidney disease with, management of,
        187–189, 188t
    transplanted kidney and, 246t
Diabetic kidney disease (DKD), 116–118
    management of, 118
    risk factors for, 117, 117t
    stages of, 116–117t, 116–117
    treatment for, 117f
Diabetic nephropathy. *See* Diabetic kidney disease
Diagnostic tests, 60–72. *See also* Urinalysis
Dialysis, 152–229
    access planning of, 167–169, 168f
    acute/chronic, indications for, 152–153, 152t
    anemia management and, 181, 181t, 182t
    bone and mineral disorders and, 184–187
    catheters in, 169–170, 169t, 170f, 170t
        infections of, 171, 171t, 172f
    chronic fluid overload and, 178–179
    dysfunction/monitoring/surveillance of,
        168–169, 169t
    for end-stage kidney disease, 164–167, 164t
    filtration fraction of, 159–162, 160f, 160t, 161f,
        162t

Dialysis *(Continued)*
  glycemia and, 188–189
  gout and, 193–194
  home hemodialysis, 199–200
  hyperglycemia and, 189, 189t, 190–191t, 192t
  hyperkalemia and, 182–184, 183t
  hyperphosphatemia and, 185, 186t
  hypertension and, 177–178t, 177–178
  hypoglycemia and, 189, 192t
  indications for, 153
  initial period of, preemptive transplantation
      versus transplantation after, 232, 232f
  intradialytic hypotension and, 179–180, 180f, 180t
  ischemic heart disease and, 176
  modalities, for acute kidney injury, 153–164
  peripheral artery disease and, 179
  peritoneal, 200–204
  pressure measurements of, 158–159
  pulmonary hypertension and, 179
  secondary hyperparathyroidism and, 184–185
  seizures and, 189, 192t
  sustained low-efficiency, 162–164, 163t
  therapeutic apheresis in, 216–217
  for urate-lowering therapy, 194
  withdrawal from, 156
Dialysis disequilibrium syndrome, 176
Dialysis Outcomes and Practice Patterns Study
    (DOPPS), 185
Dialyzer
  reactions, 174–175
  types of, 167f
Diffuse lupus nephritis, 122–123t
Dipstick test, 61–62t, 61–62
Direct-acting antivirals (DAAs), for hepatitis C
    virus, 120
Diuretics, 8t
  in hemodialysis, 177–178t
Dizziness, intradialytic hypotension and, 179
DKD. *See* Diabetic kidney disease
DOPPS. *See* Dialysis Outcomes and Practice
    Patterns Study
DPP-4 inhibitors, 190–191t
Drug clearance, dialysis and, 214t
Drug crystals
  in kidney stones, 271–273t
  in urine, 66t
Drugs
  allergy to, 13t
  side effects or overdose, 9t, 10t
Dry skin, symptoms, signs, and differential
    diagnosis of, 13, 13t
Dyslipidemia, 265

E

Early Versus Late Initiation of KRT in Critically
    Ill Patients With AKI (ELAIN), 154, 155t
Eczema, 13t
Edema
  cardiovascular, 6, 6t
  endocrine, 6, 6t
  genital, peritoneal dialysis and, 212–213t

Edema *(Continued)*
  renal, 5, 5t
  symptoms, signs, and differential
      diagnosis of, 5–13
  treatment of, 95t
Edoxaban, pharmacokinetic and pharmacodynamic
    properties of, 175t
eGFR. *See* Estimated glomerular filtration rate
ELAIN. *See* Early Versus Late Initiation of KRT
    in Critically Ill Patients With AKI
Electrolyte
  disorders, 26–48
    associated with malignancies, 119
    distribution between body
        compartments, 26, 26f
    hypercalcemia as, 37–38, 37f
    hyperkalemia as, 35–36, 36f
    hypernatremia as, 28–29, 28f
    hyperphosphatemia as, 40
    hypocalcemia as, 39
    hypokalemia as, 34–35, 34f
    hyponatremia as, 29–33, 32f
    hypophosphatemia as, 39–40, 39f
    magnesium and, 41, 41f
    plasma osmolality in, 30, 30f
    sites of electrolyte reabsorption in, 27, 27f
    volume status and urine sodium in, 30, 30f
  in peritoneal dialysis, 211, 211t, 212f
  reabsorption, sites of, 27, 27f
Emergency hypertension, 263–264
End-stage kidney disease (ESKD)
  anemia in, 181, 181t
  bone and mineral disorders in, 184
  cancer screening in, 194, 194f
  chronic fluid overload in, 178–179
  conservative management of, 165
  COVID-19 and, 194–196, 195t
  depression and, 198
  diabetes mellitus with, management of,
      187–189, 188t
  dialysis for, 152, 164–167
    appropriateness of initiation, 165
    comorbidities/coexisting conditions
        during, 176–180
    membranes, 166, 166f, 167f
    modalities of, 164t
    peritoneal, outcomes in, 213
    timing of initiation, 165
  dietary phosphate restriction for, 185
  glycemic management in, 187
  gout in, 193
  hypertension in, 177
  hypoglycemia in, 189
  ischemic heart disease in, 176
  management of patients with, 137–138
  medication management in, 213–215,
      214t, 215t
  oral hypoglycemic agents and, 189t
  pulmonary hypertension in, 179
  secondary hyperparathyroidism in, 184
  seizures in, 189, 192t

End-stage kidney disease *(Continued)*
  sleep disorders and, 198
  symptom management in, 196–198, 196t
Eosinophiluria, 68–70
  Hansel's stain with, 68–70, 70f
Epithelial cell casts, in urine, 66t
Epithelial cells, in urine, 66t
Erythropoiesis stimulating agent (ESA), 140–142
  administration, route of, 141
  for anemia, in ESKD, 181, 181t, 182t
  controversy about, 141
  dosing of, 141
  if switching from IV to SC administration in
    HD patients, 141
  indications for, 140–141
  types of, 141
ESA. *See* Erythropoiesis stimulating agent
ESKD. *See* End-stage kidney disease
Essential mixed cryoglobulinemia, 120t
Essential tremor, 266
Estimated glomerular filtration rate (eGFR)
  calculated from SCr, 64, 64–65, 65f
  chronic kidney disease and
    based on serum creatinine, 133, 134, 133–134
    based on serum cystatin C, 134
    comparison of methods to, 135
    problems with using, 134–135
    race in, controversies about, 135–136
Etelcalcetide, for secondary hyperparathyroidism,
  184
Evaluation of Cinacalcet Hydrochloride
  Therapy to Lower Cardiovascular Events
  (EVOLVE), 184
EVOLVE. *See* Evaluation of Cinacalcet
  Hydrochloride Therapy to Lower
  Cardiovascular Events
Extracorporeal treatments, for intoxication,
  215–216, 216t
Extracorporeal Treatments In Poisoning
  (EXTRIP), 215
EXTRIP. *See* Extracorporeal Treatments
  In Poisoning

F
Fabry disease, 127–128t
Fatigue
  end-stage kidney disease and, 196
  symptoms, signs, and differential diagnosis of,
    10–11, 10t
Fatty casts, in urine, 66t
Febuxostat, for urate-lowering therapy, 193–194
FENa, 77, 77t
Fentanyl, for chronic kidney disease, 197t
Ferric citrate, for hyperphosphatemia, 186t
Ferritin, 290–291t, 290–291
FGF-23, role of, in chronic kidney disease,
  143–144
Fibrosis, interstitial, 108, 108f
Filtration fraction, in dialysis, 159–162
Focal lupus nephritis, 122–123t
Focal proliferative glomerulonephritis, 95–96t

Focal segmental glomerular sclerosis (FSGS), 94t,
  98–99
  primary *versus* secondary, 99
  transplanted kidney and, 246t
Foreign body inhalation, 11–12t
Fractional excretion of sodium (FENa), 290, 290t
FSGS. *See* Focal segmental glomerular sclerosis
Fungal peritonitis, peritoneal dialysis and, 207
Fungi, in urine, 66t

G
Gastrointestinal (GI) losses, renal tubular acidosis
  versus, 52
Genital edema, peritoneal dialysis and, 212–213t
GFR. *See* Glomerular filtration rate
Glomerular disease, 92–105
  acute kidney injury and, 85–86, 85t
  hematuria and, 67t
  in HIV patients, 120–121
  IgA nephropathy, 96–97
  membranous nephropathy, 97–98
  minimal change disease, 99–100
  nephritic syndrome, 95–96t, 95–96
  nephrotic syndrome, 94–95, 94t, 95t
  presentation, 92–93t, 92–94
  serum complement components C3 and C4 of,
    93–94t, 93–94
Glomerular filtration
  autoregulation of, 16, 16f
  physiology of, 15–16, 15f
Glomerular filtration rate (GFR), 63, 291, 291t
Glomerular renal diseases, 3–4
Glomerulonephritis, 9t, 12–13t
Glucocorticoids, for acute gout flares, 193
Glucose
  in dipstick test, 61–62t
  laboratory values of, 291, 291t
Glucose intolerance, peritoneal dialysis
  and, 212–213t
Glycemia, methods of measuring, 188–189
Goodpasture's syndrome, 86
Gout, dialysis and, 193
Graft failure
  causes of, during 10 years of follow-up,
    248, 248t
  immunosuppression withdrawal
    after, 253, 253t
Granular casts, in urine, 66t
Granulomatosis with polyangiitis, 86, 246t
GST. *See* Alpha glutathione S-transferase

H
Hansel's stain, eosinophiluria with, 68–70, 70f
Hb. *See* Hemoglobin
HCO. *See* High-molecular-mass cutoff
HCO_3^-. *See* Bicarbonate
HD. *See* Hemodialysis
Heart failure, 264–265
Helper T cells (Th), 255t
Hematocrit, 292, 292t
Hematologic disorders, hematuria and, 67t

Hematopoiesis, elements of, types and origin of cells participating in immune response, 254, 254f
Hematuria, 67–68
  causes of, 67
  classification of, 67
  evaluation of, 67–68
  kidney biopsy for, 71
  symptoms, signs, and differential diagnosis of, 9, 9t
Heme pigment-induced acute kidney injury, 83, 83t
Hemodialysis (HD)
  adequacy of, 200, 201f
    in acute kidney injury, 156
  anticoagulation in, 173–174, 173t
    assessing bleeding risk during, 173t
  antihypertensive medications in, 177–178t
  catheter, complications of, 170t
  emergencies, 174–176, 175t
  home, 199–200
  in poisoning, 216t
  vascular access for, 166–167, 168f
Hemodialysis Reliable Outflow (HeRO), 166–167
Hemoglobin (Hb), 292, 292t
Hemolysis, heme pigment-induced AKI and, 83t
Hemolytic uremic syndrome, 246t
Hemoperfusion
  charcoal, 215
  in poisoning, 216t
Hemoperitoneum, in peritoneal dialysis, 212f
Henderson-Hasselbalch equation, 49
Henoch-Schönlein purpura, 246t
  treatment of, 97
Hepatitis C, kidney disease in, 120
Hepatorenal syndrome (HRS), 79, 79f
  diagnosis of, 79, 79t
  management of, 79, 79t
Hereditary nephritis, 127–128t, 246t
Hernia, peritoneal dialysis and, 212–213t
HeRO. See Hemodialysis Reliable Outflow
HHD. See Home hemodialysis
HIF-PHIs. See Hypoxic inducible factor-prolyl hydroxylase inhibitors
High-molecular-mass cutoff (HCO), in poisoning, 216t
Histocompatibility testing, 230–231t
HIV infection, kidney disease in, 120–121, 121t
HLA match, of donor, 231
Home hemodialysis (HHD), 199–200
  options of, 199, 199t
  potential advantages of, 199t
HRS. See Hepatorenal syndrome
HTN. See Hypertension
Hyaline casts, in urine, 66t
Hydromorphone, for chronic kidney disease, 197t
Hydrothorax, peritoneal dialysis and, 212–213t
Hypercalcemia, 37–38, 37f

Hypercalciuria, idiopathic, 275
Hypercoagulability, 95t
Hyperglycemia, 8t
  dialysis and
    management of, 189, 189t, 190–191t
  risk of, 189, 192t
Hyperkalemia, 35–36
  acidosis and, 57f
  acute treatment of, 36, 36f
  causes of, 35
  in chronic kidney disease, 148
  clinical manifestations of, 35–36
  management of, dialysis and, 182–184, 183t
  in peritoneal dialysis, 211t
  symptoms, signs, and differential diagnosis of, 12–13t, 12–13
Hyperlipidemia, treatment of, 95t
Hypermagnesemia, 42
Hypernatremia, 28–29
  causes of, 28, 28f
  clinical manifestations of, 28
  in peritoneal dialysis, 211t
  treatment of, 29
Hyperparathyroidism
  forms of, 144, 144t
  secondary, therapeutic options for, 144–145
Hyperphosphatemia, 40
  cases of, 40, 40t
  in CKD bone disease, 143, 143f
  management of, dialysis and, 185, 186f
Hypertension (HTN), 260–270
  blood pressure and, 261
  dialysis and, 177–178t, 177–178
  emergency, 260–261t
  in pregnancy, 126, 127, 260–261t, 260–261
  secondary causes of, evaluation of, 262, 262f
  selection of initial therapy in patients with no specific indications, 262–263
  staging of, 260, 260t
  symptoms, signs, and differential diagnosis of, 7–8t, 7–8
  treatment based on specific indications or comorbid conditions, 263–269
  urgency, 260–261t
Hypertensive nephropathy, 267
Hypertensive nephrosclerosis. See Hypertensive nephropathy
Hyperthyroidism, 7–8t
Hyperuricemia, 193
Hyperuricosuria, 276
Hypoaldosteronism, 12–13t
Hypocitraturia, 275–276
Hypoglycemic agents, oral
  characteristics of, 190–191t
  end-stage kidney disease and, 189t
Hypokalemia, 34–35, 34f
  clinical manifestations of, 35
  treatment of, 35
Hypokalemia, alkalosis and, 57f
Hypokalemia, in peritoneal dialysis, 211t

Hypomagnesemia, 41–42
  causes of, 41
  clinical manifestations of, 42
  treatment of, 42
Hyponatremia, 29–33
  clinical manifestations of, 31–32
  in peritoneal dialysis, 211t
  plasma osmolality in, 30, 30f
  treatment of, 32–33, 32f
  volume status and urine sodium in, 30, 30f
Hypophosphatemia, 39–40, 39f
Hypotension, intradialytic
  dialysis and, 179–180, 180f
  mechanism of, 179
  prevention and treatment of, 180t
Hypothyroidism, 6t, 10t
Hypoxia, tissue, lactic acidosis and, 54, 54t
Hypoxic inducible factor-prolyl hydroxylase
    inhibitors (HIF-PHIs), 141–142, 182t

I
Icodextrin, 202, 202t
IDEAL. See Initiating Dialysis Early and Late
IDH. See Intradialytic hypotension
IgA nephropathy, 96–97, 246t
  conditions associated with, 96–97
  treatment of, 97, 97t
IHD. See Intermittent hemodialysis
Immune response, lymphocytes and their role in,
    255, 255t
Immunosuppression
  of kidney transplantation, 233, 233f
  withdrawal after graft failure, 253, 253t
Immunosuppressive medications
  action of, 233, 233f
  commonly utilized, 234–238, 237f, 238f
  complications of maintenance, 238–239t,
    238–240, 239f, 240t
Imuran. See Azathioprine
Incretin mimetics, 190–191t
Infection, urinary tract, 113, 113t
Infections, dialysis catheter, 171, 171t
Inherited disorders, important, kidney and,
    127–128t, 127–128
Initiating Dialysis Early and Late (IDEAL)
    study, 165
Insulin analogues, characteristics of, 192t
Interleukin (IL)-2 inhibitors, 235–236t
Interleukin (IL)-18, urine/serum, 89t
Interlobular artery and vein, 14f
Intermittent hemodialysis (IHD)
  assessment of adequacy of, 156
  guidelines of, 153
Intermittent peritoneal dialysis (IPD), 203
International Society for Peritoneal Dialysis
    (ISPD), 204
International Society of Nephrology/Renal
    Pathology Society (ISN/RPS) 2003
    classification of lupus nephritis, 122–123t,
    122–123
Interstitial cystitis (IC), 12t

Interstitial disease, in HIV patients, 121
Interstitial fibrosis, 108, 108f
Interstitial lung disease, 11–12t
Interstitial syndromes, 3–4
Interventional therapy, for renal artery stenosis,
    266–267
Intoxication, extracorporeal treatments
    for, 215–216, 216t
Intradialytic hypotension (IDH)
  dialysis and, 179–180, 180f
  mechanism of, 179
  prevention and treatment of, 180t
Intravenous pyelography (IVP), of kidney stones, 273
Inulin clearance, for estimated glomerular filtration
    rate, 135t
IPD. See Intermittent peritoneal dialysis
Iron
  for anemia of CKD, 140f
  laboratory values of, 292, 292t
Ischemia/sepsis-associated acute tubular necrosis,
    81, 81t
Ischemic heart disease, dialysis and, 176
ISPD. See International Society for Peritoneal
    Dialysis
Itchy skin, symptoms, signs, and differential
    diagnosis of, 13, 13t
IVP. See Intravenous pyelography

K
KDIGO. See Kidney Disease: Improving Global
    Outcomes
Ketones
  in dipstick test, 61–62t
  laboratory values of, 293, 293t
Kidney, aging, with chronic kidney disease, 136f
Kidney biopsy, 71
  absolute contraindications for, 71
  complications of, 71
  indications for, 71
  relative contraindications for, 71
Kidney Disease: Improving Global Outcomes
    (KDIGO), 74, 75t, 132–133, 132f, 133f
Kidney diseases, 106–115
  acute interstitial nephritis, 106–107
  autosomal dominant tubulointerstitial kidney
      disease/medullary cystic, 111, 111t
  chronic interstitial nephritis, 107–108
  cystic, 109–111
  hypertension, 263
  interstitial fibrosis, 108, 108f
  obstructive uropathy, 111–113
  polycystic, 110–111, 110f
  role of NSAIDs in, 108–109, 109f, 109t
  urinary tract infection, 113, 113t
Kidney disorders, in other diseases, 116–131
  associated with malignancies, 118–119
  diabetic kidney disease, 116–118
    management of, 118
    risk factors for, 117, 117t
    stages of, 116–117t, 116–117
    treatment for, 117f

Kidney disorders, in other diseases *(Continued)*
 hepatitis C, 120
 HIV infection, 120–121, 121t
 inherited disorders, important, 127–128t, 127–128
 in pregnancy, 125–127
  acute renal failure, 126
  hypertension, 126, 127
  preeclampsia, 126–127
  proteinuria, 126, 126t
 systemic lupus erythematosus, 122–123
 systemic sclerosis, 124–125, 124f, 124t
 thrombotic microangiopathy, 123–124, 124t
Kidney dysfunction, 118
 malignancies and, 118–119
Kidney injury
 acute. *See* Acute kidney injury
 chronic. *See* Chronic kidney disease
 mechanism of, 267, 267f
 predictors of, 267
Kidney injury molecule-1 (KIM-1), urine/serum, 89t
Kidney replacement therapy, dialysis, 152–229
 access planning of, 167–169, 168f
 acute/chronic, indications for, 152–153, 152t
 anemia management and, 181, 181t, 182t
 bone and mineral disorders and, 184–187
 catheters in, 169–170, 169f, 170f, 170t
  infections of, 171, 171t, 172f
 chronic fluid overload and, 178–179
 dysfunction/monitoring/surveillance
  of, 168–169, 169t
 for end-stage kidney disease, 164–167, 164t
 filtration fraction of, 159–162, 160f, 160t, 161f,
  162t
 glycemia and, 188–189
 gout and, 193–194
 hyperglycemia and, 189, 189t, 190–191t, 192t
 hyperkalemia and, 182–184, 183t
 hyperphosphatemia and, 185, 186t
 hypertension and, 177–178t, 177–178
 hypoglycemia and, 189, 192t
 intradialytic hypotension and, 179–180, 180f, 180t
 ischemic heart disease and, 176
 modalities, for acute kidney injury, 153–164
 peripheral artery disease and, 179
 peritoneal, 200–204
 pressure measurements of, 158–159
 pulmonary hypertension and, 179
 secondary hyperparathyroidism and, 184–185
 seizures and, 189, 192t
 sustained low-efficiency, 162–164, 163t
 therapeutic apheresis in, 216–217
 withdrawal from, 156
Kidney stones, 9t. *See also* Nephrolithiasis
Kidney transplantation, 230–259
 2018 reference guide to the Banff Classification
  of renal allograft rejection, 242–243, 242t
 acute rejection, 241, 241f
 causes of graft failure during 10 years
  of follow-up, 248, 248t
 chronic allograft nephropathy, 244–245, 244f,
  245f

Kidney transplantation *(Continued)*
 complications of renal transplant, 243, 243f
 donor selection and role of tissue matching, 231
 early kidney transplant complications
  and allograft dysfunction, 240, 240f
 elements of hematopoiesis, 254, 254f
 factors affecting transplant graft outcome, 231
 general transplant patient management,
  253–254
 immunosuppression, 233, 233f
  withdrawal after graft failure, 253, 253t
 immunosuppressive medications
  action of, 233, 233f
  commonly utilized, 234–238, 235–236t, 237f,
   238f
  complications of maintenance, 238–239t,
   238–240, 239f, 240t
 lymphocytes and their role in immune response,
  255, 255t
 malignancies, 251, 251f
 outcomes, 248–250, 248f, 248t, 249f
 pancreas, 253, 253t
 posttransplant infectious complications
  and prophylaxis, 252, 252f
 posttransplant morbidity in, 250f, 250t
 preemptive transplantation *versus*
  transplantation after initial period
  of dialysis, 232, 232f
 risk of recurrent disease in, 245–246, 246t
 Th cells
  activation, 256–257, 256f, 257f
  role of, 255–256, 255f, 256f
 timing of, 232, 232t
 tissue typing and compatibility, 230–231, 230f
Klotho, role of, in chronic kidney disease, 144

L
Lactate, 293, 293t
Lactic acidosis
 in peritoneal dialysis, 211t
 treatment of, 55
 types of, 54–55, 54t
Lanthanum carbonate, for hyperphosphatemia, 186t
Lethargy, symptoms, signs, and differential
 diagnosis of, 10–11, 10t
Leukocyte esterase, in dipstick test, 61–62t
Light chain toxicity, 119
Light microscopy, 65
Lipid, in urine, 66t
Lithium, extracorporeal removal of, 216
Liver disease, 13t
Liver fatty-acid binding protein (L-FABP),
 urine, 89t
Liver transplant, segmental, for
 hyperoxaluria, 277
Lower urinary tract obstruction, obstructive
 uropathy and, 112
Low-protein diet, for chronic kidney disease, 147
Lupus nephritis, 246t
Lymphocyte-depleting antibodies (ATG, TMG,
 OKT3), 235–236t

M

Macroalbuminuria, 62–63, 63t
Magnesium, 293, 293t
  effects in the body, 41, 41f
  therapeutic use of, 42
Major calyx, 14f
Malignancies
  electrolyte abnormalities associated with, 119
  kidney dysfunction and, 118–119
  kidney injury associated with, 118–119
Malignant hypertension, 264
MCD. *See* Minimal change disease
MCKD. *See* Medullary cystic kidney disease
MDRD. *See* Modification of Diet in Renal Disease
Mean of urea, for estimated glomerular filtration
  rate, 135t
Medical therapy, for renal artery stenosis, 266
Medications, AKI induced by, 84, 84f
Medulla, 14f
Medullary cystic kidney disease (MCKD), 111,
  111t, 127–128t
Meglitinides, 190–191t
Membranoproliferative glomerulonephritis
  (MPGN), 95–96t, 100–101
  pathophysiology of, 101, 101f
  type I, 246t
  type II, 246t
Membranous glomerulopathy, 94t, 246t
Membranous lupus nephritis, 122–123t
Membranous nephropathy, 97–98, 98f
Mesangial proliferative glomerulonephritis, 95–96t
Mesangial proliferative lupus nephritis, 122–123t
Mesangiocapillary glomerulonephritis, 95–96t
Metabolic acidosis, 50f, 51–55, 52f
  alkalinizing therapy for, 55
  causes of, 51
  compensation for, 50t
  non-anion gap, 52, 52f
  serum osmolar gap for, 51–52
Metabolic alkalosis, 50f, 55–57, 56f
  causes of, 55–56
  compensation for, 50t
  diagnostic workup for, 56, 56f
  treatment of, 57
Metallic taste, symptoms, signs, and differential
  diagnosis of, 10, 10t
Metformin, 10t
Methadone, for chronic kidney disease, 197t
Metronidazole, 10t
MGRS. *See* Monoclonal gammopathy of renal
  significance
Microalbuminuria, 62–63, 63t
Microscopy
  preparing urine for evaluation by, 65
  techniques of, 65–66
Mineral and bone disease, in chronic kidney
  disease, 142–146
Mineralocorticoid receptor antagonists (MRAs)
  in hemodialysis, 177–178t
  for hyperkalemia, 183
Minimal change disease (MCD), 99–100

Minimal mesangial lupus nephritis, 122–123t
Minor calyx, 14f
Mixed cryoglobulinemia, 120t
Modification of Diet in Renal Disease (MDRD),
  64, 133
Monoclonal gammopathy of renal significance
  (MGRS), 119
Monoclonal immunoglobulin, 120t
MPGN. *See* Membranoproliferative
  glomerulonephritis
Muddy brown casts, in urine, 66t
Multiple myeloma, kidney disease in, 119
Muscle cramps, intradialytic hypotension and, 179
Mycophenolate mofetil (MMF) (CellCept)
  for kidney transplantation, 235–236t
  for membranous nephropathy, 98f
Myeloma, multiple, kidney disease in, 119

N

N-acetyl-beta-glucosaminidase (NAG), urine, 89t
NAT. *See* Nucleic acid test
Natural killer cells, 255t
Nausea, intradialytic hypotension and, 179
Neoral. *See* Cyclosporine
Nephritic syndrome, 3, 5t, 95–96t, 95–96
Nephrocalcinosis, 277–279
  causes of, 279
  diagnosis of, 278f, 279, 279f
  treatment of, 279
Nephrogenic diabetes insipidus, 8t
Nephrolithiasis, 271–273t, 271–279
  detection of, 273
  initial workup of, 273–274
  predisposing causes of, 275–277
    cystinuria, 276
    hypercalciuria, 275
    hyperuricosuria, 276
    hypocitraturia, 275–276
    struvite stone crystalluria, 277
  symptoms and signs of, 273
  therapy for, principles of, 274–275
Nephrology, 1–4, 1t
  common consultations, 2, 2t
  definition of, 1
  follow-up assessments of, 3
  laboratory values for, 283–298
    adrenocorticotropic hormone, 283, 283t
    albumin, 283, 283t
    albumin/creatinine ratio, 284, 284t
    aldosterone, 284, 284t
    alkaline phosphatase, 284, 284t
    amylase, 285, 285t
    angiotensin-converting enzyme, 285, 285t
    anion gap, 285, 285t
    antineutrophil cytoplasmic antibody, 286, 286t
    antinuclear antibody, 286, 286t
    bicarbonate, 287, 287t
    bilirubin, 286, 286t
    blood urea nitrogen, 287, 287t
    BUN:creatinine ratio, 287, 287t
    calcitonin, 288, 288t

Nephrology *(Continued)*
  calcium, 287–288t, 287–288
  chloride, 288–289t, 288–289
  complement (C3, C4), 289, 289t
  creatinine clearance, 289, 289t
  cystatin C, 290, 290t
  ferritin, 290–291t, 290–291
  fractional excretion of sodium, 290, 290t
  glomerular filtration rate, 291, 291t
  glucose, 291, 291t
  hematocrit, 292, 292t
  hemoglobin, 292, 292t
  iron, 292, 292t
  ketones, 293, 293t
  lactate, 293, 293t
  magnesium, 293, 293t
  osmolality, 294, 294t
  oxygen saturation, 297, 297t
  parathyroid hormone, 294, 294t
  pCO$_2$, 295, 295t
  pH, of blood, 295, 295t
  phosphorus, 296, 296t
  pO$_2$, 295, 295t
  potassium, 296, 296t
  protein/creatinine ratio, 296, 296t
  sodium, 297, 297t
  specific gravity, 297, 297t
  total iron binding capacity, 298, 298t
  transferrin saturation, 298, 298t
  uric acid, 298, 298t
  renal diseases, general overview of, 3–4
Nephron
  anatomy of, 14–15
  diuretic sites of action in, 22, 22f
  tubular function of, 16–17, 17f
Nephronophthisis (NPHP), 127–128t
Nephrosclerosis, pathology of, 267–268, 268f
Nephrotic syndrome, 3, 5t, 94–95, 94t
  treatment of, 95t
Neutrophil gelatinase-associated lipocalin
    (NGAL), urine/serum, 89t
Nitrites, in dipstick test, 61–62t
Non-anion gap metabolic acidosis, 52, 52f
Noncontrast CT, of kidney stones, 273
Nonlymphocyte-depleting antibodies, 235–236t
Nonsteroidal antiinflammatory drugs (NSAIDs)
  for acute gout flares, 193
  in kidney disease, 108–109, 109f, 109t
NPHP. *See* Nephronophthisis
NSAIDs. *See* Nonsteroidal antiinflammatory drugs
Nucleic acid test (NAT), for hepatitis C virus, 120
Nutrition, in chronic kidney disease, 147–148
  bicarbonate therapy for, 148
  nutritional needs for, 147, 147t
  potassium restriction in, 148
  role of low-protein diet in, 147
Nutritional status, peritoneal dialysis and, 205

O
Obesity, hypertension and, 266
Obstructive airways disease, 265

Obstructive uropathy, 111–113
Oral health and sinus problems, 10t
Oral hypoglycemic agents
  characteristics of, 190–191t
  end-stage kidney disease and, 189t
Osmolality, 294, 294t
Osmolar gap, serum, 51–52
Osteoblasts, 142t
Osteoclasts, 142t
Osteodystrophy, renal, 146
Osteoporosis, in chronic kidney disease,
    management of, 146, 146t
Oxycodone, for chronic kidney disease, 197t
Oxygen saturation (SaO$_2$), 297, 297t

P
PAD. *See* Peripheral artery disease
Pain, end-stage kidney disease and, 197
Pancreas transplant, 253, 253t
Papilla, 14f
Parasites, in urine, 66t
Parathyroid, activate vitamin D receptor of, 145
Parathyroid hormone (PTH), 294, 294t
  levels, high, causes of, 144
Parathyroidectomy
  for CKD, 146
  in hyperparathyroidism, 38
  for secondary hyperparathyroidism, 145
Patiromer, for hyperkalemia, 184
Pauci-immune glomerulonephritis, 102t, 103t
Paxlovid (nirmatrelvir/ritonavir), 10t
PCN. *See* Percutaneous nephrostomy
pCO$_2$, 295, 295t
PCR. *See* Protein to creatinine ratio
PD. *See* Peritoneal dialysis
Pegloticase, for urate-lowering therapy, 194
Percutaneous nephrostomy (PCN),
  for postrenal AKI, 87
Peripheral artery disease (PAD), dialysis
    and, 179
Peritoneal dialysis (PD), 200–204
  acid-base and electrolyte disturbances in, 211,
    211t, 212f
  for acute kidney injury, 164
  adequacy of, 204–205, 204t
  catheter
    in abdomen, 210f
    initiation of, 201, 202f
    removal of, 209, 209t
  complications of, 205–211, 206t, 212–213t
  disadvantage of, 200
  initiation of, 201
  outcomes of, in end-stage kidney disease, 213
  peritonitis, 205–209, 207f, 208f, 209t
  prescription of, 203
  solutions, 201–202, 202t
  technique failure in, 209–211
  techniques of, 203
  urgent-start, 205, 206t
Peritoneal equilibration test (PET), dialysis
    modality selection and, 203–204, 204t

Peritonitis, peritoneal dialysis, 205–209, 207f, 208f, 209t
PET. *See* Peritoneal equilibration test
pH, of blood, 295, 295t
Phase contrast, 65
Pheochromocytoma, 265
Phosphate, renal handling of, 23, 23f
Phosphate binders, for secondary hyperparathyroidism, 144–145
Phosphorus, 296, 296t
PKD. *See* Polycystic kidney disease
Plasma exchange, in poisoning, 216t
Plasma IL-6, 89t
Pleural effusion, 11–12t
Pneumocystis jirovecii, infection, 121
Pneumonia, 11–12t
Pneumoperitoneum, peritoneal dialysis and, 212–213t
Pneumothorax, 11–12t
pO$_2$, 295, 295t
Podocytopathy, 122–123t
Polycystic kidney disease (PKD), 110–111, 110f
    diagnosis of, 110, 110t
    treatment for, 111, 111t
Polystyrene resins, for hyperkalemia, 183
Polyuria, 8, 8t, 43, 43f, 43t
    diuretic sites of action in, 43
    diuretic therapy for edema, 44, 44f
Postrenal acute kidney injury, 87, 87t
Poststreptococcal (postinfectious) glomerulone-phritis (PSGN), 95–96t, 102
    diagnostic tests for, 102
    treatment of, 102, 102t
Posttransplant morbidity, major causes of, 250f, 250t
Potassium
    acid-base balance and, 57, 57f
    homeostasis, 20–22, 21f, 22f
    laboratory values of, 296, 296t
    restriction of, for chronic kidney disease, 148
Prednisone, for primary FSGS, 99t
Preeclampsia, 7t
    treatment of, in pregnancy, 126–127
Preformed donor antibodies, 231
Pregnancy
    hypertension in, 260–261t, 260–261, 265
    kidney disorders in, 125–127
        acute renal failure, 126
        hypertension, 126, 127
        preeclampsia, 126–127
        proteinuria, 126, 126t
    metallic taste in, 10t
    rash or itchy, dry skin in, 13t
Pressure, measurements of, in dialysis, 158–159
Primary focal segmental glomerular sclerosis, 99t
Primary hyperaldosteronism, 7–8t, 8t
Primary polydipsia, 8t
Prograf. *See* Tacrolimus
Prophylaxis
    for dialysis catheter infections, 171
    posttransplant infectious complications and, 252, 252f

Prostatic hypertrophy, 266
Protein to creatinine ratio (PCR), 62, 62t, 296, 296t
Proteins, in dipstick test, 61–62t
Proteinuria, 62–63, 63f
    degree of, in random or spot urine, 62, 62t
    kidney biopsy for, 71
    in pregnancy, 126, 126t
    treatment of, 95t
Pruritus, end-stage kidney disease and, 197
Pseudohyperkalemia, 182
Pseudohypoparathyroidism, 144t
PSGN. *See* Poststreptococcal (postinfectious) glomerulonephritis
Psoriasis, 13t
Psychogenic polydipsia, 8t
PTH. *See* Parathyroid hormone
Pulmonary embolism, 11–12t
Pulmonary hypertension, dialysis and, 179
Pulmonary-renal vasculitic syndromes, 86
Pyelography, intravenous, of kidney stones, 273
Pyelonephritis, 113t
Pyrogenic reactions, hemodialysis and, 176

R
Radiation nephropathy, 118
Radiocontrast agents, for estimated glomerular filtration rate, 135t
Radioisotopic methods, for estimated glomerular filtration rate, 135t
Rapamycin. *See* Sirolimus
Rasburicase, for urate-lowering therapy, 194
Rash, symptoms, signs, and differential diagnosis of, 13, 13t
RBC casts, in urine, 66t
Reactive airway disease, 11–12t
Recurrent disease, risk of, kidney transplantation, 245–246, 246t
Red blood cell (RBC), in urine, 66t
"Refit" formulae, 64, 136
Refractory hypertension, 260–261t, 263–264
    causes of, 261–262
    in pregnancy, 260–261t, 260–261
    secondary causes of, 262, 262f
Remdesivir, for COVID-19, 195–196
Renal acid excretion, 20, 20f
Renal allograft rejection, 2018 reference guide to the Banff Classification of, 242–243, 242t
Renal artery, 14f
Renal artery stenosis (RAS), 266–267
    causes of, 266
    evaluation of patient for, 266
    treatment of, 266–267
Renal column, 14f
Renal diseases, general overview of, 3–4
Renal failure
    acute
        kidney biopsy for, 71
        in pregnancy, 126
        risk factors for, 121, 121t
    complications of chemotherapy, 118

Renal failure *(Continued)*
    pharmacokinetic properties of anticoagulants in, 173t
Renal function, estimation of, 63–65
    Cockcroft-Gault formula for, 134, 64
    creatinine clearance in, 63
    glomerular filtration rate in, 63
Renal osteodystrophy, 146, 146t
Renal pelvis, 14f
Renal physiology, 14–25
    acid-base regulation, 19, 19f
    anatomy of kidney in, 14–24, 14f
    glomerular filtration
        autoregulation, 16, 16f
        physiology, 15–16, 15f, 16f
    of handling
        calcium, 22–23, 23f
        phosphate, 23, 23f
        sodium, 17–19, 17f, 18f, 19f
        water, 23–24, 24f
    nephron
        anatomy, 14–15, 15f
        diuretic sites of action in, 22, 22f
        tubular function, 16–17, 17f
        potassium homeostasis in, 20–22, 21f, 22f
        renal acid excretion in, 20, 20f
Renal replacement therapy (RRT), 88, 153f
Renal transplant, complications of, 243, 243f
Renal tubular acidosis (RTA)
    GI losses *versus,* 52
    types of, 53–54, 53t, 54f
Renal vein, 14f
Renin-angiotensin-aldosterone system,
    medications blocking, 268, 268f
Resistant hypertension, 260–261t, 263–264
    causes of, 261–262
    in pregnancy, 260–261t, 260–261
    secondary causes of, 262, 262f
Respiratory acidosis, 50f, 50t
Respiratory alkalosis, 50f, 50t
Restrictive lung disease, 11–12t
Reverse pseudohyperkalemia, 182
Rhabdomyolysis, heme pigment-induced
    AKI and, 83t
Rheumatoid vasculitis, 86
Rituximab, for membranous nephropathy, 98f
Rivaroxaban, pharmacokinetic
    and pharmacodynamic properties of, 175t
Roxadustat, 142, 182t
RRT. *See* Renal replacement therapy
RTA. *See* Renal tubular acidosis

S
Sandimmune. *See* Cyclosporine
SaO$_2$. *See* Oxygen saturation
Scleroderma renal crisis, 125
Sclerosing encapsulating peritonitis,
    peritoneal dialysis and, 212–213t
Sclerotic lupus nephritis, advanced, 122–123t
SCr. *See* Serum creatinine
SCUF. *See* Slow continuous ultrafiltration

Secondary focal segmental glomerular sclerosis, 99t
Secondary hyperparathyroidism, management of,
    dialysis and, 184–185
Segmental artery, 14f
Seizures, dialysis and, 189, 192t
Selective serotonin reuptake inhibitors (SSRIs), for
    end-stage kidney disease, 198
Serum creatinine (SCr)
    in AKI, 74, 74t
    equations to calculate eGFR based on, 133, 134,
        133–134
Serum cystatin C, 134, 135t
Serum osmolar gap, 51–52
Sevelamer carbonate, for hyperphosphatemia, 186t
Shortness of breath, symptoms, signs, and
    differential diagnosis of, 11–12t, 11–12
Sieving coefficient, 214
Simulect. *See* Basiliximab
Sirolimus (Rapamycin), 235–236t
SLE. *See* Systemic lupus erythematosus
SLED. *See* Sustained low-efficiency dialysis
Sleep apnea, 265
Sleep disorders, end-stage kidney disease
    and, 198
Slow continuous ultrafiltration (SCUF), 157t
Sodium
    laboratory values of, 297, 297t
    renal handling of, 17–19, 17f, 18f, 19f
Sodium phosphate, for hypercalciuria, 275
Sodium polystyrene sulfonate (SPS),
    for hyperkalemia, 183
Sodium zirconium cyclosilicate (SZC),
    for hyperkalemia, 184
SONGPD. *See* Standardized Outcomes
    in Nephrology-Peritoneal Dialysis
Specific gravity
    in dipstick test, 61–62t
    laboratory values of, 297, 297t
SPS. *See* Sodium polystyrene sulfonate
SSc. *See* Systemic sclerosis
SSRIs. *See* Selective serotonin reuptake inhibitors
Standard *versus* Accelerated Initiation of
    Renal-Replacement Therapy in Acute Kidney
    Injury (STARRT-AKI) trial, 154, 155t
Standardized Outcomes in Nephrology-Peritoneal
    Dialysis (SONGPD), 213
STARRT-AKI trial. *See* Standard *versus*
    Accelerated Initiation of Renal-Replacement
    Therapy in Acute Kidney Injury
    (STARRT-AKI) trial
Sternheimer-Malbin (SM) stain, 66
Struvite stone crystalluria, 271–273t, 277
Sucroferric oxyhydroxide, for hyperphosphatemia,
    186t
Sulfonylureas, 190–191t
Sustained low-efficiency dialysis (SLED),
    162–164, 163t
Syndrome of inappropriate antidiuretic hormone
    secretion (SIADH), 30
    differential diagnosis of, 31
Systemic disease, kidney biopsy for, 71

Systemic lupus erythematosus (SLE), 122–123
  classification of, 122–123t, 122–123
  management of, 123
Systemic sclerosis (SSc), kidney disease in,
    124–125, 124f, 124t
Systolic blood pressure (BP), 261
SZC. See Sodium zirconium cyclosilicate

T

T cell-mediated rejection (TCMR), 242–243t,
    242–243
Tacrolimus (FK506, Prograf)
  for kidney transplantation, 235–236t
  for membranous nephropathy, 98f
TCMR. See T cell-mediated rejection
Th cells
  activation, 256–257, 256f, 257f
  role of, 255–256, 255f, 256t
Therapeutic apheresis (TA), renal indications for,
    216–217, 217t
Thiazide diuretics, for hypercalciuria, 275
Thiazolidinediones, 190–191t
Thrombotic microangiopathy (TMA), kidney
    disease in, 123–124, 124t
TIBC. See Total iron binding capacity
Tidal peritoneal dialysis (TPD), 203
Tissue hypoxia, lactic acidosis and, 54, 54t
Tissue typing, for kidney transplant, 230–231t
TMA. See Thrombotic microangiopathy
TMP. See Transmembrane pressure
Total iron binding capacity (TIBC), 298, 298t
TPD. See Tidal peritoneal dialysis
Transferrin saturation, 298, 298t
Transmembrane pressure (TMP), 158, 159f
Transplant graft outcome, factors affecting, 231
Transplant kidney, kidney biopsy for, 71
Transtubular potassium gradient (TTKG), 34–35
Triple phosphate crystals
  in kidney stones, 271–273t, 277
  in urine, 66t
Trisodium citrate, 160–162
Tuberous sclerosis, 127–128t
Tubular necrosis, acute, 81–83
  biomarkers of, 89, 89t
  causes of, 81t
  in HIV patients, 121
  ischemia/sepsis-associated, 81, 81t
Tubular syndromes, 4
Tubulointerstitial lesions, 122–123t
Twenty-four-hour BP monitoring, 261
γδ T cells, 255t

U

Ultrafiltration failure, causes of, 209t
Ultrasound (US)
  of kidney stones, 273
  of nephrocalcinosis, 278f, 279
Uncomplicated urinary tract infection (UTI), 113t
Upper urinary tract obstruction, obstructive
    uropathy and, 112
Urate-lowering therapy, 193–194

Uremic arteriolopathy, calcific, 185–187, 187t
Uremic coagulopathy, 147, 147t
Uremic pruritus, treatment of, 198t
Uremic syndrome, symptoms and signs of, 152, 152t
Ureter, 14f
Ureteral stenting, for postrenal AKI, 87
Urgent-start peritoneal dialysis, 205, 206t
Uric acid
  crystals
    in kidney stones, 271–273t, 276
    in urine, 66t
  laboratory values of, 298, 298t
Urinalysis, 60–71
  dipstick test in, 61–62
  eosinophiluria in, 68–70
  estimated glomerular filtration rate in, 64–65, 65f
  estimation of renal function in, 63–65
  hematuria in, 67–68
  kidney biopsy for, 71
  microscope techniques for, 65–66
  preparing urine for evaluation by
      microscopy in, 65
  proteinuria in, 62–63
  urine color in, 60–61, 60t
  urine sediment findings in, 66, 66t
Urinary indices, in AKI, 77–78, 77t
  BUN/Cr, 78, 78t
  FENa, 77, 77t
Urinary tract infection (UTI), 9t, 12t, 113, 113t
  treatment of, 113
  types of, 113, 113t
Urination
  burning, urgency and frequency, 12, 12t
  changes in, 12
Urine
  color of, 60–61, 60t
  output, in AKI, 74, 74t
  preparing, for evaluation by microscopy, 65
  sediment findings, 66, 66t
Urologic diseases, hematuria and, 67t
US. See Ultrasound
UTI. See Urinary tract infection

V

Vadadustat, for anemia of CKD, 142
Vascular disease, 122–123t
Vascular syndromes, 3
Venous air embolism, hemodialysis and, 176
Vesicoureteral reflux, obstructive uropathy and, 112
Vitamin B12 deficiency, 10t
Vitamin D, for secondary hyperparathyroidism, 145
Vitamin D analogues, for secondary hyperparathy-
    roidism, 145, 184
Vomiting, intradialytic hypotension and, 179
von Hippel-Lindau disease, 127–128t

W

Warfarin
  pharmacokinetic and pharmacodynamic
      properties of, 175t
  side effects of, 9t

Warfarin-associated calciphylaxis, 187
Water
    disorder, 26–48
        distribution between body compartments,
            26, 26f
        hypercalcemia as, 37–38, 37f
        hyperkalemia as, 35–36, 36f
        hypernatremia as, 28–29, 28f
        hyperphosphatemia as, 40
        hypocalcemia as, 39
        hypokalemia as, 34–35, 34f
        hyponatremia as, 29–33, 32f
        hypophosphatemia as, 39–40, 39f
        magnesium and, 41, 41f
        plasma osmolality in, 30
        plasma osmolarity in, 30f
        sites of electrolyte reabsorption in, 27, 27f
        volume status and urine sodium in, 30, 30f
    renal handling of, 23–24, 24f

Waxy casts, in urine, 66t
WBC. *See* White blood cell
WBC casts, in urine, 66t
Weakness, symptoms, signs, and differential
    diagnosis of, 10–11, 10t
White blood cell (WBC), in urine, 66t
Worse Itching Intensity Numerical Rating
    Scale, 198

X
X-ray, abdominal (KUB), of kidney stones, 273

Y
Young onset hypertension, secondary causes of,
    262, 262f

Z
Zenapax. *See* Daclizumab